PUBLIC HEALTH IN THE 21ST CENTURY

CORONAVIRUS AND U.S. PUBLIC HEALTH PREPAREDNESS

PUBLIC HEALTH IN THE 21ST CENTURY

Additional books and e-books in this series can be found on Nova's website under the Series tab.

PUBLIC HEALTH IN THE 21ST CENTURY

CORONAVIRUS AND U.S. PUBLIC HEALTH PREPAREDNESS

ROGER F. MARTIN
EDITOR

snova
New York

Library of Congress Cataloging-in-Publication Data

ISBN: 978-1-53617-939-2

Published by Nova Science Publishers, Inc. † New York

CONTENTS

Preface		**vii**
Chapter 1	Overview of U.S. Domestic Response to the 2019 Novel Coronavirus (2019-nCoV) *Sarah A. Lister, Frank Gottron, Kavya Sekar, Audrey Singer and Agata Dabrowska*	**1**
Chapter 2	Another Coronavirus Emerges: U.S. Domestic Response to 2019-nCoV *Sarah A. Lister and Kavya Sekar*	**19**
Chapter 3	The Coronavirus: U.S.-China Economic Considerations *Karen M. Sutter and Michael D. Sutherland*	**23**
Chapter 4	The Wuhan Coronavirus: Assessing the Outbreak, the Response, and Regional Implications *Jennifer B. Nuzzo*	**29**
Chapter 5	What You Need to Know About Coronavirus Disease 2019 (COVID-19) *Department of Health and Human Services*	**43**
Chapter 6	Coronavirus Disease 2019 (COVID-19) Situation Summary *Centers for Disease Control and Prevention*	**47**
Chapter 7	Science and Tech Spotlight: Coronaviruses *Timothy M. Persons*	**55**
Chapter 8	COVID-19: Current Travel Restrictions and Quarantine Measures *Edward C. Liu*	**61**

Chapter 9 COVID-19: Federal Economic Development Tools and Potential Responses **67**
Michael H. Cecire

Chapter 10 COVID-2019: Global Implications and Responses **71**
Tiaji Salaam-Blyther, Susan V. Lawrence, Sara M. Tharakan and Frank Gottron

Chapter 11 Coronavirus Disease 2019 (COVID-19) Hospital Preparedness Assessment Tool **77**
Department of Health and Human Services

Chapter 12 COVID-2019: CDC Protects and Prepares Communities **81**
Department of Health and Human Services

Chapter 13 COVID-19: What to Do if You Are Sick with Coronavirus Disease 2019 (COVID-19) **83**
Department of Health and Human Services

Chapter 14 The Defense Production Act (DPA) and COVID-19: Key Authorities and Policy Considerations **87**
Michael H. Cecire and Heidi M. Peters

Chapter 15 From SARS to 2019-Coronavirus (nCoV): U.S.-China Collaborations on Pandemic Response **91**
Jennifer Bouey and The RAND Corporation

Chapter 16 Lessons from the West African Ebola Response: How to Save Lives and Protect our Nation During the Novel Coronavirus Epidemic of 2020 **107**
Ronald A. Klain

Chapter 17 The State of U.S. Public Health Bio-Preparedness: Responding to Biological Attacks, Pandemics, and Emerging Infectious Disease Outbreaks **117**
Subcommittee on Oversight and Investigations

Chapter 18 Facing 21st Century Public Health Threats: Our Nation's Preparedness and Response Capabilities, Part I **237**
Committee on Health, Education, Labor, and Pensions

Index **305**

PREFACE

Coronavirus disease 2019 (COVID-19) is a respiratory illness that can spread from person to person. The virus that causes COVID-19 is a novel coronavirus that was first identified during an investigation into an outbreak in Wuhan, China. Chapters 1-16 contain information about the science behind the virus, economic implications, global response and public safety.

Chapters 17 and 18 access the readiness of the United States Public Health System in response to emerging infectious diseases, pandemics and biological attacks.

In: Coronavirus …
Editor: Roger F. Martin
ISBN: 978-1-53617-939-2

Chapter 1

OVERVIEW OF U.S. DOMESTIC RESPONSE TO THE 2019 NOVEL CORONAVIRUS (2019-NCOV)*

Sarah A. Lister, Frank Gottron, Kavya Sekar, Audrey Singer and Agata Dabrowska

BACKGROUND

On December 31, 2019, the World Health Organization (WHO) was informed of a cluster of pneumonia cases in Wuhan City, Hubei Province of China.[1] Illnesses have since been linked to a previously unidentified strain of coronavirus, designated 2019 Novel Coronavirus, or 2019-nCoV. As of February 7, 2020, tens of thousands of people have been infected and over 500 have died, mostly in China.[2] The disease has spread to several other countries, including the United States.

---

* This is an edited, reformatted and augmented version of Congressional Research Service, Publication No. R46219, dated February 10, 2020.

[1] World Health Organization (WHO), "Novel Coronavirus (2019-nCoV)," https://www.who.int/westernpacific/emergencies/novel-coronavirus. International Health Regulations (2005) require countries to notify the World Health Organization (WHO) of events that may constitute a public health emergency of international concern (PHEIC). See CRS In Focus IF10022, *The Global Health Security Agenda and International Health Regulations*.

[2] WHO, "Novel Coronavirus (2019-nCoV) Situation Report-17," February 6, 2020, https://www.who.int/docs/defaultsource/coronaviruse/situation-reports/20200206-sitrep-17-ncov.pdf?sfvrsn=17f0dca_4.

The Response to 2019 Novel Coronavirus: Status as of February 6, 2020

International: Selected World Health Organization (WHO) Declarations

https://www.who.int/emergencies/diseases/novel-coronavirus-2019

- January 22, 2020: WHO Director-General convened Emergency Committee for Pneumonia due to the Novel Coronavirus 2019-nCoV, which agreed on the "urgency of the situation" but did not declare it a Public Health Emergency of International Concern (PHEIC).
- January 30, 2020: The Emergency Committee convened by the WHO Director-General declared the 2019-nCoV outbreak to be a PHEIC.

Domestic: Selected Events and United States Government Actions

https://www.hhs.gov/about/news/index.html; https://www.cdc.gov/coronavirus/2019-nCoV/summary.html; https://travel.state.gov/content/travel/en/traveladvisories/ea/novel-coronavirus-hubei-province—china.html; and https://www.fda.gov/emergency-preparedness-and-response/mcm-issues/novel-coronavirus-2019-ncov.

- January 7, 2020: CDC established a 2019-nCoV Incident Management Structure.
- January 21, 2020: First travel-related case of 2019-nCoV detected in the United States.
- January 21, 2020: CDC activated its Emergency Operations Center to better provide ongoing support to the 2019-nCoV response and issued updated travel guidance for China, recommending that travelers avoid all nonessential travel to all of the country.
- January 23, 2020: U.S. Department of State ordered the departure of all nonemergency U.S. personnel and their family members from Wuhan.
- January 29, 2020: President Donald Trump announced the formation of the President's Coronavirus Task Force, led by HHS and coordinated by the National Security Council.
- January 29, 2020: State Department allowed for the voluntary departure of nonemergency personnel and family members of U.S. government employees from China.
- January 30, 2020: First U.S. person-to-person transmission of 2019-nCoV.
- January 30, 2020: State Department updated the Travel Advisory for China from a Level 3: Reconsider Travel to Level 4: Do Not Travel due to novel coronavirus first identified in Wuhan, China.
- January 31, 2020: U.S. Department of Health and Human Services (HHS) Secretary Alex Azar declared the outbreak to be a Public Health Emergency pursuant to Public Health Service Act (PHSA) Section 319.
- January 31, 2020: President Trump issued a proclamation that suspends the entry of any foreign national who has been in China within the prior 14 days, subject to some exceptions.
- February 2, 2020: Travel restrictions and additional quarantine requirements on travelers from China went into effect.
- February 3, 2020: CDC submitted an Emergency Use Authorization (EUA) package to the U.S. Food and Drug Administration (FDA) for the 2019-nCoV diagnostic test—Real-Time RT-PCR Diagnostic Panel.
- February 4, 2020: FDA issued an EUA enabling emergency use of CDC's Real-Time RT-PCR Diagnostic Panel, permitting CDC to share diagnostic kit with other labs.

On January 30, 2020, the Emergency Committee convened by the WHO Director-General declared the 2019-nCoV outbreak to be a Public Health Emergency of International Concern (PHEIC).[3] The next day, on January 31, 2020, U.S. Department of

[3] WHO, "Statement on the second meeting of the International Health Regulations (2005) Emergency Committee regarding the outbreak of novel coronavirus (2019-nCoV)," January 30, 2020, https://www.who.int/news-room/detail/30-01-2020-statement-on-the-second-meeting-of-the-international-health-regulations-(2005)-

Health and Human Services (HHS) Secretary Alex Azar declared the outbreak to be a Public Health Emergency pursuant to Public Health Service Act (PHSA) Section 319, retroactively dated to January 27, 2020.[4]

As the scope of the epidemic widens in China, as of early February, U.S health officials continue to state that the immediate health risk from the new virus to the general American public is low.[5] With the situation rapidly changing, both WHO and the U.S. Centers for Disease Control and Prevention (CDC) post frequent updates.[6]

This report discusses selected actions taken by the federal government to quell the introduction and spread of 2019-nCoV in the United States. The HHS Secretary has taken several specific actions to address the 2019-nCoV threat. While some of these actions are based in generally applicable authorities of the Secretary, other authorities may be contingent upon the Secretary or another federal official making a determination or declaration, specific to that authority, regarding the existence of a public health emergency or threat. Each of the actions taken by the Secretary, its statutory basis, and any distinct declarations and determinations supporting the action is presented in this report.

2019 Novel Coronavirus (2019-nCoV)

Coronaviruses (see Figure 1) are common respiratory pathogens, usually causing mild illnesses such as the common cold; however, several strains that cause serious illness have emerged in recent years. 2019-nCoV is causing the third serious outbreak of novel coronavirus in modern times, following severe acute respiratory syndrome (SARS) in 2002 and Middle East Respiratory Syndrome (MERS) in 2012.[7] The global health community is closely monitoring 2019-nCoV because of the severity of symptoms (including death) among those infected and the speed of its spread worldwide. Experts do

---

emergency-committeeregarding-the-outbreak-of-novel-coronavirus-(2019-ncov). A PHEIC is defined in the IHR (2005) as "an extraordinary event which is determined, as provided in these Regulations: i) to constitute a public health risk to other States through the international spread of disease; and ii) to potentially require a coordinated international response." This definition implies a situation that is serious, unusual or unexpected; carries implications for public health beyond the affected State's national border; and may require immediate international action. See WHO webpage on PHEIC at https://www.who.int/ihr/procedures/pheic/en/, accessed on January 31, 2020.

4 U.S. Department of Health and Human Services (HHS), "Secretary Azar Declares Public Health Emergency for United States for 2019 Novel Coronavirus," press release, January 31, 2020, https://www.hhs.gov/ about/news/2020/01/ 31/secretary-azar-declares-public-health-emergency-us-2019-novel-coronavirus.html.

5 Centers for Disease Control and Prevention (CDC), CDC "Media Telebriefing: Update on 2019 Novel Coronavirus (2019-nCoV)," February 3, 2020, https://www.cdc.gov/media/ releases/2020/t0203-coronavirus-update.html.

6 WHO, "Novel Coronavirus (2019-nCoV) Situation Reports," https://www.who.int/emergencies/ diseases/novel-coronavirus-2019/situation-reports; and U.S. Centers for Disease Control and Prevention (CDC), "2019 Novel Coronavirus (2019-nCoV) Situation Summary," https://www.cdc.gov/coronavirus/2019-ncov/summary.html.

7 CDC, "Human Coronavirus Types," accessed February 4, 2020, https://www.cdc.gov/ coronavirus/types.html.

not know the origin of 2019-nCoV, though genetic analysis and other features suggest an animal source.[8]

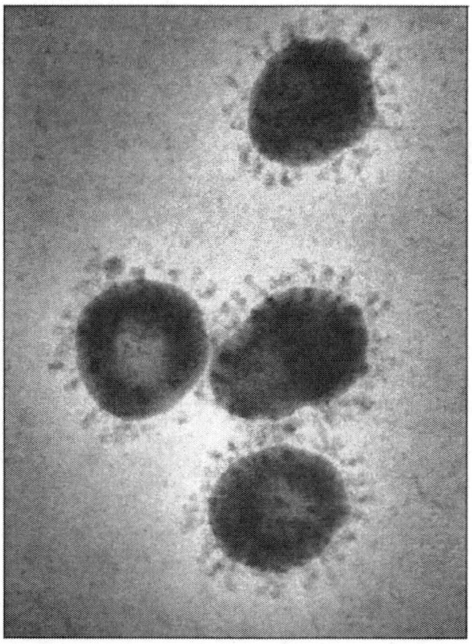

Source: CDC Public Health Image Library: https://phil.cdc.gov/Details.aspx?pid= 10270.

Note: Surface projections on the viral envelope of a poultry coronavirus form the halo or "corona" that gives this virus group its name.

Figure 1. Coronaviruses, Electron Micrograph.

Health officials and researchers are still learning about 2019-nCoV. According to CDC, 2019- nCoV typically causes respiratory infections characterized by a fever, cough, and sometimes breathing difficulty—a suite of symptoms that is common during influenza season.[9] Features that have yet to be clarified include routes of transmission (e.g., through the air, from contaminated surfaces); the incubation period (the time between infection and the onset of symptoms); and whether an infected person without symptoms can transmit infection.[10] Although it was first reported that 2019-nCoV infections resulted from an animal contact, Chinese officials confirmed person-to-person transmission on January 21, 2020.[11] Chinese officials have also reported transmission of

---

[8] Jon Cohen, "Mining Coronavirus Genomes for Clues to the Outbreak's Origins," *Science*, January 31, 2020, https://www.sciencemag.org/news/2020/01/mining-coronavirus-genomes-clues-outbreak-s-origins; and CDC, "2019 Novel Coronavirus (2019-nCoV) Situation Summary," updated February 3, 2020, https://www.cdc.gov/coronavirus/2019-nCoV/summary.html.

[9] CDC, "Symptoms—2019 Novel Coronavirus," accessed February 4, 2020, https://www. cdc.gov/coronavirus/ 2019-ncov/about/symptoms.html.

[10] CDC, "Transmission—2019 Novel Coronavirus," accessed February 4, 2020, https://www. cdc.gov/coronavirus/ 2019-ncov/about/transmission.html.

[11] Matthew Walsh and Han Wei, "Wuhan Virus Update: China Confirms Human-to-Human Transmission," *Caixin Global*, January 21, 2020, https://www.caixinglobal.com/2020-01-21/wuhan-virus-update-china-confirms-human-tohuman-transmission-101506555.html.

the virus from asymptomatic patients.[12] However, this finding has yet to be confirmed by U.S. and international health officials and other experts. While WHO and other health experts acknowledge transmission among asymptomatic individuals is possible, scientists agree that asymptomatic transmission is unlikely to be a driver of the outbreak.[13]

At this time no specific treatment or preventive vaccine exists for 2019-nCoV infections. Care for patients is supportive: maintaining hydration, preventing secondary infections, and providing respiratory support, such as use of a ventilator, if needed.[14]

DOMESTIC RESPONSE

In the United States, communicable disease control involves collaboration among federal agencies, state health departments, and international partners. Authority to compel isolation (for sick patients), quarantine (for healthy exposed persons), and disease reporting generally rests in state law.[15] The HHS Secretary and, by delegation, CDC have broad authority to assist in the control of communicable diseases through international cooperation, federal-state cooperation, and public health emergency response activities.[16] In addition, CDC (by delegation) has explicit authority to detain, examine, and release persons arriving into the United States, and traveling between states, who are suspected of having a communicable disease.[17] Other authorities, such as those in the Immigration and Nationality Act of 1952 (INA, P.L. 82-414), allow for other actions relevant to communicable disease control, such as travel restrictions.[18]

The use of federal and state disease control authorities and other key actions taken in response to the 2019-nCoV outbreak are discussed below. These activities of federal agencies in collaboration with state and local governments include, among others (1) investigation of 2019-nCoV cases and infection control measures in the community, (2) travel restrictions and/or quarantine requirements on certain travelers who have recently visited China, (3) medical countermeasure development, and (4) health system

---

[12] WHO, "Novel Coronavirus (2019-nCoV) Situation Report -12," February 1, 2020, https://www.who.int/docs/defaultsource/coronaviruse/situation-reports/20200201-sitrep-12-ncov.pdf.

[13] On January 30, details about a cluster of 2019-nCoV cases in Germany thought to have originated from an asymptomatic patient were reported in the *New England Journal of Medicine.* These findings were later questioned by observers as new information emerged about the index patient and her symptoms at the time of transmission. For further details, see "Transmission of 2019-nCoV Infection from an Asymptomatic Contact in Germany," *New England Journal of Medicine,* January 30, 2020, and Kai Kupferschmidt, "Study Claiming New Coronavirus can be Transmitted by People Without Symptoms was Flawed," *Science*, February 3, 2020, https://www.sciencemag.org/news/2020/02/paper-non-symptomatic-patient-transmitting-coronavirus-wrong.

[14] CDC, "2019 Novel Coronavirus: Information for Healthcare Professionals," https://www.cdc.gov/coronavirus/2019-nCoV/hcp/index.html.

[15] CDC, "Legal Authorities for Isolation and Quarantine," https://www.cdc.gov/quarantine/ aboutlaws regulationsquarantineisolation.html.

[16] CDC, "Selected Federal Legal Authorities Pertinent to Public Health Emergencies," August 2017, https://www.cdc.gov/phlp/docs/ph-emergencies.pdf.

[17] Interstate Quarantine regulations: 42 C.F.R. Part 70, and Foreign Quarantine regulations: 42 C.F.R. Part 71.

[18] 8 U.S.C. Chapter 12.

preparedness. Federal agencies involved include several HHS agencies, such as CDC, the Assistant Secretary for Preparedness and Response (ASPR), the National Institutes of Health (NIH), and the U.S. Food and Drug Administration (FDA), in collaboration with other agencies such as the U.S. Department of State and the Department of Homeland Security (DHS).

Investigation and Control of 2019-nCoV Cases in the Community

To curb the spread of 2019-nCoV cases in the community, state, tribal, and local health departments, with support from CDC, work to identify cases, investigate the possible spread of disease, and take infection control measures.

Case identification begins with testing for 2019-nCoV. CDC urges clinicians to consider a patient's travel and/or contact history and a 14-day incubation period when deciding whether to inform health departments and obtain patient specimens (e.g., mucus, urine) for 2019-nCoV testing. Health care providers are urged to report possible cases to state, tribal, and/or local health departments, which then report to CDC.[19]

CDC has developed a diagnostic test for the 2019-nCoV virus and initially performed all domestic testing on suspected patients.[20] On February 5, 2020, CDC announced that it would begin distributing test kits to state and local laboratories, following an authorization from the FDA (see the "Medical Countermeasures" section for more details).[21] CDC has been facilitating the collection and transport of specimens until the diagnostic test is made locally available.[22]

Once a patient is reported and in the process of having specimens tested, he or she is considered a *patient under investigation* (PUI) for 2019-nCoV. CDC has developed guidelines for isolation and other precautions for PUIs (including potential PUIs) or those receiving supportive care for 2019- nCoV infection in healthcare settings.[23] A key goal of the guidelines is the prevention of disease transmission to health care workers, who may be exposed through high-risk procedures, such as maintaining an ill patient on a ventilator.[24]

---

[19] Anita Patel, Daniel B. Jernigan, and 2019 n-CoV CDC Response Team, "Initial Public Health Response and Interim Clinical Guidance for the 2019 Novel Coronavirus Outbreak—United States, December 31, 2019–February 4, 2020," *Morbidity and Mortality Weekly Report (MMWR)*, vol. 69 (February 5, 2020).

[20] CDC, "2019 Novel Coronavirus (2019-nCoV) Situation Summary," updated February 3, 2020, https://www.cdc.gov/ coronavirus/2019-nCoV/summary.html.

[21] CDC "Media Telebriefing: Update on 2019 Novel Coronavirus (2019-nCoV)," February 5, 2020, https://www.cdc.gov/media/releases/2020/a0205-cdc-telebriefing-coronavirus-update. html.

[22] CDC, "Interim Guidance for Healthcare Professionals," updated February 2, 2020, https://www.cdc.gov/ coronavirus/2019-nCoV/hcp/clinical-criteria.html.

[23] CDC, "Interim Infection Prevention and Control Recommendations for Patients with Confirmed 2019 Novel Coronavirus (2019-nCoV) or Patients Under Investigation for 2019-nCoV in Healthcare Settings," updated February 3, 2020, https://www.cdc.gov/coronavirus/ 2019-ncov/hcp/infection-control.html.

[24] Chaolin Huang, Yeming Wang, Xingwang Li, et al., "Clinical features of Patients Infected with 2019 Novel Coronavirus in Wuhan, China," *The Lancet*, January 24, 2020.

Disease investigation for confirmed cases involves *contact tracing*—identifying and evaluating individuals who had contact with the patient to determine if transmission has occurred. These investigations are generally conducted by state, tribal, and local health officials, often with support and technical assistance from CDC.[25] As of February 3, 2020, CDC has reported two U.S. cases of person-to-person transmission of 2019-nCoV among close household contacts and has indicated that it expects to find additional cases of person-to-person transmission.[26]

As of February 3, 2020, CDC reported that it had "deployed multidisciplinary teams to Washington, Illinois, California, and Arizona to assist health departments with clinical management, contact tracing, and communications."[27] In addition, the Public Health Emergency Declaration by Secretary Azar, pursuant to PHSA Section 319, gives state, local, and tribal health departments more flexibility to reassign personnel to respond to 2019-nCoV if their salaries are funded in whole or in part by PHSA authorized programs.[28]

Travel Restrictions and Quarantine Requirements

Restrictions and Requirements in Effect

CDC and the U.S Department of State have issued advisories to avoid unnecessary travel to China, including a rare Level 4 advisory from the State Department to avoid all travel to China.[29] In addition, the Trump Administration has imposed entry restrictions and quarantine requirements in response to the entry of individuals who may pose a risk of introducing the 2019 Novel Coronavirus into the United States.

With respect to entry restrictions, President Trump issued a proclamation on January 31, 2020, that suspends the entry of any foreign national who has been in China within the prior 14 days, subject to some exceptions.[30] The exceptions cover lawful permanent residents (LPRs), most immediate relatives of U.S. citizens and LPRs, and some other

---

[25] CDC, "Transcript of 2019 Novel Coronavirus (2019-nCoV) Update," January 27, 2020, https://www.cdc.gov/media/releases/2020/t0127-coronavirus-update.html.

[26] CDC, "Transcript for CDC Telebriefing: CDC Update on Novel Coronavirus," February 3, 2020, https://www.cdc.gov/media/releases/2020/t0203-coronavirus-update.html.

[27] CDC, "2019 Novel Coronavirus (2019-nCoV) Situation Summary," updated February 3, 2020, https://www.cdc.gov/ coronavirus/2019-nCoV/summary.html.

[28] HHS, "Secretary Azar Declares Public Health Emergency for United States for 2019 Novel Coronavirus," press release, January 31, 2020, https://www.hhs.gov/about/news/2020/01/ 31/secretary-azar-declares-public-health-emergency-us-2019-novel-coronavirus.html.

[29] CDC, "Travel Health Notices: Novel Coronavirus in China," https://wwwnc.cdc.gov/travel/notices/warning/novelcoronavirus-china; and U.S. Department of State, "China Travel Advisory," February 2, 2020, https://travel.state.gov/content/travel/en/traveladvisories/ traveladvisories/china-travel-advisory.html.

[30] The White House, "Proclamation on Suspension of Entry as Immigrants and Nonimmigrants of Persons Who Pose a Risk of Transmitting 2019 Novel Coronavirus," January 31, 2020, https://www.whitehouse.gov/presidential-actions/proclamation-suspension-entry-immigrants-nonimmigrants-persons-pose-risk-transmitting-2019-novel-coronavirus/.

groups.[31] The proclamation directs the Department of State and the Department of Homeland Security (DHS) to establish procedures for implementing and enforcing the entry restrictions, which by the terms of the proclamation took effect at 5:00 p.m. (EST) on February 2, 2020. For statutory authority, the proclamation relies principally upon Section 212(f) of the INA.[32] That statute authorizes the President "to suspend the entry of all aliens or any class of aliens" whose entry he "finds ... would be detrimental to the interests of the United States."[33] The Supreme Court has held that Section 212(f) "exudes deference to the President" and gives him mostly unfettered discretion to decide "when to suspend entry," "whose entry to suspend," "for how long," and "on what conditions."[34] The presidential proclamation is in effect until terminated by the President.[35] The proclamation also directs the HHS Secretary to "recommend that the President continue, modify, or terminate this proclamation."[36] Such recommendation is required "no more than 15 days after the date of this order and every 15 days thereafter."[37]

Quarantine requirements also went into effect on February 2, 2020, according to a DHS announcement.[38] All persons, including U.S. nationals, LPRs, and their immediate families who arrive in the United States within 14 days after having been in China are to arrive and be screened at one of 11 designated arrival airports, and such persons may be subject to mandatory quarantine, pursuant to the standing quarantine authorities of the HHS Secretary under PHSA Section 361.[39] Persons showing symptoms of illness are to be evaluated by CDC staff to determine if they should be taken to a hospital for medical evaluation and to get care as needed.[40] Asymptomatic persons are generally to be held under federal quarantine for up to 14 days if they have traveled from China's Hubei province. However, asymptomatic persons who have traveled from other parts of China may be allowed to self-quarantine for 14 days.[41]

Personnel from DHS components—namely Customs and Border Protection (CBP) and the Transportation Security Administration (TSA)—are involved in excluding

---

[31] *Id.*

[32] 8 U.S.C. § 1182(f).

[33] *Id.*

[34] Trump v. Hawaii, 138 S. Ct. 2392, 2408 (2018).

[35] *Proclamation*, *supra* note 4, §5.

[36] *Id.*

[37] *Id.*

[38] Department of Homeland Security (DHS), "DHS Issues Supplemental Instructions for Inbound Flights with Individuals Who Have Been in China," press release, February 2, 2020, https://www.dhs.gov/news/2020/02/02/dhsissues-supplemental-instructions-inbound-flights-individuals-who-have-been-china.

[39] 42 U.S.C. §264. See "Domestic Quarantine and Isolation: Legal Authority and Policies," in CRS Report R43809, *Preventing the Introduction and Spread of Ebola in the United States: Frequently Asked Questions*; and CDC, "Legal Authorities for Isolation and Quarantine," https://www.cdc.gov/quarantine/aboutlaws regulationsquarantineisolation.html.

[40] CDC, "2019 Novel Coronavirus: Travelers from China Arriving in the United States," https://www.cdc.gov/coronavirus/2019-ncov/travelers/from-china.html.

[41] DHS, "DHS Issues Supplemental Instructions for Inbound Flights with Individuals Who Have Been in China," press release, February 2, 2020, https://www.dhs.gov/news/ 2020/02/02/dhs-issues-supplemental-instructions-inboundflights-individuals-who-have-been-china.

foreign nationals from entry and in assisting CDC personnel with implementation of quarantines for those who are permitted entry under these requirements.[42]

Of note, in addition to announcing the United States' use of entry restrictions and quarantine authority on January 31, HHS Secretary Azar declared the 2019-nCoV outbreak to be a Public Health Emergency, pursuant to PHSA Section 319.[43] This declaration was not statutorily required for the abovementioned entry restrictions and quarantine requirements to go into effect. Each of these authorities is independent of the others.

Potential Effects of Travel Restrictions on the Spread of 2019-nCoV

Proposals to restrict the movement of people from affected regions or countries are part of early discussions when novel communicable diseases arise. WHO generally advises against nations imposing travel restrictions on other nations, citing limited evidence of the effectiveness of such measures in controlling outbreaks and the harmful economic effects they have on nations struggling with outbreaks.[44] Voluntary movement restrictions are urged instead (see text box below).

In sum, WHO recommends exit screening—screening for symptoms of illness at the point of departure—as preferable to entry screening (i.e., at the point of arrival) as a means to prevent spread of the disease. Other than interventions for individuals who are found to be ill at exit and/or entry screening, WHO does not recommend broader travel restrictions.

The effect of travel restrictions on the spread of communicable diseases is considered poorly understood for several reasons, including (1) limited contemporary examples for study; (2) the inherent variability in the natural progression of global disease outbreaks, even those caused by the same pathogen; (3) variation in actions taken by affected countries and restrictions imposed by other countries; and (4) difficulty in accounting for the effects of nongovernmental actions such as event cancellations and airline flight adjustments. In response to the emergence of 2019- nCoV, China imposed sweeping internal movement restrictions,[45] a measure that is likely, in later analyses, to obscure or confound any additional transmission-damping effects that the U.Simposed travel restrictions may achieve.

---

[42] Ibid.

[43] HHS, "Secretary Azar Declares Public Health Emergency for United States for 2019 Novel Coronavirus," press release, January 31, 2020.

[44] See, for example, World Health Organization (WHO), "No Rationale for Travel Restrictions," May 1, 2009, in the context of the 2009 H1N1 influenza pandemic, https://www.who.int/csr/disease/ swineflu/ guidance/public_health/travel_advice/en/.

[45] Michael Levenson, "Scale of China's Wuhan Shutdown Is Believed to Be Without Precedent," *The New York Times*, January 22, 2020.

WHO Current Guidance Regarding International Travel During 2019-nCoV

"With the information currently available for the novel coronavirus, WHO advises that measures to limit the risk of exportation or importation of the disease should be implemented, without unnecessary restrictions of international traffic....

Advice for exit screening in countries or areas with ongoing transmission of the novel coronavirus 2019-nCoV (currently People's Republic of China): Conduct exit screening at international airports and ports in the affected areas, with the [aim of] early detection of symptomatic travellers for further evaluation and treatment, and thus prevent exportation of the disease, while minimizing interference with international traffic;

Advice for entry screening in countries/areas without transmission of the novel coronavirus 2019- nCoV that choose to perform entry screening: The evidence from the past outbreaks shows that effectiveness of entry screening [to prevent disease spread] is uncertain.... Temperature screening to detect potential suspect cases at Point of Entry may miss travellers incubating the disease or travellers concealing fever during travel and may require substantial investments. A focused approach targeting direct flights from affected areas could be more effective and less resource demanding....Currently the northern hemisphere (and China) is in the midst of the winter season when Influenza and other respiratory infections are prevalent. When deciding implementation of entry screening, countries need to take into consideration that travellers with signs and symptoms suggestive of respiratory infection may result from respiratory diseases other than 2019-nCoV, and that their follow-up may impose an additional burden on the health system....

WHO advises against the application of any restrictions of international traffic based on the information currently available on this event."

Source: WHO, "Updated WHO Advice for International Traffic in Relation to the Outbreak of the Novel Coronavirus 2019-nCoV," January 27, 2020, https://www.who.int/ith/2019-nCoV_advice_for_international _traffic/en/.

Several studies have examined the potential effects of travel restrictions on disease spread, particularly looking at the global spread of influenza and at the SARS outbreak in 2002-2003. Of note, these analyses sometimes indicated delays in the speed of spread of an outbreak. However, the effect of travel restrictions on the ultimate geographic spread of the outbreak—or on the reduction of overall morbidity or mortality—is unclear, and the evidence base is limited. Some studies have found no effect of travel restrictions on overall morbidity and mortality of infectious disease.[46] Others have found that very strict travel restrictions may effectively prevent the spread of disease (i.e., complete border closure) or that travel restrictions might be more effective when combined with other infection control measures, such as quarantine and isolation.[47] In particular, compulsory movement restrictions may rely on public support in order to be effective, as well as to avoid discrimination and loss of public trust. Many suggest that if public support and trust are essential in any case, enlisting movement restriction through voluntary measures may be just as effective, with less societal disruption.[48]

---

[46] Several such studies are discussed in Julia Belluz and Steven Hoffman, "The evidence on travel bans for diseases like coronavirus is clear: They don't work," *Vox*, January 23, 2020, https://www.vox.com/ 2020/1/23/21078325/wuhanchina-coronavirus-travel-ban.

[47] Sukhyun Ryu, Huizhi Gao, Jessica Y. Wong, et al., "Nonpharmaceutical Measures for Pandemic Influenza in Nonhealthcare Settings—International Travel-Related Measures," *Emerging Infectious Diseases*, vol. 26, no. 5 (May 2020).

[48] Francesca Matthews Pillemer et al., "Predicting Support for Non-pharmaceutical Interventions during Infectious Outbreaks: A Four Region Analysis," *Disasters*, vol. 39, no. 1, pp. 125-145, January, 2015, https://www. ncbi.nlm.nih.gov/pmc/articles/PMC4355939/.

In explaining the difference between the United States' response to the 2019-nCoV and the 2009 h1n1 pandemic flu, CDC official Nancy Messonnier stated that in the case of 2019-nCoV, the virus was caught early, before it spread around the world, and that CDC is taking advantage of the window of opportunity to slow its spread into the United States.[49]

Medical Countermeasures

Potential Products for Use in the 2019-nCoV Response

Medical countermeasures (MCMs) are medical products that may be used to treat, prevent, or diagnose conditions associated with emerging infectious diseases or chemical, biological, radiological, or nuclear (CBRN) threats. Examples of MCMs include biologics (e.g., vaccines, monoclonal antibodies), drugs (e.g., antimicrobials, antiretrovirals), and devices (e.g., diagnostic tests and personal protective equipment such as gloves, respirators/masks, and gowns).[50] FDA regulates MCMs domestically. Currently, there are no FDA-approved MCMs for 2019-nCoV, although FDA has authorized the use of an *unapproved* diagnostic test via an Emergency Use Authorization (EUA).[51] Federal agencies, pharmaceutical and biotech companies, nongovernmental organizations, and global regulators have been working to expedite the development and availability of MCMs for 2019-nCoV. Examples of such efforts include the following:

- Diagnostics. CDC developed the 2019-nCoV Real-Time RT-PCR Diagnostic Panel.[52] On February 4, 2020, FDA issued an EUA, which permits the distribution of the unapproved diagnostic test to and for use by state and local partners.[53] (EUAs are described in more detail below). Several federal agencies are working with industry partners to develop rapid diagnostic point-of-care tests for 2019-nCoV, including NIH, particularly through the National Institute of Allergy and Infectious Diseases (NIAID); ASPR, through the Biomedical

[49] CDC, "Transcript for CDC Telebriefing: CDC Update on Novel Coronavirus," February 5, 2020, https://www.cdc.gov/media/releases/2020/t0205-coronavirus-update.html.

[50] FDA, "What Are Medical Countermeasures?" accessed February 4, 2020, https://www. fda.gov/emergency-preparedness-and-response/about-mcmi/what-are-medical-countermeasures.

[51] FDA, "Novel coronavirus (2019-nCoV)," accessed February 4, 2020, https://www.fda.gov/ emergency-preparednessand-response/mcm-issues/novel-coronavirus-2019-ncov.

[52] Reverse transcriptase-polymerase chain reaction (RT-PCR) is a very sensitive technique that, in this use, allows the detection of otherwise undetectably low amounts of biological components specific to coronavirus.

[53] FDA, "FDA Takes Significant Step in Coronavirus Response Efforts, Issues Emergency Use Authorization for the First 2019 Novel Coronavirus Diagnostic," February 4, 2020, https://www.fda.gov/news-events/press-announcements/fda-takes-significant-step-coronavirus-response-efforts-issues-emergency-use-authorization-first.

Advanced Research and Development Authority (BARDA); and the Department of Defense (DOD).[54]

On February 5, 2020, BARDA announced an Easy Broad Agency Announcement (EZBAA) to solicit applications for development funding of 2019-nCoV molecular diagnostics. The submissions must have a viable plan to meet requirements for the FDA to consider EUA within 12 weeks of an award.[55]

- Therapeutics. Research and development into several treatment strategies for 2019-nCoV are underway by federal agencies, international partners, and industry. Drawing from research on the SARS and MERS coronaviruses, NIAID is assessing potential treatment strategies such as antiviral drugs and animal models that can be used to test potential MCMs. In addition, NIAID is developing assays and other research tools to study 2019-nCoV.[56] On February 4, 2020, BARDA announced that it would expand an existing collaboration with Regeneron Pharmaceuticals Inc. to develop monoclonal antibodies that could be used to treat 2019-nCoV infections.[57] This partnership would build upon an existing technology used to develop monoclonal antibody therapeutics to treat Ebola and MERS.

Scientists in China are testing drugs currently approved for treatment of HIV, influenza (flu), or malaria for potential effectiveness against 2019-nCoV.[58] For example, in China, AbbVie's HIV drug Kaletra has been recommended as treatment for patients who have tested positive for 2019-nCoV, while the drug undergoes clinical testing. Johnson & Johnson has reportedly provided its HIV drug Prezcobix to China to test as a potential treatment as well.[59] Scientists are also testing many experimental treatments in

[54] Dr. Anthony Fauci, Director of the National Institute of Allergy and Infectious Diseases (NIAID), HHS News Conference on Coronavirus, January 28, 2020, https://plus.cq. com/doc/newsmakertranscripts-5822133; and HHS Representative, White House Coronavirus Task Force news conference, January 31, 2020, https://plus.cq.com/doc/ newsmakertranscripts-5826415.

[55] HHS, "HHS Seeks Abstract Submissions for 2019-nCoV Diagnostics Development," press release, February 5, 2020, https://www.hhs.gov/about/news/2020/02/05/hhs-seeks-abstract-submissions-for-2019-ncov-diagnosticsdevelopment.html.

[56] Anthony Fauci, Director of the National Institute of Allergy and Infectious Diseases (NIAID), HHS News Conference on Coronavirus, January 28, 2020, https://plus.cq.com/doc/ newsmakertranscripts-5826415; and Hilary Marston, NIAID, "2019 Novel Coronavirus Stakeholder Listening Session Transcript," January 30, 2020, https://www.phe.gov/ Preparedness/nCoV/Documents/2019nCoV-Listening-Session-Transcript.pdf.

[57] HHS, "HHS, Regeneron Collaborate to Develop 2019-nCoV Treatment," February 4, 2020, https://www.hhs.gov/ about/news/2020/02/04/hhs-regeneron-collaborate-to-develop-2019-ncov-treatment.html.

[58] Manli Wang, Ruiyuan Cao, Leike Zhang, et al., "Remdesivir and chloroquine effectively inhibit the recently emerged novel coronavirus (2019-nCoV) in vitro," *Cell Research*, February 4, 2020, https://doi.org/10.1038/s41422-020-0282-0; and Panu Wongcha-um, "Cocktail of flu, HIV drugs appears to help fight coronavirus: Thai doctors," *Reuters*, February 2, 2020.

[59] Jared Hopkins, "U.S. Drugmakers Ship Therapies to China, Seeking to Treat Coronavirus," *Wall Street Journal*, January 27, 2020.

the research pipeline.[60] For example, Gilead is working with health authorities in China to determine whether its experimental antiviral drug Remdesivir can safely and effectively treat 2019-nCoV infections.[61]

- Vaccines. At least eight different 2019-nCoV vaccine development initiatives among federal agencies, industry, research institutions, and philanthropies have been announced.[62] Of note, the NIAID Vaccine Research Center (VRC) is collaborating with the drug company Moderna and the Coalition for Epidemic Preparedness Innovations (CEPI) to advance a vaccine candidate. Moderna expects this vaccine to enter phase 1 clinical testing in the spring of 2020.[63] CEPI is also supporting vaccine development by the University of Queensland (Australia) and the drug companies GlaxoSmithKline and Inovio.[64] Johnson & Johnson stated that it is mobilizing efforts to develop a possible preventive vaccine candidate against 2019-nCoV.[65]

FDA Emergency Use Authorization (EUA)

Clinical testing and the FDA review process typically take several years, so it will take time for MCMs in development to reach the commercial market. However, experimental products may become available in the United States prior to FDA approval pursuant to an EUA. FDA encourages industry and government sponsors (e.g., CDC) to engage with FDA prior to submitting a formal request for an EUA, if possible.

Under most circumstances, drugs, medical devices, and biologics may be introduced into interstate commerce only if they have been approved, cleared, or licensed by FDA. Under certain circumstances, however, FDA may permit a medical product to be provided to patients outside the standard regulatory framework, including through issuance of an EUA. In the absence of an approved MCM for 2019-nCoV, FDA may enable access to investigational MCMs by issuing an EUA, if the HHS Secretary declares that circumstances exist to justify the emergency use of an *unapproved product* or an

---

[60] Manli Wang, Ruiyuan Cao, Leike Zhang, et al., "Remdesivir and chloroquine effectively inhibit the recently emerged novel coronavirus (2019-nCoV) in vitro," *Cell Research*, February 4, 2020, https://doi.org/ 10.1038/s41422- 020-0282-0.

[61] Gilead, "Gilead Sciences Statement on the Company's Ongoing Response to the 2019 Novel Coronavirus (2019-nCoV)," January 31, 2020, https://www.gilead.com/news-and-press/ company-statements/gilead-sciences-statement-onthe-company-ongoing-response-to-the-2019-new-coronavirus.

[62] Steve Usdin and Karen Tkach Tuzman, "The Race Is on to Develop Therapies and Vaccines for the Coronavirus Outbreak," *Biocentury*, January 24, 2020, https://www.biocentury.com/ article/304290/the-coronavirus-outbreak-iscreating-a-testbed-for-new-vaccine-and-therapeutic-technologies.

[63] Moderna, "Moderna Announces Funding Award from CEPI to Accelerate Development of Messenger RNA (mRNA) Vaccine Against Novel Coronavirus," January 23, 2020, https://investors.modernatx.com/news-releases/news-release-details/moderna-announces-funding-award-cepi-accelerate-development.

[64] Coalition for Epidemic Preparedness Innovations, "CEPI and GSK announce collaboration to strengthen the global effort to develop a vaccine for the 2019-nCoV virus," February 3, 2020, https://cepi.net/ news_cepi/cepi-and-gskannounce-collaboration-to-strengthen-the-global-effort-to-develop-a-vaccine-for-the-2019-ncov-virus/.

[65] Johnson & Johnson, Novel Coronavirus, accessed February 4, 2020, https://www.jnj.com/ coronavirus.

unapproved use of an approved medical product.[66] The HHS Secretary's declaration must be based on one of four determinations; for example, a determination that there is an actual or significant potential for a public health emergency that affects or has significant potential to affect national security or the health and security of United States citizens living abroad.[67] Following the HHS Secretary's declaration, FDA, in consultation with ASPR, NIH, and CDC, may issue an EUA authorizing the emergency use of a specific drug, device, or biologic, provided that certain criteria are met (e.g., that there is no adequate, approved, and available alternative to the product).[68]

On February 4, 2020, the HHS Secretary determined that there is a public health emergency that has a significant potential to affect national security or the health and security of United States citizens living abroad, and that involves the 2019-nCoV.[69] This determination allowed FDA to assess and ultimately allow the emergency use of the CDC-developed diagnostic test for 2019- nCoV. This emergency determination by the HHS Secretary is distinct from the Public Health Emergency declaration made pursuant to PHSA Section 319.

Health System Preparedness

There is concern that if 2019-nCoV spreads widely in the community, it will overwhelm existing health care system capacity to care for patients and prevent future infections. Given that it is currently flu season, many health care facilities are already at or near patient capacity. The ASPR is the principal advisor to the HHS Secretary on the public health and medical preparedness and response for public health emergencies.[70] While 2019-nCoV has not spread widely enough to warrant broad U.S. health system

---

[66] 21 U.S.C. §360bbb-3. For additional information, see CRS In Focus IF10745, *Emergency Use Authorization and FDA's Related Authorities*.

[67] 21 U.S.C. §360bbb-3(b)(1). A determination by the Secretary of Homeland Security that there is an actual or significant potential for a domestic emergency involving a heightened risk of attack with one or more CBRN agents; a determination by the Secretary of Defense that there is an actual or significant potential for a military emergency involving a heightened risk of attack with either with one or more CBRN agents, or with one or more agents that may cause or are associated with an imminently life-threatening and specific risk to United States military forces; a determination by the HHS Secretary that there is an actual or significant potential for a public health emergency that affects or has significant potential to affect national security or the health and security of United States citizens living abroad, and that involves one or more CBRN agents; or the identification by Secretary Homeland Security of a material threat pursuant to Public Health Service Act §319F-2.

[68] 21 U.S.C. §360bbb-3(c).

[69] This determination, made pursuant to Section 564(b)(1)(C) of the Federal Food, Drug, and Cosmetic Act (21 U.S.C. §360bbb-3(b)(1)(C)), is noted on page 1 of the letter of authorization from FDA to CDC, advising of the authorization for emergency use of the CDC-developed diagnostic test. This letter is available at "Novel coronavirus (2019-nCoV) EUA Information" on the FDA webpage "Emergency Use Authorization," https://www.fda.gov/emergencypreparedness-and-response/mcm-legal-regulatory-and-policy-framework/emergency-use-authorization. See also footnote 53.

[70] HHS, "2019 Novel Coronavirus," https://www.phe.gov/Preparedness/nCoV/ Pages/default.aspx. See also CRS Insight IN11038, *U.S. National Health Security: Homeland Security Issues in the 116th Congress*.

response activities, ASPR and CDC have indicated the following actions in preparation for the potential spread of 2019-nCoV:

- Capacity assessment and monitoring. ASPR and CDC are projecting the potential long-term impact of 2019-nCoV and assessing the capacity of the health care system to respond to a larger outbreak. A sustained response could engage the Regional Treatment Network for Ebola and Other Special Pathogens, a tiered health system response network developed with funding provided by Congress for response to the Ebola outbreak in 2015.[71]
- Supply chain management. Both ASPR and CDC have indicated that they are working with health care and industry partners to ensure an adequate supply of medical products needed to contain the outbreak, such as personal protective equipment (PPE; e.g., surgical masks). A chief concern in supply chain management is that many medical products or drugs are manufactured, at least in part, in China, the epicenter of the current outbreak.[72]
- Strategic National Stockpile (SNS). The SNS, managed by ASPR, provides select medicines and medical supplies during public health emergencies when local supply chains are disrupted.[73] ASPR states it is working to ensure the adequacy of SNS supplies to prepare for the possible spread of 2019-nCoV.
- Mobilization of health care surge capacity. ASPR has indicated that it is working to ensure the availability of additional HHS health care support, such as deployment of the National Disaster Medical System (NDMS), in the event that local health care systems require augmentation to respond to the 2019-nCoV outbreak.[74]

Response Funding

CDC and other federal agencies may have the authority needed to respond to the 2019-nCoV epidemic, but their ability to act may be affected by the availability of appropriations. Annual appropriations and standing transfer authority provide the HHS

---

[71] HHS, "HPP Funds Regional Treatment Network for Ebola and Other Special Pathogens," https://www.phe.gov/Preparedness/planning/hpp/Pages/hpp-pathogens.aspx.

[72] Robert Kadlec, HHS Assistant Secretary for Preparedness and Response (ASPR), "2019 Novel Coronavirus Stakeholder Listening Session Transcript," January 30, 2020, https://www.phe. gov/Preparedness/nCoV/Documents/2019nCoV-Listening-Session-Transcript.pdf; and CDC, "CDC Update on Novel Coronavirus," February 5, 2020, https://www.cdc.gov/ media/releases/2020/t0205-coronavirus-update.html.

[73] HHS, "Strategic National Stockpile," https://www.phe.gov/about/sns/Pages/default.aspx.

[74] The National Disaster Medical System is described in CRS Report R43560, *Deployable Federal Assets Supporting Domestic Disaster Response Operations: Summary and Considerations for Congress*; and HHS Assistant Secretary for Preparedness and Response (ASPR), "2019 Novel Coronavirus Stakeholder Listening Session Transcript," January 30, 2020, https://www.phe.gov/Preparedness/nCoV/Documents/2019nCoV-Listening-Session-Transcript.pdf.

Secretary with some flexibility.[75] Upon a declaration of a Public Health Emergency pursuant to PHSA Section 319—which HHS Secretary Azar made on January 31, 2020—HHS may access a Public Health Emergency Fund,[76] but the fund does not have an available balance at this time. Separately, funding has generally not been available under the Robert T. Stafford Disaster Relief and Emergency Assistance Act (the Stafford Act) for the response to infectious disease outbreaks. As a result, Congress and the President provided supplemental appropriations for the response to the recent Ebola and Zika virus outbreaks in FY2015 and FY2016.[77]

In 2018, Congress established an Infectious Diseases Rapid Response Reserve Fund (IDRRRF) for CDC, providing appropriations of $50 million for FY2019 (P.L. 115-245) and $85 million for FY2020 (P.L. 116-94), available until expended.[78] These funds may be made available for an infectious disease emergency if the HHS Secretary either (1) declares a Public Health Emergency pursuant PHSA Section 319, or (2) determines that the infectious disease outbreak has significant potential to occur and, if it occurs, the potential to affect national security or the health and security of U.S. citizens, both domestically and abroad.

Before HHS Secretary Azar declared the 2019-nCoV outbreak to be a Public Health Emergency under PHSA Section 319, he issued a determination on January 25, 2020, allowing the allotment of $105 million from the IDRRRF for the 2019-nCoV response.[79] Secretary Azar had previously determined that the U.S. response to the Ebola outbreak in the Democratic Republic of Congo allowed the use of up to $30 million from the IDRRRF. If both the Ebola and 2019-nCoV amounts are fully used, all funds currently in the IDRRRF would be exhausted.[80] On February 2, 2020, HHS reportedly notified Congress of its intention to use the Secretary's standing authority to transfer up to $136

---

[75] Annual appropriations acts give the HHS Secretary limited authority to transfer funds from one budget account to another within the department. For instance, a provision in the FY2020 HHS appropriations act (P.L. 116-94, Division A, Title II, §205) generally allows the Secretary to transfer up to 1% of the funds from any given account. However, in general, a recipient account may not be increased by more than 3%. Congressional appropriators must be notified in advance of any transfer. Another FY2020 appropriations provision (P.L. 116-94, Division A, Title V, §514) addresses the Secretary's authority to reprogram funds from one program, project, or activity in a given budget account to a different program, project, or activity within the same budget account. This provision places certain limits on such actions and clarifies the circumstances in which appropriations committees must be consulted in advance. (See P.L. 115-245).

[76] See HHS, "Legal Authority with Declaration of Public Health Emergency," https://www.phe. gov/ Preparedness/support/secauthority/Pages/default.aspx#phe.

[77] Rebecca Katz, Aurelia Attal-Juncqua, and Julie E. Fischer, "Funding Public Health Emergency Preparedness in the United States," *American Journal of Public Health*, vol. 107, suppl. 2, pp. S148-S152, September, 2017, https://www.ncbi.nlm.nih.gov/pmc/articles/PMC55 94396/.

[78] The IDRRRF authority is codified at 42 U.S.C. §247d-4a.

[79] CQ Newsmaker Transcripts, "Health and Human Services Secretary Azar Holds News Conference on Coronavirus," January 28, 2020, https://www.phe.gov/Preparedness/support/secauthority/Pages/ default .aspx#phe.

[80] Communication with CDC, January 28, 2020.

million for 2019-nCoV response efforts, of which $75 million would be made available to CDC, $52 million for ASPR, and $8 million for the HHS Office of Global Affairs.[81]

CDC has an additional source of emergency support through the CDC Foundation, a 501(c)(3) public charity established by Congress "to support and carry out activities for the prevention and control of diseases, disorders, injuries, and disabilities, and for promotion of public health."[82] The CDC Foundation activated its Emergency Response Fund (ERF) to support 2019-nCoV response on January 27, 2020, as requested by CDC.[83] Funds have been donated to the ERF for this response by the Robert Wood Johnson Foundation, among others. Although the support provided by the foundation for outbreak response has been modest compared with supplemental appropriations, the foundation has greater spending flexibility and can sometimes procure response supplies and services more quickly than CDC through federal procurement processes.[84]

The trajectory of the 2019-nCoV outbreak is uncertain. If the United States experiences sustained person-to-person transmission of the novel virus in the future, the nation's public health and health care systems could be stretched to respond, and resources mobilized from the IDRRRF, HHS transfer authority, and the CDC Foundation may potentially be insufficient. Some Members of Congress have suggested that the Trump Administration consider a request for supplemental funding.[85]

---

[81] Yasmeen Abutaleb and Erica Werner, "HHS Notifies Congress that it May Tap Millions of Additional Dollars for Coronavirus Response," *Washington Post*, February 3, 2020. Likely the authority described in footnote 75.

[82] Public Health Service Act Section 399G, 42 U.S.C. §280e–11. See "National Foundation for the Centers for Disease Control and Prevention" in CRS Report R46109, *Agency-Related Nonprofit Research Foundations and Corporations*.

[83] CDC Foundation, "Responding to Coronavirus," https://www.cdcfoundation.org/coronavirus.

[84] See, for example, CDC Foundation, "2018 Ebola Outbreak," https://www.cdcfoundation. org/2018-ebola-outbreak.

[85] Andrew Siddons, "HHS Chases Virus Treatment as Congress Weighs Additional Funds," CQ, February 4, 2020.

In: Coronavirus …
Editor: Roger F. Martin
ISBN: 978-1-53617-939-2

Chapter 2

ANOTHER CORONAVIRUS EMERGES: U.S. DOMESTIC RESPONSE TO 2019-NCOV*

Sarah A. Lister and Kavya Sekar

THE EMERGENCE OF 2019-NCOV

On December 31, 2019, the World Health Organization (WHO) was informed of a cluster of pneumonia cases in Wuhan, China. Illnesses have since been linked to a previously unidentified strain of coronavirus, designated 2019 novel Coronavirus, or 2019-nCoV. To date, thousands have been infected, mostly in China, and over 100 have died. The disease has spread to several other countries, including the United States. As the scope of the epidemic widened in China, the U.S. Centers for Disease Control and Prevention (CDC) stated on January 27, 2020, that "the immediate health risk from the new virus to the general American public is low currently." With the situation rapidly changing, both WHO and CDC post frequent updates.

Coronaviruses (see *Figure 1*) are common respiratory pathogens, usually causing mild illnesses such as the common cold. The global health community is closely monitoring 2019-nCoV because of the severity of symptoms (including death) among those infected, and the speed of its spread worldwide. 2019-nCoV is causing the third-serious novel coronavirus outbreak in modern times, following severe acute respiratory syndrome (SARS) in 2002 and Middle East Respiratory Syndrome (MERS) in 2012. Experts do not know the origin of 2019-nCoV, though genetic analysis and other features suggest an animal source.

---

* This is an edited, reformatted and augmented version of Congressional Research Service Publication No. IN11212, dated January 29, 2020.

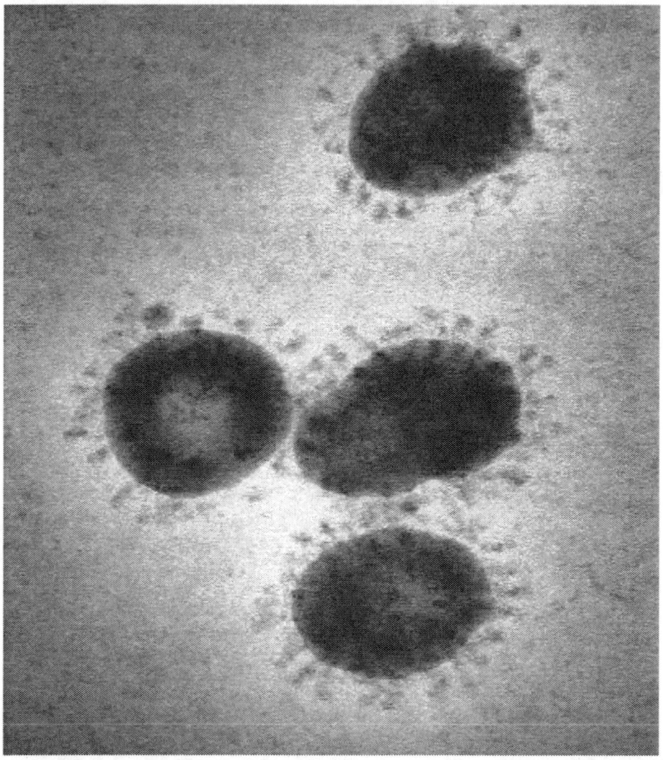

Source: CDC Public Health Image Library: https://phil.cdc.gov/Details.aspx?pid =10270.

Note: Surface projections on the viral envelope of a poultry coronavirus form the halo or "corona" that gives this virus group its name.

Figure 1. Coronaviruses, Electron Micrograph.

INFECTION AND TRANSMISSION

Health officials and researchers are still learning about 2019-nCoV. According to CDC, 2019-nCoV typically causes respiratory infections characterized by a fever, cough, and sometimes breathing difficulty—a suite of symptoms that is common during influenza season. Features that have yet to be clarified include routes of transmission (e.g., through the air, from contaminated surfaces), the incubation period (the time between infection and the onset of symptoms), and whether an infected person without symptoms can transmit infection. Although it was first thought that all 2019-nCoV infections resulted from an animal contact, Chinese officials recently reported evidence of person-to-person transmission.

The U.S. Domestic Response

In the United States, communicable disease control involves collaboration among federal agencies, state health departments, and international partners. Authority to compel isolation (for sick patients), quarantine (for healthy exposed persons), and disease reporting generally rest in state law. The Secretary of Health and Human Services (HHS) and, by delegation, CDC have broad authority to assist in the control of communicable diseases through international cooperation, federal-state cooperation, and public health emergency response activities. In addition, CDC (by delegation) has explicit authority to detain, examine, and release persons arriving into the United States, and traveling between states, who are suspected of having a communicable disease.

Case Identification and Investigation

CDC has developed a diagnostic test for the 2019-nCoV virus, but it is not widely available. At this time, all testing is being done by CDC, which has announced plans to share the test with domestic and international public health partners. Until local testing is available, CDC urges clinicians to consider a patient's travel history and a 14-day incubation period in deciding whether to obtain patient specimens (e.g., blood, urine) for testing. Health care providers are urged to report possible cases to state and local health departments, which then report to CDC. CDC is facilitating the collection and transport of specimens.

Although CDC reports that no person-to-person transmission has been confirmed in the United States, disease investigation for confirmed cases involves *contact tracing*—identifying and evaluating individuals who had contact with the patient to determine if transmission has occurred. These investigations are generally conducted by state and local health officials.

Clinical Guidance

No vaccine or specific treatment exists for 2019-nCoV infection at this time. Based on knowledge of the novel virus and other coronaviruses, CDC has developed guidance for isolation and other precautions for *patients under investigation* or receiving supportive care for 2019-nCoV infection. A key goal is the prevention of disease transmission to health care workers, who may be exposed through high-risk procedures such as maintaining an ill patient on a ventilator.

Travel Notices and Entry Screening

CDC and the State Department have issued advisories to reconsider or avoid unnecessary travel to China, including a rare Level 4 advisory from the State Department to avoid all travel to Hubei Province. In collaboration with U.S. Customs and Border Protection, CDC is screening passengers returning on flights from certain areas of China at 20 U.S. airports, looking for symptoms of illness and disseminating information. On January 29, a U.S. government-chartered flight from Wuhan, China, repatriated 201 Americans, who have been screened for illness and advised on procedures to follow should symptoms arise in the coming weeks.

Medical Countermeasures

CDC and the National Institutes of Health (NIH) continue to study the virus to inform response efforts. NIH reports that a vaccine candidate is in development and could be available for initial clinical trials within three months.

Considerations for Congress

CDC and other federal agencies may have the authority needed to respond to the 2019-nCoV epidemic, but they may lack available funds to support their efforts. Annual appropriations and standing transfer authority provide the HHS Secretary with some flexibility. Under certain circumstances the Secretary may access a Public Health Emergency Fund, but the fund does not have an available balance at this time.

Generally, funding has not been available under the Robert T. Stafford Disaster Relief and Emergency Assistance Act (the Stafford Act) for the response to infectious disease outbreaks. As a result, Congress provided supplemental appropriations for the response to the recent Ebola and Zika virus outbreaks.

Subsequently in 2018, Congress established an Infectious Disease Rapid Response Reserve Fund (IDRRRF) for CDC, providing $50 million for FY2019 (P.L. 115-245) and $85 million for FY2020 (P.L. 116-94), available until expended. These funds can be made available for an infectious disease emergency if the HHS Secretary either (1) declares a Public Health Emergency or (2) determines that the infectious disease outbreak has significant potential to occur and, if it occurs, the potential to affect national security or the health and security of U.S. citizens, both domestically and abroad. HHS Secretary Alex Azar has not declared the 2019-nCoV outbreak to be a Public Health Emergency, but has issued a determination allowing the allotment of $105 million from the IDRRRF for the 2019-nCoV response.

The trajectory of the 2019-nCoV outbreak is unknown at this time. Congress may choose to conduct oversight of federal response efforts, and monitor the expenditure of funds, as the situation progresses.

In: Coronavirus …
Editor: Roger F. Martin

ISBN: 978-1-53617-939-2

Chapter 3

THE CORONAVIRUS: U.S.-CHINA ECONOMIC CONSIDERATIONS*

Karen M. Sutter and Michael D. Sutherland

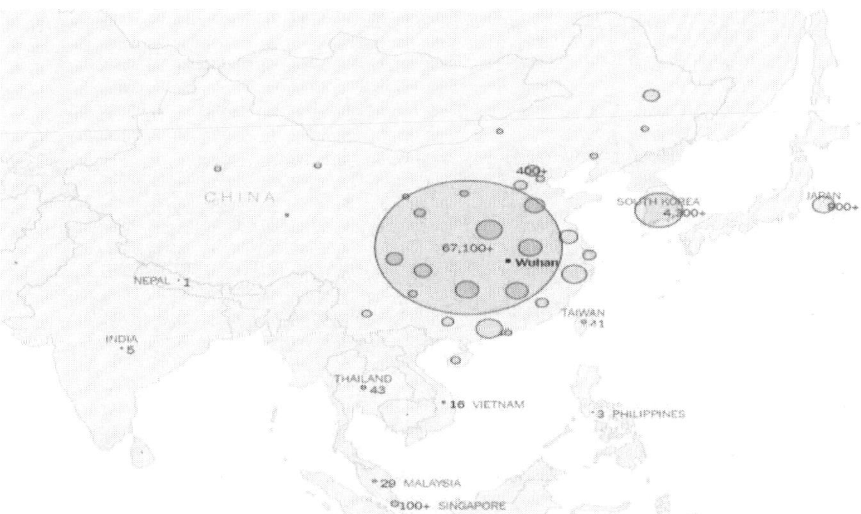

Source: New York Times, "Coronavirus Map: Tracking the Spread of the Outbreak," March 2, 2020.

Figure 1. COVID-19 Regional Case Map.

The novel coronavirus outbreak (COVID-19) is slowing economic activity in China and raising concerns about potential U.S. supply chain vulnerabilities in a range of sectors that rely directly and indirectly on China-based suppliers. These sectors include medical supplies, pharmaceuticals, auto parts, microelectronics, and strategic raw materials. Similar to the outbreak of severe acute respiratory syndrome (SARS) in China

* This is an edited, reformatted and augmented version of Congressional Research Service Publication No. IF11434, Updated March 2, 2020.

in 2002-2003, most cases so far are concentrated in China, but the current number of infections is already an order greater and every Chinese province is affected. U.S. senior officials have expressed concerns about the completeness and timeliness of the information China is reporting, complicating assessments of the scope, trajectory, and economic impact of the outbreak. The Chinese government has also imposed tight content controls on media reporting and placed Sina Weibo, Tencent, ByteDance, and other Internet firms under "special supervision" of the Cyberspace Administration of China, further limiting coverage of the outbreak.

Economic Outlook

The coronavirus is hitting China during an economic downturn as the government grapples with U.S. tariffs and China's counter tariffs, rising consumer inflation due in part to domestic pork shortages resulting from African swine fever, and efforts to rein in local government spending and shadow lending. China's economic growth could go negative in the first quarter of 2020 and fall below 5% for the year, with more serious effects if the outbreak continues beyond March. In a sign the slowdown could last past March, the Chinese government cancelled several spring meetings: the State Council's China Development Forum, the National People's Congress annual legislative session, and the Canton Trade Fair.

A key factor affecting the economic outlook in China is the ability of businesses to resume operations after the Lunar New Year was extended from late January until February 10, 2020. Business reopening has been uneven across sectors and locations in China. Many firms are awaiting government approvals to reopen and are facing difficulties in meeting new operating requirements, such as providing masks for employees. Foxconn, a Taiwan electronics firm that produces for Apple, has applied to reopen in early March. Resumption of transportation and travel appears to be a major obstacle. Chinese media has reported on employees struggling to return to work amid transportation shutdowns and contagion concerns. The American Chamber of Commerce in Shanghai reported on February 17, 2020, that most companies surveyed do not yet have sufficient staff to run a production line and face numerous logistics constraints. Almost half of the companies surveyed report that their global operations are already affected by the outbreak. These companies expect demand to be lower over the next several months.

The Chinese government has locked down cities in China's provinces of Hubei (e.g., Wuhan, Ezhou) and Zhejiang (e.g., Wenzhou, Hangzhou, Ningbo, and Taizhou). In total, an estimated 90 cities across China face some form of restrictions. The Chinese government has leaned on online delivery services and the military for logistics support, and is restricting consumer activity across multiple cities.

Domestic and global transportation links have been significantly curtailed with ramifications for trade. Air services face reduced capacity with the canceling of passenger travel and restrictions on pilots and flight staff on cargo flights to third countries. Cargo operations in China depend on port staffing and are reportedly operating at significantly reduced capacity. While most businesses typically plan for a shut down during the Lunar New Year, including some stockpiling, companies are now likely to experience more serious shortages. Cargo shipments from China to the United States typically take approximately three weeks; slowdowns in maritime shipping could affect a wide range of industrial and consumer goods.

The Chinese government is trying to encourage economic activity, but restrictions on business reopening, travel, and transportation are hampering its support efforts. Unlike other types of economic slowdowns, government stimulus cannot generate real economic activity on its own if business operations remain partially or completely shut down. The Chinese government is issuing economic support measures such as tax exemptions and special- purpose bonds. City governments in Beijing, Qingdao, Shanghai, and Suzhou are offering small- and medium- sized businesses in hard-hit industries support to reduce loans and delay payments for rent and social security. With a priority on social stability, localities are also offering preferences to companies that retain workers. In early February, China's central bank pumped $57 billion into the banking system, capped banks' interest rates on loans for major firms, and extended deadlines for banks to curb shadow lending. The central bank has been setting the reference rate for China's currency stronger than its official close rate to keep it stable.

There have been press reports of shortages of medical supplies—N95 respirator masks, medical protective equipment, antiviral drugs—and food. In response, the government has repurposed some production facilities to meet health and medical needs, including the facilities of U.S. firms such as General Motors (GM) and 3M. In early February, the Commerce Ministry directed local governments to increase imports of medical supplies, production materials, and agricultural products, potentially providing U.S. export opportunities in these sectors.

GLOBAL ECONOMIC IMPACT

China's economy is globally connected through trade, investment, and tourism, and any slowdown and persistent travel and transportation restrictions beyond March are likely to pressure global supply chains and potentially create worldwide economic fallout. Measures to contain the outbreak have significantly curtailed domestic and global transportation links, preventing the transport of many products and manufacturing inputs. Passenger air traffic has slowed significantly, taking offline significant air cargo capacity for microelectronics and other products that ship by air. Production has slowed across

China, with sharp slowdowns in sectors concentrated in Hubei, such as auto parts, LCD panels, and pharmaceuticals. Manufacturing that recently shifted offshore to other parts of Asia still often depends on intermediate inputs from China and thus is not insulated from China's production slowdown.

Disruptions in Chinese supply chains are expected to have a limited macroeconomic effect on developed markets in the short term but developing markets and Asia's developed economies, are more vulnerable. Vietnam, Taiwan, Malaysia, South Korea, Japan, Thailand, and Singapore all have strong supply chain links with China and are reporting supply shortages. South Korea's Hyundai and Kia, for example, announced production slowdowns in response to problems in securing auto parts from China. While developed economies might be insulated in the short term, the economic risks grow the longer the outbreak continues.

At the firm level, companies in sectors such as technology and autos or that are exposed to China's tourism, retail, or other services businesses could take a significant hit.

According to the United Nations World Tourism Organization, China's outbound tourism spending in 2018 was $277 billion, of which an estimated $36 billion was in the United States. U.S. business will likely be affected by China's slowdown, including through shortages of inputs, the cancelation of some commercial activity, and potential increased costs related to a strengthening U.S. dollar.

China's Commerce Ministry is helping firms obtain free *force majeure* certifications—which allow firms to opt out of contractual obligations without legal recourse because of developments beyond their control—and China National Offshore Oil Company declared *force majeure* in cancelling some LNG imports.

BROADER CONSIDERATIONS FOR CONGRESS

Phase One Trade Deal

The crisis is calling into question China's ability to implement the U.S.-China phase one trade deal signed in January 2020. Transportation constraints and a slowdown in demand could affect China's import levels. The agreement has a *force majeure* provision that could give China flexibility in implementing its commitments. The deal was finalized in December 2019, when Chinese officials reportedly knew about the outbreak, which raises questions about the rationale and timing of the decision to include the *force majeure* provision. As part of the phase one trade deal, China and the United States on February 14, 2020, cut by 50% the tariffs they imposed in September 2019. China also announced a tariff exemption process for 700 tariff lines that include some agriculture, medical supplies, raw materials, and industrial inputs.

Pharmaceutical Market Access and IP

Pharmaceuticals are a component of *Made in China 2025* industrial plans that aim to create competitive advantages for China in certain strategic industries. The Chinese government restricts market access for foreign pharmaceutical firms, including the disclosure of proprietary information for drug trials and sales. The Wuhan Institute of Virology and China's military recently applied to patent an adaption of an antiviral drug developed by California-based Gilead Sciences, Remdesivir. Also, Chinese firm BrightGene Bio- Medical Technology Co. announced it can produce a generic alternative to Remdesivir, potentially complicating Gilead's way forward in China. Gilead's patent application in China for Remdesivir use in coronaviruses has been pending since 2016. The Chinese government is also conducting an antitrust review of AbbVie's acquisition of Allergan, Inc. and could set terms for the use or transfer of AbbVie's antiviral intellectual property to benefit Chinese industry. China has required technology transfer in other antitrust reviews of foreign firms in *China 2025* sectors.

Table 1. Select U.S. Imports of healthcare products from China

Product	2019 value U.S.$	2019 % of U.S. imports
Antibiotics	$302,866,251	35%
PPE	$1,852,214,083	30%
Medical Devices	$3,911,308, 981	8.6%

Source: U.S. International Trade Commission, Assessed Customs Value.

Supply Chain Vulnerabilities

China's role as a global supplier of medical personal protective equipment (PPE), medical devices, antibiotics, and active pharmaceutical ingredients means reduced production or exports from China could lead to shortages and increased costs of critical medical supplies in the United States. The outbreak is also likely to create shortages in China-sourced raw materials, manufacturing inputs, microelectronics, and finished goods.

In: Coronavirus …
Editor: Roger F. Martin
ISBN: 978-1-53617-939-2

Chapter 4

THE WUHAN CORONAVIRUS: ASSESSING THE OUTBREAK, THE RESPONSE, AND REGIONAL IMPLICATIONS*

Jennifer B. Nuzzo

Good afternoon, Chairman Bera, Ranking Member Yoho, and Members of the Committee. Thank you for giving me the chance to appear before you today to discuss the emergence and global spread of the 2019 novel coronavirus (2019 nCoV).

I am an Associate Professor in the Departments of Environmental Health and Engineering and Epidemiology at Johns Hopkins Bloomberg School of Public Health. I am also a Senior Scholar at the Johns Hopkins Center for Health Security. *The opinions expressed herein are my own and do not necessarily reflect the views of The Johns Hopkins University.* Our Center for Health Security's mission is to protect people's health from major epidemics and disasters and build resilience. We study the organizations, systems, and tools needed to prepare and respond. At the Center, I direct the Outbreak Observatory, which conducts operational research to improve outbreak response. My testimony is also influenced by my previous experiences as a public health practitioner. I have also served as a public health epidemiologist for New York City, where I conducted surveillance for infectious diseases.

My colleagues and I at the Johns Hopkins Center for Health Security have spent close to twenty years analyzing infectious disease outbreaks, including epidemics and pandemics, in attempt to better understand the resources, practices and policies that are

* This is an edited, reformatted and augmented version of United States House of Representatives Committee on Foreign Affairs Subcommitee on Asia, The Pacific, and Nonproliferation Publication, dated February 5, 2020.

need to prevent, mitigate and contain them. Like many others, we've been closely following novel coronavirus outbreak since it was first announced in China at the end of December. We've been trying to analyze and understand the risk the virus poses to the United States (US) and other countries around the world and to make recommendations to policy-makers, legislators and practitioners about what should be done to respond to this epidemic.

I have two caveats regarding my testimony today. First, I have not been involved in the on-the- ground public health response to 2019 nCoV. My knowledge and assessment of this epidemic comes from my analysis of publicly shared information and conversations I have had with individuals and organizations that are closely involved in the response. Second, as you have likely heard, this is an evolving situation. Our knowledge of the virus is growing and changing as more data become available. What I offer you today is my best interpretation and judgment given the facts known at the time this testimony was prepared.

WHAT DO WE KNOW ABOUT 2019 NCOV?

The ongoing epidemic of 2019 nCoV was first recognized in the Wuhan city, Hubei Province, China. On December 31, 2019, health officials in Wuhan announced that they were investigating an outbreak of viral pneumonia involving 27 hospitalized cases in the city. Though the finding of viral pneumonia patients in any hospital during flu season is not by itself cause for alarm, health authorities were alerted to these cases by clinicians who noted the shared a common occupational exposure to the Huanan Seafood Wholesale Market. Wuhan health officials launched epidemiologic and environmental investigations. An official statement provided by the Wuhan Municipal Health Commission noted that all patients were treated in isolation and that there was no clear evidence of person-to-person transmission. Health officials closed the Huanan seafood market on January 1. One week later, health authorities in China announced that a novel coronavirus had been isolated from the viral pneumonia patients and the viral sequence was shared publicly.

Since the identification of 2019 nCoV as the likely cause of the viral pneumonia outbreak in Wuhan, we have learned several important things about the virus. First, the virus appears to be capable of sustained human-to-human transmission. Though it was initially thought that 2019 nCoV infection was limited to individuals with a history of exposure to the Huanan seafood market, cases have been found in individuals who reported never having visited markets in Wuhan. The appearance in other countries of multiple generations of 2019 nCoV cases who have not traveled to China provides additional evidence of sustained human to human transmission.

This finding differentiates the virus from the Middle East Respiratory Syndrome coronavirus (MERS-CoV), for which only limited human-to-human transmission has been reported.

Second, though severe illness and deaths have been reported, virus appears to be capable of causing a spectrum of disease. The emergence 2019 nCoV was first recognized among patients who were hospitalized with viral pneumonia. Since then 2019 nCoV cases with milder disease presentations have since been reported. Hospitalized patients also have a varied clinical picture—ranging from relatively mild symptoms to critical illness.

There is evidence that the virus jumped from animals and may have caused human infections earlier than initially recognized. A study published in the *Lancet* has shown some evidence the initial outbreak of 2019 nCoV may have started at the beginning of December or earlier--weeks before the outbreak was first recognized. It is not known when the virus became adapted to humans and capable to being spread via person-to person transmission.

Since the first report of human 2019 nCoV cases, more than 17,000 cases and 300 deaths (as of February 3, 2020) have been recorded in 23 countries. China accounts for the vast majority of cases. Cases have spread well beyond Wuhan—every province in China has since reported cases. From public reports and limited scientific studies published to-date, it appears as though the majority of reported deaths have occurred among elderly individuals and individuals with underlying medical conditions—patient groups known to be at risk for severe illness and death from other respiratory infections.

All deaths have occurred in China, with the exception of a death in the Philippines. The WHO has said that the deceased, who tested positive for nCoV, had also been infected with influenza and pneumococcus, a bacterium that causes pneumonia, bloodstream infections and meningitis. Outside of China, reported cases have so far been described as having mild disease presentations.

What is Unknown?

Size and Scope of the Epidemic

What is not yet known is the true size and geographic scope of this epidemic. Though countries are quickly ramping up surveillance for this virus, it is likely that many lack the capacity to actively search for cases. Even countries that have mobilized surveillance programs are likely missing cases. Surveillance in China seem to be heavily focused on cases that show up at hospitals or clinics. Though this makes sense given limited testing capabilities, what it means is that individuals who don't seek medical attention for their infections are likely not being captured by existing surveillance in China. Outside of

China, countries have, for the most part, only been testing people who have travelled to Wuhan or, in some cases, broader China.

Countries are not, as a matter of routine, looking for local cases that may resulted from infected individuals who entered the country before travel screening began.

Another complicating factor for surveillance is the occurrence of mild cases. Though there have been a concerning number of deaths and severe illnesses reported, the continued finding of mild cases raises the possibility that many more cases have occurred than have been detected. Mild cases are difficult to spot because their non-specific symptoms make them difficult to differentiate from other common respiratory illnesses. If individuals with mild symptoms don't seek medical attention, which is likely, and aren't tested, their infections will not be detected by most surveillance systems.

Hospitalization statistics are not reliable indicators of the burden of severe illness. China and other countries have been hospitalizing infected patients regardless of the severity of their symptoms. Infected patients are also remaining in hospitals until they are free of the virus, which may be well after patients' symptoms disappear.

Current US guidelines for testing for 2019 nCoV among individuals who are not contacts of confirmed cases are contingent on patients' symptoms and to travel to China. According to current guidelines from the US Centers for Disease Control and Prevention (CDC), individuals would likely not be tested for 2019 nCoV infection unless they are a symptomatic contact of a known case; traveled to Wuhan and experience fever and lower respiratory illness; or, traveled to broader China and are hospitalized for a lower respiratory infection. It is not clear whether and how these testing criteria will change now that all provinces in China and more than 20 countries are reporting cases.

Severity

We don't yet have a clear understanding regarding the severity of illnesses caused by 2019 nCoV. The reasons for the observed discrepancies in severe illness and deaths inside and outside of China is not yet known. Though a concerning number of severe and critically ill patients and deaths have been reported, the frequency with which infected people get critically ill and die is not yet understood. But the apparent discrepancy in between the severity of symptoms and number of deaths among cases in China versus other countries raises the possibility that outbreaks in other countries may be less severe and/or comparable to other respiratory viruses, such as influenza.

The way most countries are conducting surveillance for nCoV will not allow us to directly estimate the percentage of infected individuals that develops severe illness and die. A key reason is that we are likely missing many cases, and, in particular mild cases. An outbreak caused by a new pathogen, like 2019 nCoV, is often not recognized until an unusual cluster of severely ill patients turn up in hospitals or an increase in deaths is noted and people launch an investigation to figure out why. As we stand up surveillance for novel viruses, such as 2019 nCoV, and begin to look for cases more broadly, we may identify milder cases in individuals who either didn't seek medical attention or whose symptoms were misdiagnosed. We may be vastly underestimating the total number of infected individuals, which means it is not accurate to estimate severity from the total number of reported cases and deaths. Nonetheless, people have been attempting to determine the severity by doing crude estimates with the limited information available. These crude estimates show that the percentage of deaths among total reported cases may be falling, which, if true, would be consistent with what we've observed in previous emerging infectious disease outbreaks.

Asymptomatic Spread

There have been a few case reports that have raised the possibility that individuals who experience no symptoms (asymptomatic) or have not yet developed symptoms (presymptomatic) may be capable of transmitting their infection to others. In addition, virus has been detected in patients after their symptoms went away, which raises the possibility of post-symptomatic spread. The extent to asymptomatic or presymptomatic cases are contributing to the larger epidemic is not known and the evidence supporting this is weak. If significant level of asymptomatic or presymptomatic transmission is occurring, this will make it harder to interrupt disease spread. However, the World Health Organization has said that asymptomatic patients are not likely to be the main driver of disease spread.

International Response

On January 30, the WHO declared the epidemic to be a Public Health Emergency of International Concern (PHEIC). This is the sixth time the WHO has designated an infectious disease event a PHEIC since the 2005 International Health Regulations (IHRs) gave the organization this power. This most recent declaration means that WHO is currently involved in the response to three simultaneous PHEICs— 2019 nCoV, Ebola in the Democratic Republic of Congo, and international spread of poliovirus.

In announcing that the global spread of 2019 nCoV constituted a PHEIC, the WHO Director General Tedros Ghebreyesus made clear that countries should respond with "facts, not fear." The WHO has said that it does not recommend that countries implement travel or trade restrictions to prevent the importation of the virus. WHO has cautioned that countries that do take these measures could accelerate the spread of the virus by hindering the ability of responders and supplies to travel to where they are needed and by diverting public health resources from local disease control efforts. Nonetheless, many countries are implementing measures that the WHO has specifically advised against. Many countries, including the United States, have announced suspension of travelers from China, and an intention to quarantine travelers returning from China for up to 14 days. The IHRs were created to define the maximum measures countries could take to prevent the importation of disease; countries that take measures that are above what the WHO recommends do so in contravention of the IHRs.

But despite these unfortunate developments, I see in countries' initial response to this nCoV epidemic some important signs for optimism. First, I must commend the astute clinicians in Wuhan, China who first recognized this unusual event. Front-line clinicians are our first defense against infectious disease outbreaks. That they recognized that their patients shared an unusual commonality—a link to the seafood market—is possibly the only reason why this outbreak was detected when it was and not later. This points to the importance of having well-trained clinicians who can recognize and rapidly report unusual events.

Second, I am greatly encouraged by the speed with which health authorities are expanding laboratory testing for a never-before-detected virus. This includes China, which isolated, identified and published the sequence of the novel coronavirus quickly, enabling other countries to develop their own laboratory tests. This also includes other countries, who immediately began screening and testing symptomatic travelers from China for a completely new virus. It is important to point out this rapid surveillance work reflects advanced laboratory capabilities that require investment, training and sustainment.

In addition, epidemiological investigations conducted in and shared by other countries have improved our understanding of the virus and its transmission. Thailand identified a 2019 nCoV case in a traveler from Wuhan who reported not having exposure to the initially implicated seafood market. This epidemiological finding first raised the possibility of infection among those without a connection to the Huanan market. The first evidence that this virus was capable of human-to-human transmission was provided by health officials in Vietnam, who identified and investigated a 2019 nCoV case in a 27-year old man who had not visited China, but had been caring for his sick father who had recently travelled from Wuhan.

Each of the above examples illustrates why it is so essential that countries have the public health capacities to prevent, detect and respond to infectious disease emergencies. The sharing of detailed surveillance and case reports from Vietnam, Thailand, and other countries that are now reporting cases is indispensable for global efforts to control the spread of this disease. It is also how, in the face of scientific uncertainties about the virus, WHO makes a determination of the global risk posed by the virus and how countries like the US gather the information they need to make decisions about how to protect their own citizens.

We should not take for granted the response successes that have occurred to date. The astute clinicians and the capacities to screen, diagnose and isolate patients with a novel virus and identify and monitor their contacts represent important global health security capacities— laboratory-based surveillance, trained epidemiologic workforce, infection prevention and control practices—that needed to be developed and maintained so that they could function in this epidemic. The speed with which countries have gathered and shared key epidemiological data has enabled others to better gauge risks posed by this virus and enhance response plans.

Comparing the 2019 nCoV epidemic to prior novel coronavirus outbreaks illustrates some of the progress that has been made in strengthening countries' global health security. In 2003, it took months before a novel coronavirus was identified as the cause of Severe Acute Respiratory Syndrome (SARS) as compared with weeks in the current epidemic. In 2015, the Republic of Korea experienced a large outbreak of Middle East Respiratory Syndrome coronavirus (MERS- CoV), in part due to delayed recognition and nosocomial spread of the virus. However, in 2019 Korea quickly detected and isolated an imported case with mild symptoms and became the third country outside of China to report cases. Korea and other countries that have experienced infectious disease challenges have done the hard work of improving their public health capacities deserve our recognition and gratitude.

The fact that countries are able to conduct surveillance for and epidemiological investigations of 2019 nCoV cases is the result of hard work and sustained investment, both by the countries themselves and by international donors. US technical and financial support has been critical to the development of surveillance systems and trained workforce in a number of countries now reporting 2019 nCoV cases. In the case of Thailand, US support spanned decades. Thailand now has a world class epidemiologic workforce and is a leader in global health security. In Vietnam, sustained US support and assistance have enabled the development an early warning surveillance system, which includes a network of emergency operations centers and enhancement of field epidemiology workforce training. These resources were used to support Vietnam's detection and response to Zika virus and are likely a supporting the country's on-going response to 2019 nCoV.

Worrisome Trends in Global Readiness for Epidemics and Pandemics

Much of the world is not fully prepared to respond to serious infectious disease epidemics or pandemics. Though there are positive examples of countries like Thailand and Vietnam rapidly responding to infectious disease threats, there are critical gaps in worldwide capacities that can inhibit the responses of many countries to this epidemic and others.

In October, my colleagues and I at the Johns Hopkins Center for Health Security and the Nuclear Threat Initiative, together with the research power of the Economist Intelligence Unit, released the Global Health Security Index (GHS Index), a first-ever assessment of 195 countries' global health security. The first GHS Index was the result of a sustained effort to define a framework to comprehensively and reproducibly understand and compare global health security at the national level and to collect and measure the extent to which countries' show evidence of having the capacities and capabilities required to respond to an epidemic or pandemic. The GHS Index builds on peer evaluations conducted by the WHO but covers all un members, including China, and is regularly repeatable to measure progress. What we found is that no country, including the US, is fully prepared for significant infectious disease outbreaks. There is even less evidence that countries have demonstrated the ability to exercise these capacities or use them in an actual emergency. How unprepared is the globe as a whole? Out of a possible score of 100 points, we found that the average GHS Index score across 195 countries was just 40.2. Even countries with more resources are not ready, as the majority of high- and middle-income countries do not score above 50. What these results tell us is that action is urgently needed to improve countries' readiness for high-consequence infectious disease outbreaks.

In declaring the 2019 nCoV epidemic a PHEIC, WHO Director General Tedros Ghebreyesus said that a key reason for the declaration was a concern about the weakness of health systems in much of the globe. I share his worries. Among each of the 6 categories measured in our GHS Index, countries' scores were lowest (the average score was 26.4 out of in the category that examined the readiness of national health systems to treat the sick and protect health workers.

This finding tracks with observed challenges in recent epidemics, such as the on-going epidemic of Ebola in Democratic Republic of Congo (DRC), which represents one of the three on-going PHEICs to which the WHO is currently responding. Though DRC has prior experience and success in containing Ebola outbreaks, disease transmission occurring in unprepared health facilities has played an important role in exacerbating the spread of disease. Transmission in healthcare facilities also occurred during the 2003 SARS epidemic and during outbreaks of MERS in 2015.

What this tells us is that there may be critical gaps in hospitals and other health facilities that will likely be the on the front-lines of responding to the 2019 nCoV epidemic. Many countries— including well-resourced ones like the US, may experience difficulties in responding to a surge of patients infected with 2019 nCoV. If the virus produces more severe illnesses than have been seen outside of China to-date, then the challenges of safely treating these patients will be even greater. The recent report of a healthcare worker in France who became infected with nCoV is a concerning development that speaks to the challenges that even well-resourced countries are likely to face in responding to this disease.

My worries about these identified weaknesses in national capacities to respond to epidemics and pandemics is increased by the lack of resources allocated to address them. The GHS Index showed that only 5% of countries—fewer than 10 countries overall—scored above 66.7 out of 100 points for financing health security. Prioritizing health security, especially in the strengthening of foundational health systems, will be critical in helping to control this epidemic, but also in addressing future infectious disease emergencies.

Recommendations to Improve US Readiness for Continued Spread of 2019 nCoV

The ultimate trajectory of the 2019 nCoV epidemic is hard to predict with certainty, but there are increasing signs that it may not be possible to contain the disease. We must plan for the possibility that 2019 nCoV will result in a global pandemic. My recommended priority actions to improve preparedness for global spread of 2019 nCoV are divided between international engagement and domestic readiness.

International engagement recommendations:

1. Halt the current US policy of denying visas to travelers from China and quarantining Americans returning from China.
2. Engage in a productive, collaborative dialogue with China to in order to ensure continued access to data and critical medical supplies

Domestic response recommendations:

1. Ensure health departments have the resources they need to conduct surveillance to promote proven mitigation measures, such as case isolation outside a hospital to the extent possible.
2. Ensure hospitals and other health facilities have the resources needed to safely treat a surge of patients.
3. Facilitate the development of medical countermeasures, such as diagnostics, vaccines, therapeutics.

The current US policy to deny visas to travelers from China and to quarantine returning Americans is not the right approach to controlling the spread of 2019 nCoV and may make us less safe. These measures are unlikely to keep the virus out of our country.

The virus is spreading too quickly and too quietly for us to possibly know where all cases are. We do not have a complete picture of where in the world the virus is spreading to be able to stop infected people from coming to the US. It is also possible that unrecognized infections are occurring in US. In the weeks before the US began to screen travelers and airlines began reducing flights, thousands of people traveled to the US from China each day. And just because we are only looking for cases among people with a connection to China doesn't mean that those are the only individuals who are infected. As global case counts continue to grow and as more and more countries report cases, it will raise the question as to whether we should continue to focus on travel to Wuhan or broader China as criteria for testing. It is unlikely that we would be able to maintain our current approach to quarantine returning Americans and screen travelers if we needed to include additional countries or regions of the world.

I am deeply concerned that these measures will make us less safe by diverting public health resources from higher priority disease mitigation approaches that I describe below. It is not yet clear which agencies will have the responsibility of caring for and monitoring returning travelers who have been placed into quarantine. It is possible that local health authorities would play a lead role, as they did in monitoring travelers returning from West Africa during the Ebola epidemic of 2014, which required considerable resources that had to be diverted from other public health activities. Caring for and monitoring even small numbers of quarantined individuals would likely be a challenge for many health departments and would require a large investment of resources.

By singling out China for travel bans, we are, effectively penalizing it for openly reporting and sharing data about the epidemic. Our ability to respond to epidemics depends on having access to epidemiological information generated by other countries. Geographically-targeted measures may exacerbate the social and economic tolls of this epidemic and send a signal to countries that it may not be in their best interests to be forthcoming about disease outbreaks. This could diminish countries' willingness to be transparent about outbreaks and allow diseases to spread before outbreaks are uncovered, which would make everyone less safe. We should reward countries that report cases through offers of help and assistance.

It is in our best interest to maintain a productive and collaborative relationship with China and to help it better respond to the spread of 2019 nCoV disease. To appropriately gauge how the US should respond to this evolving health threat, it will be critical to continue to have access to data from China. Just prior to the US's announcement of travel bans, China indicated that it would allow US scientists in to participate in the epidemic response. This was an important development and may have led to an improved understanding of the current epidemic. But it is now questionable whether this offer is still viable, given the on-going travel restrictions.

It is essential that we maintain positive relationships with China to ensure the continued availability of essential goods. China is a major producer of the medical resources which the US will need to respond to this epidemic, such as surgical masks and other personal protective equipment. Our dependence on medical supplies from China is not just restricted to products needed for responding to this epidemic. For example, China is a major global producer of raw materials for commonly-used medicines, such as the blood thinner heparin. The US recently experienced shortages in its supplies of heparin, which is derived from pigs, due to China's efforts to cull pigs in order to control the spread of African Swine Fever. What this example should indicate to us that should help China respond to 2019 nCoV to ensure that the actions it takes do not interrupt the production and distribution of essential goods. There are already reports suggesting that China's massive efforts to restrict the movements of tens of millions of individuals may interrupt the production of goods. China needs our help and it is in our best interest to provide it.

We must now contemplate the possibility of pandemic spread of 2019 nCoV and must plan for how we will mitigate the impacts of the virus. In my view, it is highly likely that the United States will continue to see cases of 2019 nCoV, despite the recently implemented travel bans and quarantines. Though there are still important unknowns, this epidemic bears a number of similarities to the 2009 influenza A/H1N1 pandemic. It is essential that we plan for the possibility that the 2019 nCoV virus will follow a similar pattern to the 2009 pandemic. If the virus continues to circulate and cases keep climbing, the probability of community-wide transmission will increase. Responding to a novel virus for which no specific therapy or vaccine yet exists leaves only the possibility of mitigating the disease spread. What measures we take to find cases and mitigate disease spread will be determined by the observed severity and the availability of resources. If there continue to be concerns about the severity of the virus, our priority should be to rapidly detect and isolate of cases and identify and monitor their close contacts for signs of illness. Communities will likely consider other mitigation strategies, such as limiting public gatherings and closing schools, but the operational feasibility of these measures must be examined, and potential adverse consequences (e.g., reduced availability of healthcare personnel due to childcare obligations) should be considered. If the disease continues to demonstrate mild tendencies in cases outside of China, we may consider focusing efforts on protecting those most likely to become ill and preventing deaths.

We must ensure that responding agencies have the resources necessary to respond to 2019 nCoV cases across the country. Each of the above scenarios requires that health departments and hospitals have the resources they need to conduct surveillance to promote proven mitigation measures, such as case isolation. Unless patients require medical attention, they should be isolated outside of a hospital to reduce the possibility that they infect healthcare workers and other patients. Hospitals and other health facilities will need resources to safely treat a surge of patients.

If the number of 2019 nCoV cases in the US continues to grow, the US Congress will likely be called to appropriate emergency funds to enable states to respond to the virus.

During the 2009 pandemic, the Ebola epidemic of 2014, and the response to the Zika pandemic, the US Congress approved emergency supplemental funding that went to support state and local response efforts. The current fiscal outlook in states is such that they will be unable to fully respond without additional federal funding. Federal agencies such as HHS and CDC, which have been responding to multiple on-going disease emergencies, such as Ebola in DRC, have already indicated that they may need additional emergency response funds to support the 2019 nCoV response.

Government leadership is needed to facilitate the development of medical countermeasures, including diagnostics. Though a number of efforts to develop a vaccine have been announced, it is likely that a usable vaccine will not be available for some time. Research is also being conducted to develop therapeutic medicines, which may help those with severe illness and prevent deaths. Enhanced diagnostic tools are essential to the use of both vaccine and therapeutics, yet comparatively less attention has been given to the need to accelerate the development of new diagnostic tools. CDC is currently conducting all of the testing for 2019 nCoV in the US, but has plans to roll out testing capabilities to state public health labs. This will be important to reduce current lag times in getting test results for persons under investigation for 2019 nCoV and to meet a likely increase in the demand for testing as case counts rise. However, there is also a need for diagnostics in clinical settings. If more patients seek care at healthcare facilities, there will be an increased need for diagnostic tools to help clinicians rule out infection with nCoV, make decisions about cohorting or isolating patients, and to determine course of therapy.

CONCLUSION

The points I have raised today hopefully paint a picture of an epidemic that is in many ways complex and evolving, but for which we are increasingly gaining clarity. International collaboration will be essential for continuing to monitor and learn about the virus and the epidemic it is causing. Even amid uncertainty, we should root our response in evidence. Without evidence to guide our actions, we may inadvertently exacerbate the toll of this epidemic. In evaluating how we should respond to this public health emergency, we must consider not only whether the measures will work, but also whether the ends justify the means. While we want to do the utmost to protect health, we don't want to pursue measures that will extract a greater toll on societies and our economy than the virus would alone. We must continually assess whether our response strategies are matched to the level of threat that the virus poses and adapt our approach as new information becomes available. With evidence mounting of continued global spread despite aggressive actions being taken by countries, it is becoming clear that a change of course may be needed. Instead of trying to implement measures that likely will not work to prevent the virus from entering out country, we should focus on efforts that we know will help to lessen its impacts, such as ensuring that federal, state and local health agencies, and hospitals and health clinics have the resources they need to diagnose, isolate and safely treat cases, and to promote feasible approaches to community mitigation that are most likely to mitigate disease spread. For this we will need government leadership and additional investments.

In: Coronavirus …
Editor: Roger F. Martin
ISBN: 978-1-53617-939-2

Chapter 5

WHAT YOU NEED TO KNOW ABOUT CORONAVIRUS DISEASE 2019 (COVID-19)*

Department of Health and Human Services

WHAT IS CORONAVIRUS DISEASE 2019 (COVID-19)?

Coronavirus disease 2019 (COVID-19) is a respiratory illness that can spread from person to person. The virus that causes COVID-19 is a novel coronavirus that was first identified during an investigation into an outbreak in Wuhan, China.

CAN PEOPLE IN THE U.S. GET COVID-19?

COVID-19 is spreading from person to person in China, and limited spread among close contacts has been detected in some countries outside China, including the United States. At this time, however, this virus is NOT currently spreading in communities in the United States. Right now, the greatest risk of infection is for people in China or people who have traveled to China. Risk of infection is dependent on exposure. Close contacts of people who are infected are at greater risk of exposure, for example health care workers and close contacts of people who are infected with the virus that causes COVID-19. CDC continues to closely monitor the situation.

* This is an edited, reformatted and augmented version of Department of Health and Human Services Publication, No. CS 314937-A 02, dated February 21, 2020.

Have There Been Cases of COVID-19 in the U.S.?

Yes. The first case of COVID-19 in the United States was reported on January 21, 2020. The current count of cases of COVID-19 in the United States is available on CDC's webpage at https://www.cdc.gov/coronavirus/ 2019-ncov/cases-in-us.html.

How Does COVID-19 Spread?

The virus that causes COVID-19 probably emerged from an animal source, but now it seems to be spreading from person to person. It's important to note that person-to-person spread can happen on a continuum. Some diseases are highly contagious (like measles), while other diseases are less so. At this time, it's unclear how easily or sustainably the virus that causes COVID-19 is spreading between people. Learn what is known about the spread of newly emerged coronaviruses at https://www.cdc.gov/ coronavirus/2019-ncov/about/ transmission.html.

What Are the Symptoms of COVID-19?

Patients with COVID-19 have had mild to severe respiratory illness with symptoms of

- fever
- cough
- shortness of breath

What Are Severe Complications from This Virus?

Many patients have pneumonia in both lungs.

How Can I Help Protect Myself?

The best way to prevent infection is to avoid being exposed to the virus that causes COVID-19.

There Are Simple Everyday Preventive Actions to Help Prevent the Spread of Respiratory Viruses. These Include

- Avoid close contact with people who are sick.
- Avoid touching your eyes, nose, and mouth with unwashed hands.
- Wash your hands often with soap and water for at least 20 seconds. Use an alcohol-based hand sanitizer that contains at least 60% alcohol if soap and water are not available.

If You Are Sick, to Keep from Spreading Respiratory Illness to Others, You Should

- Stay home when you are sick.
- Cover your cough or sneeze with a tissue, then throw the tissue in the trash.
- Clean and disinfect frequently touched objects and surfaces.

What Should I Do if I Recently Traveled to China and Got Sick?

If you were in China within the past 14 days and feel sick with fever, cough, or difficulty breathing, you should seek medical care. Call the office of your health care provider before you go, and tell them about your travel and your symptoms. They will give you instructions on how to get care without exposing other people to your illness. While sick, avoid contact with people, don't go out and delay any travel to reduce the possibility of spreading illness to others.

Is There a Vaccine?

There is currently no vaccine to protect against COVID-19. The best way to prevent infection is to avoid being exposed to the virus that causes COVID-19.

IS THERE A TREATMENT?

There is no specific antiviral treatment for COVID-19. People with COVID-19 can seek medical care to help relieve symptoms.

In: Coronavirus …
Editor: Roger F. Martin
ISBN: 978-1-53617-939-2

Chapter 6

CORONAVIRUS DISEASE 2019 (COVID-19) SITUATION SUMMARY*

Centers for Disease Control and Prevention

This is an emerging, rapidly evolving situation and CDC will provide updated information as it becomes available, in addition to updated guidance.

BACKGROUND

CDC is responding to an outbreak of respiratory disease caused by a novel (new) coronavirus that was first detected in China and which has now been detected in almost 70 locations internationally, including in the United States. The virus has been named "SARS-CoV-2" and the disease it causes has been named "coronavirus disease 2019" (abbreviated "COVID-19").

On January 30, 2020, the International Health Regulations Emergency Committee of the World Health Organization declared the outbreak a "public health emergency of international concernexternal icon" (PHEIC). On January 31, 2020, Health and Human Services Secretary Alex M. Azar II declared a public health emergency (PHE) for the United States to aid the nation's healthcare community in responding to COVID-19.

---

* This is an edited, reformatted and augmented version of Centers for Disease Control and Prevention Publication, Updated March 3, 2020.

SOURCE AND SPREAD OF THE VIRUS

Coronaviruses are a large family of viruses that are common in people and many different species of animals, including camels, cattle, cats, and bats. Rarely, animal coronaviruses can infect people and then spread between people such as with MERS-CoV, SARS-CoV, and now with this new virus (named SARS-CoV-2).

The SARS-CoV-2 virus is a betacoronavirus, like MERS-CoV and SARS-CoV. All three of these viruses have their origins in bats. The sequences from U.S. patients are similar to the one that China initially posted, suggesting a likely single, recent emergence of this virus from an animal reservoir.

Early on, many of the patients at the epicenter of the outbreak in Wuhan, Hubei Province, China had some link to a large seafood and live animal market, suggesting animal-to-person spread. Later, a growing number of patients reportedly did not have exposure to animal markets, indicating person-to-person spread. Person-to-person spread was subsequently reported outside Hubei and in countries outside China, including in the United States. Some international destinations now have apparent community spread with the virus that causes COVID-19, including in some parts of the United States. Community spread means some people have been infected and it is not known how or where they became exposed. Learn what is known about the spread of this newly emerged coronaviruses.

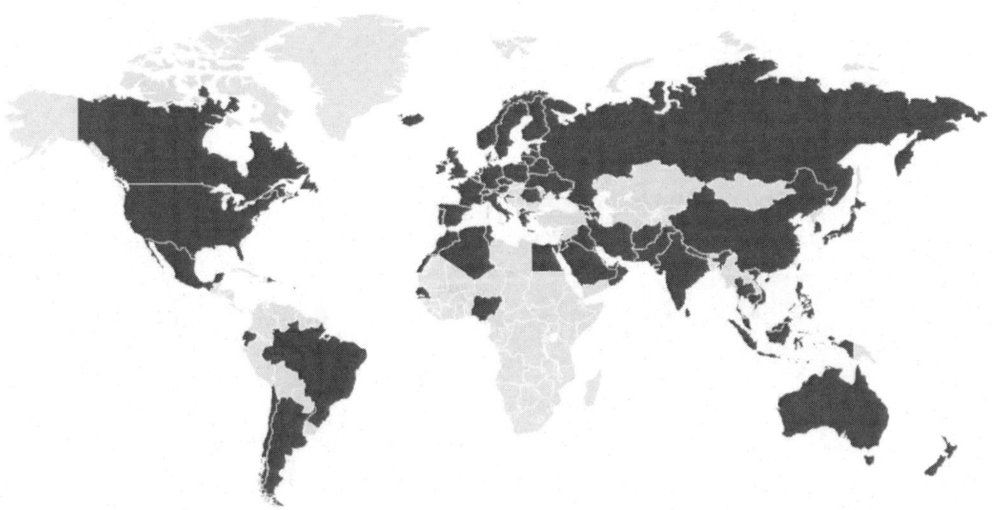

Confirmed COVID-19 Cases Global Map.

View larger image and see a list of locations

COVID-19 CASES IN THE U.S.

Situation in U.S.

- Imported cases of COVID 19 in travelers have been detected in the U.S.
- Person-to-person spread of COVID-19 was first reported among close contacts of returned travelers from Wuhan.
- During the week of February 23, CDC reported community spread of the virus that causes COVID-19 in California (in two places), Oregon and Washington. Community spread in Washington resulted in the first death in the United States from COVID-19, as well as the first reported case of COVID-19 in a health care worker, and the first potential outbreak in a long-term care facility.

Illness Severity

Both MERS-CoV and SARS-CoV have been known to cause severe illness in people. The complete clinical picture with regard to COVID-19 is not fully understood. Reported illnesses have ranged from mild to severe, including illness resulting in death. While information so far suggests that most COVID-19 illness is mild, a reportexternal icon out of China suggests serious illness occurs in 16% of cases. Older people and people with certain underlying health conditions like heart disease, lung disease and diabetes, for example, seem to be at greater risk of serious illness.

Learn more about the symptoms associated with COVID-19.

There are ongoing investigations to learn more. This is a rapidly evolving situation and information will be updated as it becomes available.

RISK ASSESSMENT

Outbreaks of novel virus infections among people are always of public health concern. The risk from these outbreaks depends on characteristics of the virus, including how well it spreads between people, the severity of resulting illness, and the medical or other measures available to control the impact of the virus (for example, vaccine or treatment medications). The fact that this disease has caused illness, including illness resulting in death, and sustained person-to-person spread is concerning. These factors meet two of the criteria of a pandemic. As community spread is detected in more and more countries, the world moves closer toward meeting the third criteria, worldwide spread of the new virus.

Reported community spread of COVID-19 in parts of the United States raises the level of concern about the immediate threat for COVID-19 for those communities. The potential public health threat posed by COVID-19 is very high, to the United States and globally.

At this time, however, most people in the United States will have little immediate risk of exposure to this virus. This virus is NOT currently spreading widely in the United States. However, it is important to note that current global circumstances suggest it is likely that this virus will cause a pandemic. This is a rapidly evolving situation and the risk assessment will be updated as needed.

Current risk assessment:

- For most of the American public, who are unlikely to be exposed to this virus at this time, the immediate health risk from COVID-19 is considered low.
- People in communities where ongoing community spread with the virus that causes COVID-19 has been reported are at elevated, though still relatively low risk of exposure.
- Healthcare workers caring for patients with COVID-19 are at elevated risk of exposure.
- Close contacts of persons with COVID-19 also are at elevated risk of exposure.
- Travelers returning from affected international locations where community spread is occurring also are at elevated risk of exposure.

CDC has developed guidance to help in the risk assessment and management of people with potential exposures to COVID-19.

WHAT MAY HAPPEN

More cases of COVID-19 are likely to be identified in the coming days, including more cases in the United States. It's also likely that person-to-person spread will continue to occur, including in communities in the United States. It's likely that at some point, widespread transmission of COVID-19 in the United States will occur.

Widespread transmission of COVID-19 would translate into large numbers of people needing medical care at the same time. Schools, childcare centers, workplaces, and other places for mass gatherings may experience more absenteeism. Public health and healthcare systems may become overloaded, with elevated rates of hospitalizations and deaths. Other critical infrastructure, such as law enforcement, emergency medical services, and transportation industry may also be affected. Health care providers and hospitals may be overwhelmed. At this time, there is no vaccine to protect against

COVID-19 and no medications approved to treat it. Nonpharmaceutical interventions would be the most important response strategy.

CDC Response

Global efforts at this time are focused concurrently on containing the spread and mitigating the impact of this virus. The federal government is working closely with state, local, tribal, and territorial partners, as well as public health partners, to respond to this public health threat. The public health response is multi-layered, with the goal of detecting and minimizing introductions of this virus in the United States. CDC is operationalizing all of its pandemic preparedness and response plans, working on multiple fronts to meet these goals, including specific measures to prepare communities to respond to local transmission of the virus that causes COVID-19. There is an abundance of pandemic guidance developed in anticipation of an influenza pandemic that is being repurposed and adapted for a COVID-19 pandemic.

Highlights of CDC's Response

- CDC established a COVID-19 Incident Management System on January 7, 2020. On January 21, CDC activated its Emergency Operations Center to better provide ongoing support to the COVID-19 response.
- The U.S. government has taken unprecedented steps with respect to *travel* in response to the growing public health threat posed by this new coronavirus:
    - Effective February 2, at 5pm, the U.S. government suspended entry of foreign nationals who have been in China within the past 14 days.
        - U.S. citizens, residents, and their immediate family members who have been in Hubei province and other parts of mainland China are allowed to enter the United States, but they are subject to health monitoring and possible quarantine for up to 14 days.
    - On February 29, the U.S. government announced it was suspending entry of foreign nationals who have been in Iran within the past 14 days.
    - CDC has issued the following travel guidance related to COVID-19:
        - China — Level 3, Avoid Nonessential Travel — updated February 22;
        - Hong Kong — Level 1, Practice Usual Precautions — issued February 19;
        - Iran — Level 3, Avoid Nonessential Travel — updated February 28;
        - Italy — Level 3, Avoid Nonessential Travel — updated February 28;

        - Japan — Level 2, Practice Enhanced Precautions — updated February 22;
        - South Korea — Level 3, Avoid Nonessential Travel — updated February 24.
    - CDC also recommends that all travelers reconsider cruise ship voyages into or within Asia at this time.
- CDC is issuing clinical guidance, including:
    - On January 30, CDC published guidance for healthcare professionals on the clinical care of COVID-19 patients.
    - On February 3, CDC posted guidance for assessing the potential risk for various exposures to COVID-19 and managing those people appropriately.
    - On February 27, CDC updated its criteria to guide evaluation of persons under investigation for COVID-19.
    - On February 28, CDC issued a Health Alert Network (HAN): Update and Interim Guidance on Outbreak of COVID-19.
- CDC has deployed multidisciplinary teams to support state health departments case identification, contact tracing, clinical management, and communications.
- CDC has worked with the Department of State, supporting the safe return of Americans who have been stranded as a result of the ongoing outbreaks of COVID-19 and related travel restrictions. CDC has worked to assess the health of passengers as they return to the United States and provided continued daily monitoring of people who are quarantined.

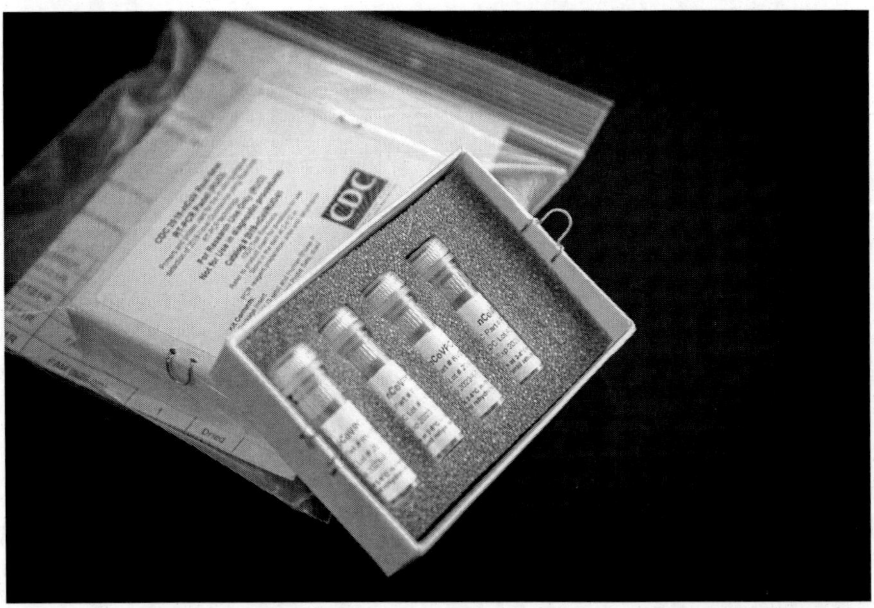

This is a picture of CDC's laboratory test kit for severe acute respiratory syndrome coronavirus 2 (SARS-CoV-2). CDC is shipping the test kits to laboratories CDC has designated as qualified, including U.S. state and local public health laboratories, Department of Defense (DOD) laboratories and select international laboratories. The test kits are bolstering global laboratory capacity for detecting SARS-CoV-2.

- An important part of CDC's role during a public health emergency is to develop a test for the pathogen and equip state and local public health labs with testing capacity.
  - After distribution of a CDC rRT-PCR test to diagnose COVID-19 to state and local public health labs started, performance issues were identified related to a problem in the manufacturing of one of the reagents. Laboratories were not able to verify the test performance.
  - CDC worked on two potential resolutions to this problem.
    - CDC developed a new protocol that uses two of the three components of the original CDC test kit to detect the virus that causes COVID-19 after establishing that the third component, which was the problem with the original test, can be excluded from testing without affecting accuracy. CDC is working with FDA to amend the existing Emergency Use Authorization (EUA) for the test, but in the meantime, FDA granted discretionary authority for the use of the original test kits.
    - Public health laboratories can use the original CDC test kit to test for the virus that causes COVID-19 using the new protocol.
    - Further, newly manufactured kits have been provided to the International Reagent Resourceexternal icon for distribution.
  - Combined with other reagents that CDC has procured, there are enough testing kits to test more than 75,000 people.
  - In addition, CDC has two laboratories conducting testing for the virus that causes COVID-19. CDC can test approximately 350 specimens per day.
  - Commercial labs are working to develop their own tests that hopefully will be available soon. This will allow a greater number of tests to happen close to where potential cases are.
  - CDC has grown the COVID-19 virus in cell culture, which is necessary for further studies, including for additional genetic characterization. The cell-grown virus was sent to NIH's BEI Resources Repositoryexternal iconexternal icon for use by the broad scientific community.

CDC RECOMMENDS

- Everyone can do their part to help us respond to this emerging public health threat:
    - It's currently flu and respiratory disease season and CDC recommends getting a flu vaccine, taking everyday preventive actions to help stop the spread of germs, and taking flu antivirals if prescribed.
    - If you are a healthcare provider, be on the look-out for:
        - People who recently traveled from China or another affected area and who have symptoms associated with COVID-19, and
        - People who have been in close contact with someone with COVID-19 or pneumonia of unknown cause. (Consult the most recent definition for patients under investigation [PUIs].)
    - If you are a healthcare provider or a public health responder caring for a COVID-19 patient, please take care of yourself and follow recommended infection control procedures.
    - If you are a close contact of someone with COVID-19 and develop symptoms of COVID-19, call your healthcare provider and tell them about your symptoms and your exposure.
- If you are a resident in a community where person-to-person spread of COVID-19 has been detected and you develop COVID-19 symptoms, call your healthcare provider and tell them about your symptoms.
- For people who are ill with COVID-19, but are not sick enough to be hospitalized, please follow CDC guidance on how to reduce the risk of spreading your illness to others. People who are mildly ill with COVID-19 are able to isolate at home during their illness.
- If you have been in China or another affected area or have been exposed to someone sick with COVID-19 in the last 14 days, you will face some limitations on your movement and activity for up to 14 days. Please follow instructions during this time. Your cooperation is integral to the ongoing public health response to try to slow spread of this virus.

In: Coronavirus …
Editor: Roger F. Martin
ISBN: 978-1-53617-939-2

Chapter 7

SCIENCE AND TECH SPOTLIGHT: CORONAVIRUSES*

Timothy M. Persons

WHY THIS MATTERS

Coronaviruses can spread rapidly and cause outbreaks with high mortality rates. They were not considered a major risk for humans until the SARS outbreak in 2002. Since then, there have been multiple highly contagious outbreaks originating in animals and spreading to humans—most recently the outbreak in Wuhan, China of Coronavirus Disease 2019 (COVID-19).

THE SCIENCE

What Is It?

While the outbreak of COVID-19 in China has brought the term coronavirus into daily usage, coronaviruses can vary in severity. They can cause respiratory issues, such as pneumonia, and are believed to be one cause of the common cold. According to the Centers for Disease Control and Prevention (CDC), most people will be infected by a coronavirus at some point in their lifetimes. As of March 2020, seven coronaviruses have been identified that can cause illness in humans. Most infections result in mild to

---

* This is an edited, reformatted and augmented version of the United States Government Accountability Office Publication, No. GAO-20-472SP Coronaviruses, dated March 2020.

moderate symptoms, such as runny nose, headache, cough, sore throat, fever, and a run-down feeling.

Coronaviruses are most commonly transmitted by coughing, sneezing, person-to-person contact, and touching objects that have viral particles on them, according to CDC. The best prevention is washing hands with soap and avoiding contact with people who are sick or work in quarantine areas. Current treatment methods are limited, and research is being fast-tracked to develop a vaccine against existing and emerging coronaviruses.

Recent high-profile coronavirus outbreaks have raised new concern because of high mortality rates relative to the coronaviruses that cause the common cold. In addition, the severe coronaviruses can cause both upper- and lower-respiratory-tract infections, including pneumonia.

Since 2002, there have been three severe outbreaks of respiratory illness caused by coronaviruses, all three originating in animals. In 2002, an outbreak of Severe Acute Respiratory Syndrome (SARS) began in China and had a mortality rate of approximately 10 percent. In 2012, an outbreak of Middle East Respiratory Syndrome (MERS) had a mortality rate reported as high as 34 percent. Most recently, a December 2019 outbreak of a new coronavirus, SARS-CoV-2—which causes COVID-19—has seen a high infection rate, with over 70,000 infected and over 2,600 deaths—a mortality rate of approximately 3 percent as of February 24th, 2020, according to the World Health Organization (WHO). Estimates of the reproductive ratio, or R_0, for COVID-19 have also indicated that it has the potential to spread rapidly. These estimates are tentative, however, because the R_0 is a complex epidemiologic measure that is context-specific and affected by numerous biological, behavioral, and environmental factors.

How Does It Work?

Coronaviruses are believed to work in similar ways. Viral particles attach themselves to specific molecules, known as receptors, on the surface of a human or animal cell, allowing the virus to enter. Once inside, the virus discards its outer coating, releasing its genetic material into the host cell. This can occur in many cells at the same time. The virus can then use the cell's own mechanisms—for example, the mechanism to produce proteins based on genetic code—to replicate itself. The hijacking of the cell's functions causes the release of new viral particles and restarting the process, either in more cells of the same host or in another host that becomes infected.

Coronaviruses mutate rapidly compared to other viruses, enabling them to adapt to new environments. Coronaviruses are ribonucleic acid (RNA) viruses, which are more prone to random mutations than deoxyribonucleic acid (DNA) viruses. Because DNA viruses, like chickenpox and many others, are more stable, it is easier to create long term effective vaccines against them. In contrast, RNA viruses, like flu, may regularly require new vaccines.

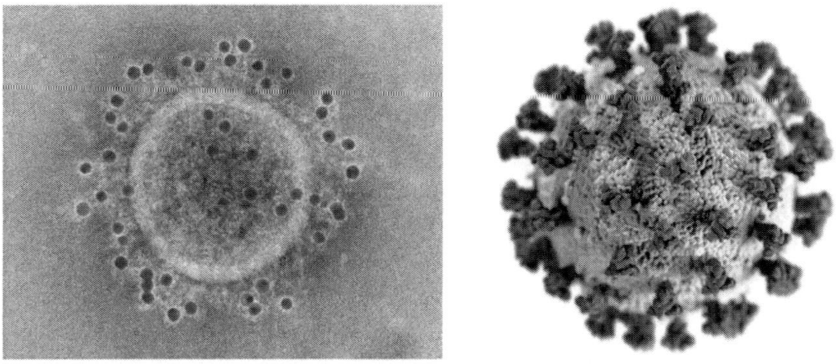

Sources (left to right): National institute of Allergy and Infectiious Diseases; Centers for Disease Control and Prevention, Alissa Eckert, Dan Higgins. | GAO-20-472SP.

Figure 1. Electron microscope image and schematic of coronavirus particles (Middle East Respiratory Syndrome Coronavirus and general coronavirus respectively).

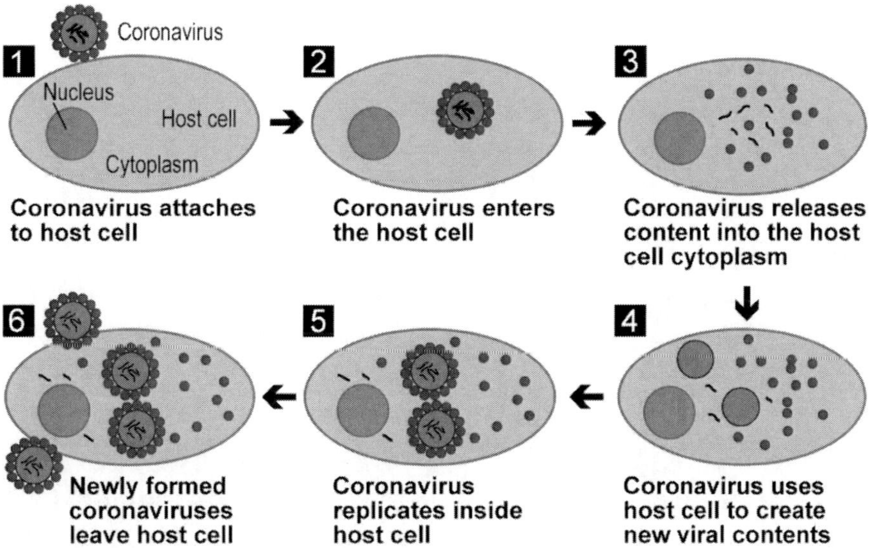

Source: GAO analysis of Fenner's Veterinary Virology edited by N. James MacLachlan and Edward J. Dubovi. | GAO-20-472SP.

Figure 2. Schematic of how a coronavirus infects host cells. This process is similar for all RNA viruses, the large class to which coronaviruses belong.

Generally, coronaviruses originate in animals, with the most likely origin being bats, and can spread from animal to animal. In environments where humans and multiple animal species mix, such as live animal markets and farms, there is an increased likelihood that a coronavirus can mutate and spread into humans. The original animal vector for SARS-CoV-2 has not yet been determined.

How Mature Is It?

Several procedures, including diagnostic testing, are available to address coronaviruses, and are being used in the U.S. response. However, vaccines and therapies are not yet mature.

In the wake of the COVID-19 outbreak, Chinese researchers isolated the virus, sequenced its genome, and shared the results with the scientific community. The sequencing allowed CDC to develop a diagnostic test that is now being distributed to local labs. Also, based on genetic similarities, a vaccine developed for SARS has been recommended by researchers as a possible option for SARS-CoV-2. And researchers are drawing on the SARS-CoV-2 genome to help determine which aspects of the coronavirus might be used to develop a more specific vaccine against it.

For those already infected, doctors are trying a drug originally made to treat Ebola that also works against SARS and MERS. The first U.S. patient diagnosed with COVID-19 was treated with this drug under compassionate use (a policy allowing some use of non-approved drugs), and additional antivirals are being tested.

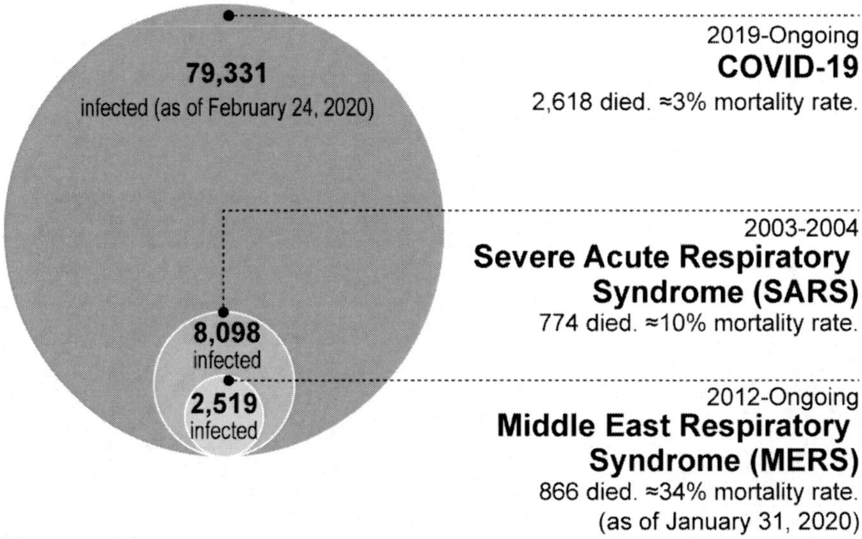

Source: World Health Organization (WHO). | GAO-20-472SP.

Figure 3. The recent outbreaks of coronavirus-caused diseases known to infect humans (COVID-19 numbers are confirmed and as reported by China).

Opportunities

- Identification of common targets in coronaviruses to develop
- vaccines against all coronaviruses.

- Increased coordination by industry, academia, and government could improve awareness of treatment options for future outbreaks.
- Advances in predictive infectious disease modelling to better inform decisions about interventions in future outbreaks.

Challenges

- For rapid deployment, potential treatments need to be prepared prior to an outbreak despite limited information and incentives.
- Development of vaccines for RNA viruses requires frequent evaluation and reformulation. It is complex, costly, and time consuming.
- Outbreak detection requires constant monitoring and coordination among nations, which can be impeded by more closed societies.
- Global economic consequences of such outbreaks can be serious. According to multiple economic forecasting models, SARS cost the global economy $30-100 billion.

Policy Context and Questions

- To what extent are surveillance and clinical data, computational models, and information sharing mechanisms in place to promote agile and effective risk management during disease outbreaks?
- What policies and mechanisms are in place or needed to help maintain medical supply chains during global disease outbreaks?

Selected References

Centers for Disease Control and Prevention
https://www.cdc.gov/ coronavirus/index.html
World Health Organization
https://www.who.int/health-topics/ corona virus

In: Coronavirus ...
Editor: Roger F. Martin
ISBN: 978-1-53617-939-2

Chapter 8

COVID-19: CURRENT TRAVEL RESTRICTIONS AND QUARANTINE MEASURES*

Edward C. Liu

The United States, along with many countries, is responding to an outbreak of a respiratory disease, now referred to as COVID-19, which is caused by a novel coronavirus first detected in mainland China's Hubei Province in late 2019. Cases of COVID-19 have now been detected in several countries, including the United States.

To date, the federal government has taken two key actions to deter persons with suspected COVID-19 infection from entering the country or spreading the virus to persons within the United States. First, the federal government has restricted many non-U.S. nationals (aliens) who recently travelled to mainland China or Iran from entering the United States. Second, the federal government has imposed a quarantine requirement on all persons entering the United States, regardless of citizenship status, who have recently been to mainland China. This Legal Sidebar examines the legal authorities underlying these actions, as well as possible legal challenges to their use.

ENTRY RESTRICTIONS

To deter the entry of aliens into the United States who may have been exposed to COVID-19, President Trump has invoked his authority over alien entry under Section 212(f) of the Immigration and Nationality Act (INA). That provision allows the President

* This is an edited, reformatted and augmented version of Congressional Research Service Publication No. LSB10415, dated March 5, 2020.

to "suspend the entry of all aliens, or any class of aliens" whose entry he "finds . . . would be detrimental to the interests of the United States." Under this authority, President Trump issued a Proclamation on January 31, 2020, generally suspending the entry of any foreign national who had been in mainland China at some point within the prior 14 days. But lawful permanent residents (LPRs), most immediate relatives of U.S. citizens and LPRs, and some other groups, such as some airplane and ship crew members, are exempted from this restriction, as are those with prior presence in Hong Kong or Macau. On February 29, 2020, President Trump issued a second Proclamation that similarly suspends the entry of any foreign national who has been in Iran within the prior 14 days, in addition to making minor amendments to the earlier Proclamation.

While this appears to be the first time Section 212(f) has been used to control the spread of acommunicable disease, the provision has been previously invoked to restrict foreign travelers from coming into the United States. Perhaps most notably, Section 212(f) provided the legal basis for the Trump Administration's imposition of the so-called "travel ban" on certain foreign nationals from designated countries. In the context of a challenge to that invocation of Section 212(f), the Supreme Court held that the provision "exudes deference to the President in every clause" and gives him mostly unfettered discretion to decide "when to suspend entry," "whose entry to suspend," "for how long," and "on what conditions." In light of the deference afforded to the President's determinations over these matters, coupled with the amount of evidence demonstrating the communicability of COVID-19, it seems unlikely that a court would find that the Proclamations issued with respect to mainland China and Iran exceed the scope of the President's authority under Section 212(f).

QUARANTINE AND ISOLATION

The Administration's January 31, 2020, Proclamation also directed the Secretary of Homeland Security "to regulate the travel of persons and aircraft to the United States to facilitate the orderly medical screening and, where appropriate, quarantine of persons who enter the United States and who may have been exposed to the virus." To this end, on February 2, 2020, the U.S. Department of Homeland Security (DHS) imposed screening and quarantine rules for persons – including U.S. nationals, LPRs, and their immediate family members – who arrive in the United States within 14 days after having been in mainland China. Those persons travelling by air must arrive at one of 11 designated airports where they will be screened. On March 2, 2020, DHS imposed similar requirements for air travelers who were recently present in Iran. Screened persons will be taken to a medical facility for isolation and treatment if fever, cough, or difficulty breathing is detected. Asymptomatic persons are generally to be held under federal quarantine for 14 days from the time they left mainland China if they visited Hubei

Province. But asymptomatic persons whose recent travel did not include Hubei Province are asked to self-quarantine for 14 days. State and local health authorities are to provide oversight of individuals who self-quarantine.

Authority for these quarantine rules comes from Section 361 of the Public Health Service Act, which authorizes the U.S. Department of Health and Human Services (HHS) to promulgate and enforce regulations "necessary to prevent the introduction, transmission, or spread of communicable diseases from foreign countries into the States or possessions, or from one State or possession into any other State or possession." Besides authorizing the apprehension and examination of "any individual reasonably believed to be infected with a communicable disease in a qualifying stage" who is "moving or about to move from a State to another State," Section 361 also authorizes the apprehension and quarantine of persons who are not engaged in interstate travel, but are reasonably believed "to be a probable source of infection to individuals who, while infected with such disease in a qualifying stage, will be moving from a State to another State." To facilitate these quarantine requirements, HHS promulgated an interim final rule, effective February 7, 2020, requiring airlines with flights arriving in the United States to transmit to HHS's Centers for Disease Control and Prevention (CDC) identifying information about passengers or crew who may be at risk of exposure to communicable disease.

In addition to federal quarantine authority, states may quarantine or isolate persons as public health risks using their police powers. State mandatory quarantine laws vary, with some implemented through public health orders issued by state health departments, and others effectuated through court orders authorizing the detention of an individual upon some evidentiary showing that the person poses a public health risk.

Possible Constitutional Challenges

Because quarantine requirements involve a deprivation of a person's liberty to move freely, they have occasionally been challenged on constitutional grounds. Specifically, the Supreme Court "repeatedly has recognized that civil commitment for any purpose constitutes a significant deprivation of liberty that requires due process protection." Accordingly, quarantine measures may be challenged as violating the Constitution's *substantive* or *procedural* due process protections.

Substantive due process challenges center on whether a governmental action "is so egregious, so outrageous, that it may fairly be said to shock the contemporary conscience," without regard to "the fairness of the procedures used to implement" the action. Recent challenges to quarantine and isolation for public health reasons have borrowed from substantive due process precedents involving involuntary commitment. In that context, substantive due process challenges question whether the government has set forth an adequate justification to support the deprivation of liberty effected by a quarantine policy (a type of challenge that might also be viewed through an equal protection rather than a due process lens). In either case, a substantive due process challenge to quarantine policies affecting those suspected of COVID-19 seems unlikely to succeed given the degree of public health risk posed by the virus. Courts have recognized that expeditious actions by government officials are frequently required to protect public health or safety, and have been reluctant to find substantive due process violations even if those actions are found to be erroneous after the fact.

There might also be concerns as to whether a quarantine policy satisfies the Constitution's *procedural due process* requirements. These requirements concern whether the *process* attending a particular deprivation by the government – in this case the restraint on liberty during the quarantine period – is fair. The degree of protection required by procedural due process is a "flexible" concept, requiring an examination of the private interests at stake; the risk of an erroneous deprivation of such interest and the probable value of additional safeguards; and the government's interests. In the context of state action, the Supreme Court has said that the Due Process Clause typically "requires some kind of a hearing *before* the State deprives a person of liberty," but has also held that the "necessity of quick action by the State or the impracticality of providing any predeprivation process" may mean that a *post-deprivation* remedy is constitutionally adequate. Here, the government may argue that the contagiousness of the COVID-19 virus may make predeprivation process impractical before requiring the quarantine of a person suspected of COVID-19 infection.

In 2014, a federal district court applying this standard in the context of a Friday-to-Monday quarantine of a nurse who had recently been in contact with Ebola patients found that the lack of a predeprivation hearing was not a clear violation of due process because quarantine is "necessarily prophylactic and peremptory." However, the court noted that the relatively short duration of the quarantine (80 hours) also factored into its conclusion. Moreover, to the extent that post-deprivation procedural due process claims may be made, government actors may still enjoy qualified immunity to civil liability if the action "does not violate clearly established statutory or constitutional rights of which a reasonable person would have known."

OTHER LEGAL ISSUES

Federal officials have warned that as the United States begins to see "community spread" of COVID-19, actions taken to limit entry of persons into the country may be less important than domestic quarantine and isolation of persons already present in the United States. Shifts in the types of actions taken in response to the disease may also present distinct legal issues from those discussed above. For example, questions have arisen regarding the employment protections that workers may have under federal laws, such as the Family and Medical Leave Act (or perhaps under state laws), if those workers fall ill, are placed under mandatory quarantine, or choose to stay home voluntarily to avoid exposure to themselves or others or to take care of an infected family member.

The federal government may also seek to facilitate the distribution of medical countermeasures to COVID-19 as they continue to develop through the issuance of emergency use authorizations (EUA) under Section 564 of the Federal Food, Drug, and Cosmetic Act. One such EUA was issued on February 4, 2020, to enable emergency use of the CDC's real-time COVID-19 diagnostic test. On February 29, 2020, FDA issued additional guidance stating that it would not object to the use of certain diagnostic tests prior to issuance of an EUA. In addition, the federal government has the authority to waive liability for manufacturers, distributors, and providers of such countermeasures, under the Public Readiness and Emergency Preparedness Act, which it most recently invoked with respect to Ebola countermeasures.

In: Coronavirus …
Editor: Roger F. Martin
ISBN: 978-1-53617-939-2

Chapter 9

COVID-19: FEDERAL ECONOMIC DEVELOPMENT TOOLS AND POTENTIAL RESPONSES*

Michael H. Cecire

The current coronavirus disease (COVID-19) outbreak has led to tens of thousands of cases and thousands of deaths worldwide. In addition to the disease's mortality and public health effects, it may have potentially significant economic implications, including productivity losses, supply chain disruptions, labor dislocation, and potential financial pressure on businesses and households. Relatively few federal programs are available to provide timely economic relief to affected businesses. This Insight considers the outbreak's economic development implications and policy considerations for Members of Congress who have shown interest in addressing the economic dimensions of this public health issue.

COVID-19 ECONOMIC DEVELOPMENT IMPLICATIONS

COVID-19 is a newly designated disease caused by a previously undetected coronavirus. Most cases have been reported in China, with additional cases on every inhabited continent. Clusters of illness have occurred in South Korea, Japan, Singapore, Italy, and Iran. For more information on the health and epidemiological aspects of COVID-19, see CRS products R46219 and IF11421.

* This is an edited, reformatted and augmented version of Congressional Research Service Publication No. IN11228, dated February 28, 2020.

The COVID-19 outbreak is foremost a public health issue. However, the epidemic itself and containment measures in China and elsewhere could have significant economic implications for the United States and globally. In the short-term, the COVID-19 outbreak is primarily a threat to businesses dependent on supply chains in China, or for exports there. However, many economists have warned that a more prolonged crisis may see broader economic disruptions if workplaces and schools are closed to contain the outbreak, and medical and food supplies dwindle due to disrupted supply and increased demand.

In China, mass containment measures have disrupted global supply chains and capital markets. In the near term, the outbreak's effects on the U.S. economy could be limited to localized disruptions for businesses and workers—particularly in communities dependent on technology manufacturing and tourism. In certain cases, supply chain issues may stall production, prevent companies from fulfilling orders, and potentially impact firm revenues.

In a prolonged or wider epidemic, supply chain issues may further compound. Growth could slow further, and affected companies may be forced to furlough or lay off workers, and others may slow hiring. As demonstrated in China and elsewhere, social distancing measures can effectively stop local economic activity, which may impact localized labor markets, household finances, and governmental tax revenues and service delivery. Additional considerations include potential shortages of medical supplies and foodstuffs, other ancillary health effects, and the U.S. medical and public health system's ability to cope with a significant outbreak.

CONSIDERATIONS FOR CONGRESS

Many Members of Congress have heard concerns from constituents affected by supply chain-, exports-, and tourism-related disruptions from the outbreak. Relatively few federal programs exist to provide timely relief to businesses for outbreak-related disruptions. Some programs include

- The Small Business Administration (SBA) administers disaster and non-disaster loans for small businesses and organizations, and supports an extensive network of SBA-affiliated resource partners who provide management and technical assistance to small businesses;
- The Department of the Treasury's Community Development Financial Institution Fund supports organizations that provide loans to businesses, homebuyers, community developers, and investors in distressed areas; and
- The Department of Agriculture's (USDA) Rural Development program offers limited services to support rural businesses to create or retain jobs.

In the event that disruptions continue and grow, public and non-profit organizations may consider tapping various federal economic development resources, including

- The Department of Housing and Urban Development's Community Development Block Grant (CDBG) program may be used for technical assistance, community assets, and workforce development;
- The Department of Commerce's Economic Development Administration programs may be used to diversify local economic bases;
- USDA programs can provide technical assistance and infrastructure support; and
- Federal regional commissions and authorities support economic diversification, workforce development, and technical assistance in their service areas.

Federal economic development programs are generally not equipped to provide rapid support to firms or communities affected by public health emergencies, though unemployment compensation programs have the ability to rapidly respond and provide immediate income support. In response to a COVID-19 outbreak, Congress may consider measures used in past disasters or economic crises:

- CDBG authorities for disaster recovery (CDBG-DR) could be utilized to address the outbreak's economic impact. Previous CDBG-DR uses included loans and grants to small and medium-sized enterprises (SMEs), workforce development, and community stabilization.
- Public health-related disruption eligibility for SBA's Economic Injury Disaster Loans (EIDLs) could be made explicit. EIDLs provide up to $2 million to small businesses that suffer economic injury following disasters such as hurricanes. EIDLs may be awarded if the President issues a disaster or emergency declaration, or a disaster declaration by the SBA administrator upon request from a state governor.
- In response to the 2007-2009 recession, federal measures included direct interventions to stabilize industries and markets. A similar effort could support affected industries or supply chains, and/or federal loan guarantees to assist affected SMEs.
- In the recession, Unemployment Compensation benefits were temporarily augmented and extended, with some costs temporarily assumed by the federal government. Disaster Unemployment Assistance, which provides federally funded unemployment benefits to those unable to work as a result of a federally declared disaster and otherwise ineligible for regular benefits, could be a model for responding to public health emergencies.

- Following a federally declared disaster, the Internal Revenue Service (IRS) can provide tax relief to affected individuals. The IRS could provide such allowances to affected individuals and SMEs affected by a public health emergency.

Other federal emergency authorities could be utilized in more severe scenarios for individual and public assistance. In such cases, localities with major revenue shortfalls from federally declared disasters—such as those highly dependent on a dislocated industry, such as tourism—could utilize Community Disaster Loans, which provide up to $5 million in liquidity and are potentially forgivable. The President may also call upon the Defense Production Act (DPA) to mobilize key segments of the economy in response to the outbreak. In major national emergencies, DPA authorities may be used to rebalance disrupted critical supply chains, and to allocate and procure emergency supplies.

In: Coronavirus …
Editor: Roger F. Martin
ISBN: 978-1-53617-939-2

Chapter 10

COVID-2019: GLOBAL IMPLICATIONS AND RESPONSES*

Tiaji Salaam-Blyther, Susan V. Lawrence, Sara M. Tharakan and Frank Gottron

OVERVIEW

As of February 27, 2020, the novel coronavirus first identified in patients in Wuhan, China, in early January 2020 had spread to over 45 countries, including the United States. Daily new cases reported outside China now exceed those reported in China. The World Health Organization (WHO) has declared the outbreak a Public Health Emergency of International Concern but has resisted labeling it a "pandemic." WHO Director-General Tedros Adhanom Ghebreyesus stated on February 26 that using the word "pandemic" could "signal that we can no longer contain the virus, which is not true." WHO has named the new virus "severe acute respiratory syndrome coronavirus 2" (SARS-CoV-2) and the disease that it causes "coronavirus disease 2019" (COVID-19).

THE VIRUS

Coronaviruses are a large family of zoonotic viruses (viruses transmissible between animals and humans) that can cause illness ranging from the common cold to more severe

* This is an edited, reformatted and augmented version of Congressional Research Service Publication No. IF11421, Updated February 27, 2020.

diseases such as Middle-East Respiratory Syndrome (MERS) and Severe Acute Respiratory Syndrome (SARS). The most common symptoms among confirmed COVID-19 patients include fever, dry cough, and shortness of breath. As of February 26, 2020, WHO reported more than 80,000 confirmed COVID-19 cases globally, including more than 2,700 deaths. All but 5% of the cases and 60 of the deaths were in mainland China, and over 80% of cases in mainland China were reported in Hubei Province, whose capital is Wuhan. Of confirmed COVID-19 patients in China, about 80% experienced only mild symptoms, 13% experienced severe symptoms, and 6% became critically ill. Outside mainland China, the jurisdictions with the highest reported caseloads were South Korea, Italy, Japan, and Iran. More than 700 cases have been detected from the Diamond Princess cruise ship, docked alongside Yokohama, Japan. In addition to China, the United States and Germany have confirmed community transmission of COVID-19, indicating the global response may need to move from a containment strategy to one of mitigation.

Within days of Chinese scientists' sequencing the virus, scientists around the globe developed lab tests to diagnose COVID-19. Current diagnostic supplies are insufficient to meet global demand, however. While trying to increase supply of these tests, developers are also trying to create faster, cheaper, and more easily administered tests. No specific treatments or vaccines for COVID-19 exist. The U.S. National Institutes of Health (NIH) indicated in late January that a candidate vaccine for COVID-19 could be ready for early-stage human testing within three months, compared to the 20 months it took to begin early-state development of an investigational SARS vaccine.

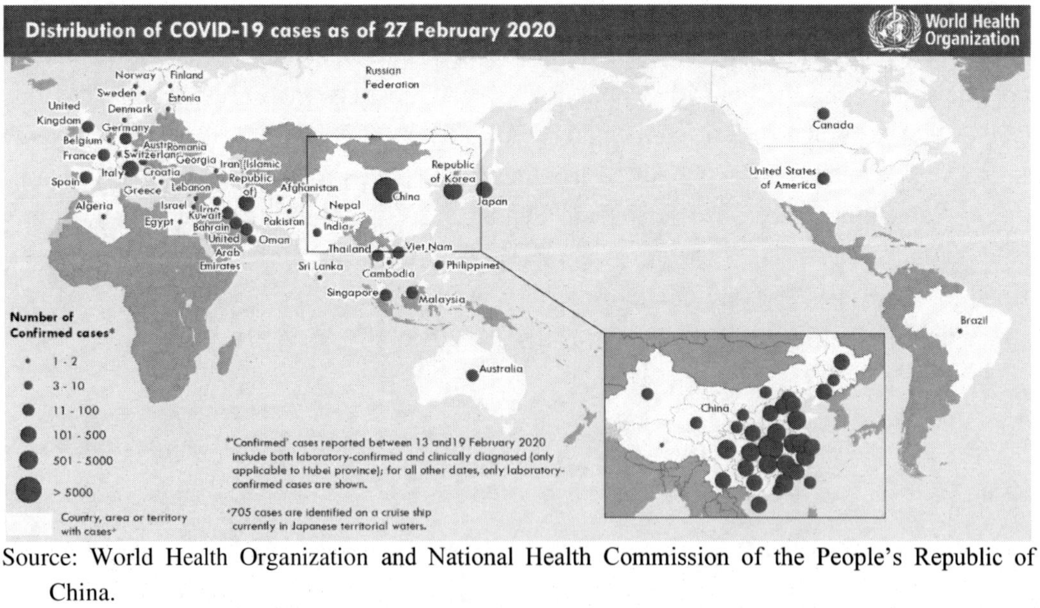

Source: World Health Organization and National Health Commission of the People's Republic of China.

Figure 1. Locations with Confirmed COVID-19 Cases Globally, as of February 27, 2020.

Developments in China

China first reported cases of pneumonia of an unknown cause to the WHO on December 31, 2019. Chinese scientists isolated the virus on January 7, 2020, and shared its genetic sequence with the world on January 12. China's government did not raise the alarm to its own people until January 20, however. Before then, the government appears to have worked to suppress information about the outbreak. Observers have suggested that by withholding information, the government may have squandered an early window of opportunity to stem the virus's spread.

After January 20, Chinese authorities began taking aggressive actions to prevent the virus from spreading further. By February 20, they had imposed *cordon sanitaires*, or restrictions on movement in and out of defined areas, on as many as 760 million people. Human rights groups and others have questioned such measures. Bruce Aylward, the Canadian co-team leader of a WHO- China Joint Mission on COVID-19, praised China, however, for a "bold approach" that "changed the course" of the epidemic and prevented "probably hundreds of thousands of cases of COVID-19 in China."

The WHO-China Joint Mission, which included representatives from the U.S. Centers for Disease Control and Prevention (CDC) and NIH, carried out an on-the-ground investigation of the outbreak in China from February 16 to 24. The mission concluded that the epidemic in China peaked and plateaued between January 23 and February 2, and has been waning since. Aylward acknowledged that the outbreak is not yet controlled in Wuhan, and he warned of the risk that the epidemic could "come back up again as people start to move again, the shops start to open, restaurants open, schools open." He said that risk was "being managed very carefully."

WHO Response

PHEIC

Following the emergence of a disease that might be deemed a Public Health Emergency of International Concern (PHEIC), WHO convenes an advisory group, the IHR Emergency Committee, to review data and make recommendations to the WHO Director-General. At its second meeting, on January 30, WHO's 15-member IHR Emergency Committee for Pneumonia due to the Novel Coronavirus COVID-19 concluded the outbreak had become a PHEIC. That day, WHO Director-General Tedros issued a PHEIC declaration, prompting countries to take specific actions, including heightening surveillance and reporting of the disease. In the case of the United States, Department of Health and Human Services (HHS) Secretary Alex Azar declared "a public health emergency for the entire United States." A PHEIC declaration can prompt countries to provide additional resources for global and domestic response and enable WHO to access certain emergency funding, such as from the United Nations Central Emergency Response Fund (CERF) and the World Bank Pandemic Emergency Financing Facility (PEF).

Pandemic Designation Debate

Some observers have questioned why WHO has not labeled the global COVID- 19 outbreak a pandemic. On February 26, WHO Director- General Tedros defended WHO's caution, arguing, "For the moment, we are not witnessing sustained and intensive community transmission of this virus, and we are not witnessing large-scale severe disease or death." He nonetheless urged countries to "prepare for a potential pandemic," stating, "Every country needs to be ready to detect cases early, to isolate patients, trace contacts, provide quality clinical care, prevent hospital outbreaks, and prevent community transmission."

WHO Funds

On February 5, WHO announced a $675 million COVID-19 preparedness plan for February through April. It aims to provide international coordination and operational support, bolster country readiness and response capacity (particularly in low-resource countries), and accelerate relevant research and innovation. As of February 26, six donors had pledged to provide $30.0 million in support of the plan and WHO had received $1.4 million.

U.S. Response

Leadership

On January 29, President Donald J. Trump announced the formation of the President's Coronavirus Task Force, led by HHS and coordinated by the National Security Council. On February 27, the President appointed Vice President Mike Pence as the Administration's COVID-19 task force leader, and the Vice President subsequently appointed President's Emergency Plan for AIDS Relief (PEPFAR) Ambassador Deborah Birx as the "White House Coronavirus Response Coordinator."

Funds for Global COVID-19 Control

On February 7, the Department of State and the U.S. Agency for International Development committed to use up to $100 million of existing funds to assist China and other affected countries with COVID-19 responses. HHS has made available up to $105 million from the Infectious Disease Rapid Response Reserve Fund for domestic and international COVID-19 responses. In late February, the Administration stated those funds would be exhausted by the end of the month. On February 24, the Administration asked Congress for an emergency supplemental appropriation of $1.25 billion for COVID-19 response efforts. The Administration also asked Congress to allow repurposing of another $1.25 billion in existing funds from across the government, including HHS funds for current Ebola response activities.

Travel Issues and Evacuations

On January 31, 2020, the President suspended the entry into the United States of any foreign national who has been in China within the prior 14 days. On February 2, the Department of Homeland Security issued instructions subjecting returning U.S. citizens with recent travel to Hubei Province to mandatory quarantine of up to 14 days. The State Department has issued a Level 4 ("Do Not Travel") advisory for China and evacuated U.S. citizens and others from Wuhan. The Department ordered the mandatory departure of nonemergency U.S. personnel and their families from the U.S. consulate in Wuhan, and the voluntary departure of nonemergency U.S. personnel and their families from other diplomatic posts in China. The U.S. government also repatriated U.S. citizens from the *Diamond Princess* cruise ship in Japan.

In: Coronavirus …
Editor: Roger F. Martin
ISBN: 978-1-53617-939-2

Chapter 11

Coronavirus Disease 2019 (COVID-19) Hospital Preparedness Assessment Tool*

Department of Health and Human Services

All U.S. hospitals should be prepared for the possible arrival of patients with Coronavirus Disease 2019 (COVID-19). All hospitals should ensure their staff are trained, equipped and capable of practices needed to:

- Prevent the spread of respiratory diseases including COVID-19 within the facility
- Promptly identify and isolate patients with possible COVID-19 and inform the correct facility staff and public health authorities
- Care for a limited number of patients with confirmed or suspected COVID-19 as part of routine operations
- Potentially care for a larger number of patients in the context of an escalating outbreak
- Monitor and manage any healthcare personnel that might be exposed to COVID-19
- Communicate effectively within the facility and plan for appropriate external communication related to COVID-19

The following checklist does not describe mandatory requirements or standards; rather, it highlights important areas for hospitals to review in preparation for potential arrivals of COVID-19 patients.

---

* This is an edited, reformatted and augmented version of Department of health and Human Services Publication.

Elements to be assessed

1. Infection prevention and control policies and training for healthcare personnel (HCP):

- Facility leadership including the Chief Medical Officer, quality officers, hospital epidemiologist, and heads of services (e.g., infection control, emergency department, environmental services, pediatrics, critical care) has reviewed the Centers for Disease Control and Prevention's COVID-19 guidance. https://www.cdc.gov/coronavirus/2019-nCoV/guidance-hcp.html ☐
- Facility provides education and job-specific training to HCP regarding COVID-19 including: ☐
  - Signs and symptoms of infection
  - How to safely collect a specimen
  - Correct infection control practices and personal protective equipment (PPE) use
  - Triage procedures including patient placement
  - HCP sick leave policies and recommended actions for unprotected exposures (e.g., not using recommended PPE, an unrecognized infectious patient contact)
  - How and to whom COVID-19 cases should be reported

2. Process for rapidly identifying and isolating patients with confirmed or suspected COVID-19:

- Signs are posted at entrances with instructions to individuals with symptoms of respiratory infection to: immediately put on a mask and keep it on during their assessment, cover their mouth/nose when coughing or sneezing, use and dispose of tissues, and perform hand hygiene after contact with respiratory secretions. ☐
- Facemasks are provided to coughing patients and other symptomatic individuals upon entry to the facility. ☐
- Signs are posted in triage areas (e.g., ED entrances) advising patients with fever or symptoms of respiratory infection and recent travel outside the US, specifically to China, to immediately notify triage personnel so appropriate precautions can be put in place. ☐
- Alcohol based hand sanitizer for hand hygiene is available at each entrance and in all common areas. ☐
- Facility provides tissues and no-touch receptacles for disposal of tissues in waiting rooms and in common areas. ☐
- Facility has a separate well-ventilated space that allows waiting patients to be separated by 6 or more feet, with easy access to respiratory hygiene and cough etiquette supplies. ☐
- Facility has a process to ensure patients with confirmed or suspected COVID-19 are rapidly moved to an Airborne Infection Isolation Room (AIIR). ☐
- Alternatively, for patients that cannot be immediately placed in a room for further evaluation, a system is provided that allows them to wait in a personal vehicle or outside the facility (if medically appropriate) and be notified by phone or other remote methods when it is their turn to be evaluated. ☐
- Triage personnel are trained on appropriate processes (e.g., questions to ask and actions to take) to rapidly identify and isolate suspect cases. ☐
- Facility has a process that occurs after a suspect case is identified to include immediate notification of facility leadership/infection control. ☐
- Facility has a process to notify local or state health department of a suspect case soon after arrival. ☐
- Facility has a process for receiving suspect cases arriving by ambulance. ☐

3. Patient placement:

- Confirm the number and location of Airborne Infection Isolation Rooms (AIIRs) available in the facility (ideally AIIRs will be available in the emergency department and on inpatient units) ☐
- Document that each AIIR has been tested and is effective (e.g., sufficient air exchanges, negative pressure, exhaust handling) within the last month. The AIIR should be checked for negative pressure before occupancy. ☐

continue on next page

cont.

- Verify each AIIR meets the following criteria: ☐
  - Minimum of 6 air changes per hour (12 air changes per hour are recommended for new construction or renovation).
  - Air from these rooms should be exhausted directly to the outside or be filtered through a high-efficiency particulate air (HEPA) filter before recirculation.
  - Room doors should be kept closed except when entering or leaving the room, and entry and exit should be minimized.
  - When occupied by a patient, the AIIR is checked daily for negative pressure.
- A protocol is established, which specifies that aerosol-generating procedures that are likely to induce coughing (e.g., sputum induction, open suctioning of airways) are to be performed in an AIIR using appropriate PPE. ☐
- Facility has plans to minimize the number of HCP who enter the room. Only essential personnel enter the AIIR. Facilities should consider caring for these patients with dedicated HCP to minimize risk of transmission and exposure to other patients and HCP. ☐
- Facility has a process (e.g., a log, electronic tracking) for documenting HCP entering and exiting the patient room. ☐
- Facility has policies for dedicating noncritical patient-care equipment to the patient. ☐

4. Transmission-Based Precautions (use Standard, Contact, Airborne Precautions plus eye protection for patients with confirmed or suspected COVID-19 cases):

- Personal protective equipment (PPE) and other infection prevention and control supplies (e.g., hand hygiene supplies) that would be used for both healthcare personnel (HCP) protection and source control for infected patients (e.g., facemask on the patient) are located in sufficient supply including at patient arrival, triage, and assessment locations. ☐
- Facility has a respiratory protection program. Appropriate HCP have been medically cleared, fit-tested, and trained for respirator use. ☐
- HCP receive appropriate training, including "just in time" training on selection and proper use of (including putting on and removing) PPE, with a required demonstration of competency. ☐
- Facility has a process for auditing adherence to recommended PPE use by HCP. ☐

5. Movement of patients with confirmed or suspected COVID-19 within the facility:

- Patient movement outside of the AIIR will be limited to medically-essential purposes. ☐
- A protocol is in place to ensure that, if the patient is being transported outside of the room, HCP in the receiving area are notified in advance. ☐
- Patients transported outside of their AIIR will be asked to wear a facemask and be covered with a clean sheet during transport. ☐

6. Hand hygiene (HH):

- HH supplies, including alcohol-based hand sanitizer are readily accessible in patient care areas, including areas where HCP remove PPE. ☐
- Facility has a process for auditing adherence to recommended hand hygiene practices by HCP. ☐

7. Environmental cleaning:

- Facility has a plan to ensure proper cleaning and disinfection of environmental surfaces and equipment in the patient room. ☐
- If environmental services personnel are given this responsibility, they should be appropriately trained and fit-tested. ☐
- All HCP with cleaning responsibilities understand the contact time for selected products. ☐
- Facility has a process to ensure shared or non-dedicated equipment is cleaned and disinfected after use according to manufacturer's recommendations. ☐
- Facility uses an EPA-registered hospital-grade disinfectant with EPA-approved emerging viral pathogens claims on hard non-porous surfaces. ☐
  - If there are no available EPA-registered products that have an approved emerging viral pathogen claim for COVID-19, products with label claims against human coronaviruses should be used according to label instructions.

8. Monitoring and managing HCP:

- The facility follows the local/state public health authority's policies and procedures for monitoring and managing HCP with potential for exposure to COVID-19, including ensuring that HCP have ready access, including via telephone, to medical consultation. ☐
- Facility has a process to track exposures and conduct active- and/or self-monitoring of HCP if required by public health. ☐
- Facility has a process to conduct symptom and temperature checks prior to the start of any shift of asymptomatic, exposed HCP that are not work restricted. ☐

9. Visitor access and movement within the facility:

- Plans for visitor access and movement within the facility have been reviewed and updated within the last 12 months. ☐
- Visitors are screened for symptoms of acute respiratory illness before entering the hospital. ☐
- Facility has a plan to restrict visitation to rooms of patients with confirmed or suspected COVID-19. ☐
- If visitors are allowed to enter the room of a confirmed or suspected COVID-19 patient, the facility will: ☐
  - Enact a policy defining what PPE should be used by visitors.
  - Provide instruction to visitors before they enter a patient room, on hand hygiene, limiting surfaces touched, and use of PPE according to current facility policy.
  - Maintain a record (e.g., a log with contact information) of all visitors who enter and exit the room.
  - Ensure that visitors limit their movement within facility (e.g. avoid the cafeteria).

10. Facility regularly monitors the situation on CDC's coronavirus disease (COVID-19) web page. www.cdc.gov/COVID19 ☐

In: Coronavirus …
Editor: Roger F. Martin

ISBN: 978-1-53617-939-2
© 2020 Nova Science Publishers, Inc.

Chapter 12

COVID-2019: CDC PROTECTS AND PREPARES COMMUNITIES*

Department of Health and Human Services

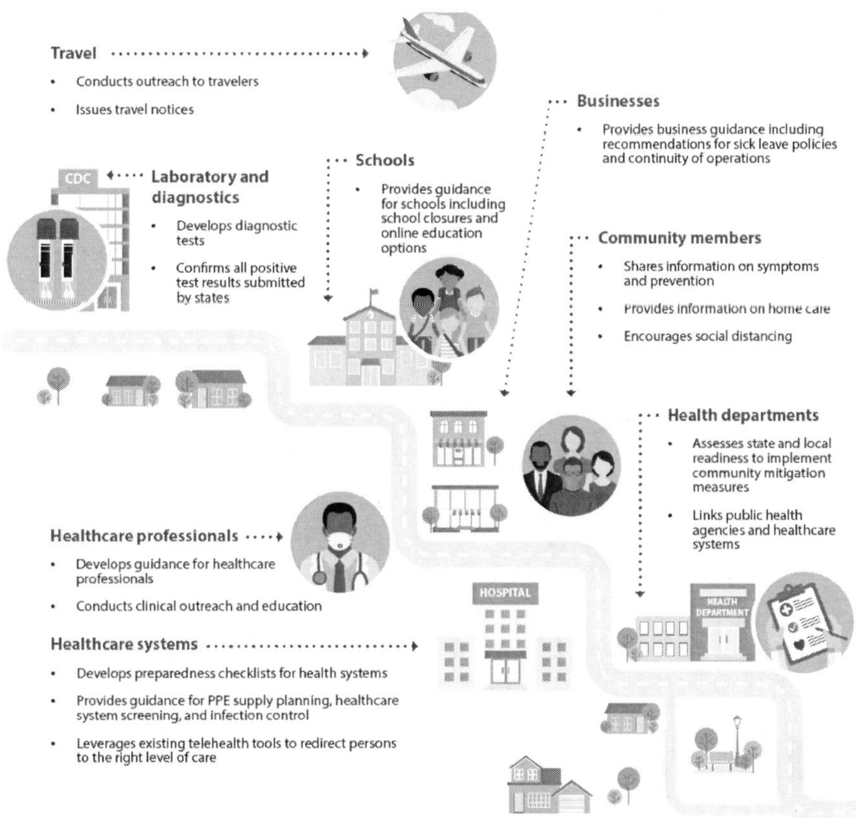

* This is an edited, reformatted and augmented version of Department of Health and Human Services Publication No. CS 315454-A, dated February 25, 2020.

CDC Protects and Prepares Communities

CDC is aggressively responding to the global outbreak of COVID-19 and preparing for the potential of community spread in the U.S.

For more information: www.cdc.gov/COVID19.

In: Coronavirus …
Editor: Roger F. Martin
ISBN: 978-1-53617-939-2

Chapter 13

COVID-19: WHAT TO DO IF YOU ARE SICK WITH CORONAVIRUS DISEASE 2019 (COVID-19)*

Department of Health and Human Services

If you are sick with COVID-19 or suspect you are infected with the virus that causes COVID-19, follow the steps below to help prevent the disease from spreading to people in your home and community.

STAY HOME EXCEPT TO GET MEDICAL CARE

You should restrict activities outside your home, except for getting medical care. Do not go to work, school, or public areas. Avoid using public transportation, ride-sharing, or taxis.

SEPARATE YOURSELF FROM OTHER PEOPLE AND ANIMALS IN YOUR HOME

- People: As much as possible, you should stay in a specific room and away from other people in your home. Also, you should use a separate bathroom, if available.

* This is an edited, reformatted and augmented version of Department of Health and Human Services, Publication No. CS 314937-D, dated February 24, 2020.

- Animals: Do not handle pets or other animals while sick. See COVID-19 and Animals for more information.

Call Ahead Before Visiting Your Doctor

If you have a medical appointment, call the healthcare provider and tell them that you have or may have COVID-19. This will help the healthcare provider's office take steps to keep other people from getting infected or exposed.

Wear a Facemask

You should wear a facemask when you are around other people (e.g., sharing a room or vehicle) or pets and before you enter a healthcare provider's office. If you are not able to wear a facemask (for example, because it causes trouble breathing), then people who live with you should not stay in the same room with you, or they should wear a facemask if they enter your room.

Cover Your Coughs and Sneezes

Cover your mouth and nose with a tissue when you cough or sneeze. Throw used tissues in a lined trash can; immediately wash your hands with soap and water for at least 20 seconds or clean your hands with an alcohol-based hand sanitizer that contains at least 60 to 95% alcohol, covering all surfaces of your hands and rubbing them together until they feel dry. Soap and water should be used preferentially if hands are visibly dirty.

Avoid Sharing Personal Household Items

You should not share dishes, drinking glasses, cups, eating utensils, towels, or bedding with other people or pets in your home. After using these items, they should be washed thoroughly with soap and water.

Clean Your Hands Often

Wash your hands often with soap and water for at least 20 seconds. If soap and water are not available, clean your hands with an alcohol-based hand sanitizer that contains at least 60% alcohol, covering all surfaces of your hands and rubbing them together until they feel dry. Soap and water should be used preferentially if hands are visibly dirty. Avoid touching your eyes, nose, and mouth with unwashed hands.

Clean All "High-Touch" Surfaces Every Day

High touch surfaces include counters, tabletops, doorknobs, bathroom fixtures, toilets, phones, keyboards, tablets, and bedside tables. Also, clean any surfaces that may have blood, stool, or body fluids on them. Use a household cleaning spray or wipe, according to the label instructions. Labels contain instructions for safe and effective use of the cleaning product including precautions you should take when applying the product, such as wearing gloves and making sure you have good ventilation during use of the product.

Monitor Your Symptoms

Seek prompt medical attention if your illness is worsening (e.g., difficulty breathing). Before seeking care, call your healthcare provider and tell them that you have, or are being evaluated for, COVID-19. Put on a facemask before you enter the facility. These steps will help the healthcare provider's office to keep other people in the office or waiting room from getting infected or exposed.

Ask your healthcare provider to call the local or state health department. Persons who are placed under active monitoring or facilitated self-monitoring should follow instructions provided by their local health department or occupational health professionals, as appropriate.

If you have a medical emergency and need to call 911, notify the dispatch personnel that you have, or are being evaluated for COVID-19. If possible, put on a facemask before emergency medical services arrive.

DISCONTINUING HOME ISOLATION

Patients with confirmed COVID-19 should remain under home isolation precautions until the risk of secondary transmission to others is thought to be low. The decision to discontinue home isolation precautions should be made on a case-by-case basis, in consultation with healthcare providers and state and local health departments.

For more information: www.cdc.gov/COVID19.

In: Coronavirus …
Editor: Roger F. Martin

ISBN: 978-1-53617-939-2

Chapter 14

THE DEFENSE PRODUCTION ACT (DPA) AND COVID-19: KEY AUTHORITIES AND POLICY CONSIDERATIONS*

Michael H. Cecire and Heidi M. Peters

As the coronavirus (COVID-19) outbreak develops, the United States faces drug and medical supply scarcities due to disrupted supply chains and increased demand. In response, the President may exercise emergency authorities under the Defense Production Act of 1950 (DPA; 50 U.S.C. §§4501 et seq.) to address supply shortages and economic development impacts, and may have begun the process of doing so. This Insight considers DPA authorities that may be used to address domestic essential goods and materials shortages caused by the outbreak, and explores potential policy considerations for Congress.

DPA PROVISIONS AND RECENT USE

The DPA confers broad presidential authorities to mobilize domestic industry in service of the *national defense*, defined in statute as various military activities and "homeland security, stockpiling, space, and any directly related activity" (50 U.S.C. §4552.) including emergency preparedness activities under the Stafford Act, which has

* This is an edited, reformatted and augmented version of Congressional Research Service Publication No. IN11231, dated March 6, 2020.

been used for public health emergencies. Many of these authorities are delegated to executive agencies under Executive Order 13603.

Current DPA authorities include, but are not limited to:

- *Title I: Priorities and Allocations*, which allows the President to require persons (including businesses and corporations) to (1) prioritize and accept government contracts for materials and services, and (2) allocate or control the general distribution of materials, services, and facilities as necessary to promote the national defense. Title I prioritization authorities are regularly utilized by the Department of Defense (DOD) to acquire critical military capabilities and less frequently by the Department of Homeland Security (DHS) for disaster response and preparedness needs. The allocations authority has not been invoked since the Cold War, such as to promote energy development in 1974.
- *Title III: Expansion of Productive Capacity and Supply*, which allows the President to provide economic incentives to secure domestic industrial capabilities essential to meet national defense and homeland security requirements. DPA Title III is specifically intended to "create, maintain, protect, expand, or restore domestic industrial base capabilities" (50 U.S.C. §4533). Authorized incentives include loans, loan guarantees, direct purchases and purchase commitments, and the authority to procure and install equipment in private industrial facilities. DOD regularly utilizes Title III authorities and operates a standing DPA Title III program funded by annual congressional appropriations.
- *Title VII: General Provisions,* which includes key definitions and other distinct authorities. These provisions grant the President the authority to establish voluntary agreements with private industry; the authority to block proposed or pending foreign corporate mergers, acquisitions, or takeovers that threaten national security; and the authority to employ persons of outstanding experience and ability and to establish a volunteer pool of industry executives who could be called to government service in the interest of the national defense.

For a more in-depth discussion of DPA authorities, see CRS Report R43767.

DPA AUTHORITIES AND COVID-19

As the DPA's definition of national defense encompasses homeland security issues, the DPA could potentially be used to respond to public health emergencies, though this has not occurred before. At the President's discretion, DPA authorities could be employed to address concerns over medical supplies shortages due to the COVID-19 outbreak.

Case Study: Using DPA to Expand Medical Protective Gear Production

As an example of how DPA authorities could be exercised, consider the availability of personal protective equipment (PPE), such as respirator masks, amid the outbreak. Reported PPE shortages may be due to significantly increased consumer demand related to the outbreak itself, and supply chain disruptions resulting from containment measures in China and elsewhere.

Under Title I, the President could prioritize domestic production of PPE to ensure sufficient national stockpiles, and allocate them according to the needs of the emergency. Under Title III, the federal government could use authorized incentives to expand domestic capacity for PPE manufacturing to meet the needs of the emergency. Under Title VII, the President could establish voluntary agreements with private industry—which might normally be subject to anti-trust statutes—to coordinate industry PPE production.

Policy Implications for Congress

The decision whether to employ DPA authorities generally lies with the President. However, in addition to Congress's inherent oversight authority, the DPA statute outlines several specific congressional equities:

1. Title I authorities can only be used for wage and price controls if accompanied by a joint resolution of Congress (50 U.S.C. §4514). This could be applicable in this case in the production and sale of PPE, drug treatments or vaccines, or other necessary goods, and would require coordination between the Administration and Congress.
2. Budget authority for Title III direct loans and guarantees must be specifically included in an appropriations act passed by Congress (50 U.S.C. §4531).
3. Title III projects that cumulatively cost more than $50 million must be authorized by an act of Congress, and the President is required to notify the committees of jurisdiction (the House Committee on Financial Services and the Senate Committee on Banking, Housing, and Urban Affairs), and provide 30 days for comment (50 U.S.C. §4533). A large-scale effort to expand outbreak-related production capacity may require sums far greater than $50 million.

However, the DPA confers broad waivers to its Title III requirements:

> During a period of national emergency declared by Congress or the President; or upon determination by the President, on a nondelegable basis, that action is necessary to avert an industrial resource or critical technology item shortfall that would severely impair national defense capability. (50 U.S.C. §4531(d)(1)(B))

Another area of possible congressional interest is DPA funding, which is appropriated annually. The FY2020 appropriation to the DPA fund was $64.4 million; the President's FY2021 budget requested $182 million for the DPA fund (p. 276). DPA appropriations could also be made as part of a supplemental appropriations package if the DPA fund is exhausted and/or to provide resources for other DPA authorities.

In: Coronavirus …
Editor: Roger F. Martin

ISBN: 978-1-53617-939-2

Chapter 15

FROM SARS TO 2019-CORONAVIRUS (NCOV): U.S.-CHINA COLLABORATIONS ON PANDEMIC RESPONSE*

Jennifer Bouey[1] and The RAND Corporation[2]

Chairman Bera, Ranking Member Yoho, and members of the subcommittee, thank you for inviting me to testify about U.S.-China collaboration on pandemic response, especially in light of the recent novel coronavirus outbreak. First, I will describe the 2002–2003 outbreak of severe acute respiratory syndrome (SARS) and the global response. Next, I will discuss U.S.-China collaboration from 2003–2012, followed by developments in the years prior to the current coronavirus outbreak. Lastly, I will analyze the characteristics of 2019-nCoV and China's early responses, and offer policy recommendations.

---

* This is an edited, reformatted and augmented version of United States House of Representatives Testimony presented before the House Foreign Affairs Subcommittee on Asia, the Pacific, and Nonproliferation, Publication No. CT-523, dated February 5, 2020.

[1] The opinions and conclusions expressed in this testimony are the author's alone and should not be interpreted as representing those of the RAND Corporation or any of the sponsors of its research.

[2] The RAND Corporation is a research organization that develops solutions to public policy challenges to help make communities throughout the world safer and more secure, healthier and more prosperous. RAND is nonprofit, nonpartisan, and committed to the public interest.

2002–2003: SARS

Almost 17 years ago, a novel coronavirus was silently causing deadly pneumonia outbreaks—which later became known as SARS—in China. The index case of the SARS outbreak occurred in the city of Foshan in Guangdong Province, China, on November 16, 2002. Neither this case nor a few other cases in December attracted any notice from the public. A public health expert team from the province, which included a few representatives from the national Ministry of Health, went to one of the cities in Guangdong province in January 2003 to investigate. The team concluded that the atypical pneumonia diagnoses were probably caused by a virus. The team then suggested in a "top-secret" report that the provincial health bureau should establish a case-reporting system. This reasonable—although rather feeble—suggestion was expressed in a news bulletin for local health care professionals but fell on deaf ears during the Chinese New Year. The world did not find out for another two months that this was severe acute respiratory syndrome (SARS), a viral pneumonia that would infect more than 8,000 people globally and lead to 774 deaths.

At that time, China lacked a national center for disease control, which would have been responsible for maintaining a robust surveillance system for detecting emerging diseases. It also lacked a national case-reporting system. In addition, according to the *Implementing Regulations of the Law of the People's Republic of China on Guarding State Secrets* regarding the handling of public health-related information, any occurrence of infectious disease should be classified as a state secret before it is "announced by the Ministry of Health."[3] No physician or journalist can alert the public without breaking the law. With no information from government or media, the Chinese public was unaware of the outbreak until cell phone messages about a "deadly flu" started to circulate in early February 2003 in Guangzhou. A widespread panic caused residents to clear out antibiotics and flu medicines in pharmacies. Prompted by the public panic, the Guangdong health officials finally held a press conference on February 11 to announce the 305 atypical pneumonia cases in the province. China submitted the case report to the World Health Organization (WHO) as *atypical pneumonia*, probably caused by chlamydia or a virus around the same time. Afterward, information about the disease was reported on the news media, but the flow of information stopped on February 23. The news blackout from February 23 continued during the run-up to the National People's Congress in March, and the government shared little with the public until early April.[4]

Meanwhile, a "super-spreading" chain of transmission emerged at the end of the January and lasted until March, causing international attention on the outbreak: A patient

[3] Yanzhong Huang, "The SARS Epidemic and Its Aftermath in China: A Political Perspective," in Stacey Knobler, Adel Mahmoud, Stanley Lemon, Alison Mack, Laura Sivitz, and Katherine Oberholtzer, eds., Learning from SARS: Preparing for the Next Disease Outbreak: Workshop Summary, Washington, D.C.: The National Academies Press, 2004.

[4] Huang, 2004 ibid.

with pneumonia in Guangdong was transferred between three different hospitals, ultimately infecting 200 people, including a doctor from Zhongshan Hospital. The doctor traveled to Hong Kong and infected 12 people in a hotel, and these 12 people then carried the virus to Singapore, Vietnam, Canada, Ireland, and the United States.[5]

By mid-March 2003, SARS clusters started to appear in Vietnam, Hong Kong, Singapore, and Canada. The WHO subsequently picked up the alerts from the Global Outbreak Alert and Response Network (GOARN) and issued a global alert about a new infectious disease of unknown origin. Between March 16 and March 21, the WHO started to suspect that the more than 300 cases from February—which China had labeled "atypical pneumonia" in its report— were actually SARS cases. At China's request, the WHO sent a team to China on March 23. On March 27, the WHO team concluded that the "atypical pneumonia" cases were same as SARS, and China announced 792 cases and 31 deaths.6 Under intense international pressure to mobilize against the pandemic threat, the Chinese government publicly acknowledged the SARS outbreak at the end of March and undertook a series of responsive actions in the following weeks, including

- establishment of new rules requiring all local health officials to report the number of cases daily, with severe penalties for noncompliance
- streamlining of interdepartmental communication and cooperation on the crisis
- creation of national and provincial interdepartmental SARS task forces
- dedication of over $1 billion to treating the patients and controlling the epidemic.[7]

In late April 2003, China's health minister and Beijing's mayor were fired one day after the Chinese Premier announced severe consequences for local officials who failed to report SARS cases in a timely and accurate manner. (That same day, the number of cases in Beijing jumped from 37 to 407.) By the end of May, more than 1,000 officials were fired or penalized for their "slack" responses to SARS.[8] The remaining officials, driven by political zeal, began to seal off villages, apartment complexes, and university campuses; quarantined tens of thousands of people; and set up checkpoints to take temperatures. A new hospital was built within 20 days in Beijing to accommodate and quarantine SARS patients. The epidemic started to subside in late May. By June 27, the

[5] Institute of Medicine, "Summary and Assessment," in Stacey Knobler, Adel Mahmoud, Stanley Lemon, Alison Mack, Laura Sivitz, and Katherine Oberholtzer, eds., *Learning from SARS: Preparing for the Next Disease Outbreak: Workshop Summary*, Washington, D.C.: The National Academies Press, 2004.

[6] World Health Organization, "Severe Acute Respiratory Syndrome (SARS) Multi-Country Outbreak – Update 10: Disease Outbreak Reported," news alert, March 26, 2003. As of February 3, 2020: https://www.who.int/csr/don/2003_03_26/en/.

[7] Yanzhong Huang, "The SARS Epidemic and Its Aftermath in China: A Political Perspective," in Stacey Knobler, Adel Mahmoud, Stanley Lemon, Alison Mack, Laura Sivitz, and Katherine Oberholtzer, eds., *Learning from SARS: Preparing for the Next Disease Outbreak: Workshop Summary*, Washington, D.C.: The National Academies Press, 2004.

[8] Huang, 2004.

WHO announced that China was "SARS-free." On August 16, the last two SARS patients were discharged from a Beijing hospital.

SARS revealed the state of China's unprepared public health system. It led the country to significantly rethink its approach to both domestic and global health. The government soon invested 6.8 billion renminbi (RMB) (850 million U.S. dollars [USD]) for the construction of a three-tiered network of disease control and prevention. The outbreak also spurred China to strengthen its relationships with the United States and the wider international community around issues of public health concerns. The change in China was welcomed and enthusiastically supported by governments and scientists around the world.

2003–2013: U.S.-China Collaborations and China's Public Health Restructuring and Capacity-Building

Increased U.S.-China collaboration on global health was an important result of the SARS response. In October 2003, three months after the conclusion of the SARS pandemic, U.S. Secretary of Health and Human Services Tommy Thompson visited China and signed a multiyear partnership with the Chinese Ministry of Health to develop a more robust public health infrastructure in China. Thompson also established an HHS health attaché at the U.S. embassy in Beijing. The following month, U.S. Secretary of State Colin Powell noted that

> It is upon such concrete forms of cooperation on issues of regional and global importance that a 21st century U.S.-China relationship will be built, issue by issue, experience by experience, challenge by challenge, initiative by initiative, program by program.[9]

H5N1: 2003–2009

Not long after the SARS pandemic, China and the international community confronted another complex challenge with the H5N1 influenza virus—commonly known as "avian flu" or "bird flu" because it infects and spreads largely through birds. Cases of bird-to-human transmission were discovered in Fujian Province in 2003. In 2004, the Chinese National Influenza Center and the U.S. Centers for Disease Control and Prevention (CDC) initiated cooperative agreements to build Chinese capacity in influenza surveillance. The two agencies collaborated on 1) developing technical

[9] Colin L. Powell, "Remarks at Conference on China-U.S. Relations," College Station, Tex., November 5, 2003.

expertise in virology and epidemiology in China; 2) developing a comprehensive influenza surveillance system by enhancing influenza-like illness reporting; 3) strengthening analysis, utilization, and dissemination of surveillance data; and 4) improving early response to influenza viruses with pandemic potential. In 2005, both governments inaugurated the Collaborative Program on Emerging and Re-emerging Infectious Diseases, which turned into the CDC's China Center. That same year, both countries established the U.S.-China Health Care Forum to address bilateral commercial, trade, and policy issues relating to health. Additionally, U.S. President George W. Bush announced the International Partnership on Avian and Pandemic Influenza—an ongoing framework for U.S.-China cooperation around the issue—in an address to the United Nations (UN).[10] In 2006, the U.S. Department of Health and Human Services (HHS) and China's Ministry of Health (MOH) further expanded their collaboration on biomedical research with a memorandum of understanding on research, technology, training, and personnel exchange.

H1N1: 2009

The capacity-building and infrastructure put into place to monitor the continuing threat from avian flu served China and the United States well when another novel influenza strain—H1N1, commonly known as "swine flu"—emerged in 2009. The epicenter was in the United States and Mexico, but the flu soon spread across the globe. American and Chinese health authorities shared information and technology to facilitate national monitoring of H1N1's spread and to develop a vaccine; China subsequently became the first country to mass-produce an H1N1 vaccine. During the summer lull in the 2009 pandemic, the two countries strengthened their bilateral health communications through the U.S.-China Strategic Economic Dialogue. As then–U.S. President Barack Obama visited China in November 2009 in the midst of the H1N1 outbreak, the two countries addressed global public health in a joint statement, pledging to "deepen cooperation on global public health issues, including Influenza A (H1N1) prevention, surveillance, reporting and control, and on avian influenza, HIV/AIDS, tuberculosis, and malaria."[11]

---

[10] George W. Bush, statement delivered to the 2005 World Summit of the United Nations, High Level Plenary Meeting, New York, September 14, 2005. As of February 3, 2020: http://www.un.org/webcast/summit2005/statements/usa050914.pdf.

[11] The White House, Office of the Press Secretary, "U.S.-China Joint Statement," statement by U.S. President Barack Obama and Chinese President Hu Jintao, November 17, 2009. As of February 3, 2020: https://obamawhitehouse.archives.gov/realitycheck/the-press-office/us-china-joint-statement.

China's National Influenza Center Expansion: 2010–2014

From 2010 to 2014, China expanded the Chinese National Influenza Center (CNIC) to include 408 laboratories and 554 sentinel hospitals, and it trained 2,500 public health staff. CNIC became the fifth WHO Collaborating Centre for Reference and Research on Influenza. CNIC established viral drug resistance surveillance and platforms for gene sequencing, reverse genetics, serological detection, and development of vaccine strains. CNIC also built a bioinformatics platform to strengthen data analysis, publishing weekly online influenza surveillance reports in English and Chinese. The surveillance system now collects between 200,000 and 400,000 specimens and tests more than 20,000 influenza viruses annually, which provide valuable information for WHO influenza vaccine strain recommendations. CNIC now provides training for other countries to improve global capacity for influenza control.[12]

H7N9: 2013

CNIC was fully functional when another novel strain of avian influenza, H7N9, emerged in eastern China in 2013. This form of avian influenza has a high fatality rate, of 30 percent (similar to Middle East Respiratory System [MERS]), but human-to-human transmission proved extremely rare, allowing the outbreak to remain in check with effective public health measures.

This time, China quickly reported the new viral strain to the WHO after only three cases were detected, and it also posted the full viral genome sequences of these cases in a public international database to facilitate research around the world. The outbreak plateaued in June at around 130 confirmed cases with more than 40 confirmed deaths, but, as expected, the virus reemerged the following winter, with more than 100 confirmed cases and 20 deaths in China in January 2014 alone.

China's domestic response to the H7N9 outbreak prevented the virus from spreading beyond mainland China, save for a handful of cases in Hong Kong, Taiwan, and Malaysia. Chinese scientific cooperation with the international community also allowed other countries to prepare for further spread of the virus. Chinese scientists developed a vaccine in October 2013—the first influenza vaccine developed entirely in China—and shared their method with the world, facilitating vaccine development efforts by the U.S. CDC and private pharmaceutical companies. The Chinese and American CDCs collaborated throughout the H7N9 outbreak by sharing epidemiological data and

[12] Yuelong Shu, Ying Song, Dayan Wang, Carolyn M. Greene, Ann Moen, C. K. Lee, Yongkun Chen, Xiyan Xu, Jeffrey McFarland, Li Xin, Joseph Bresee, Suizan Zhou, Tao Chen, Ran Zhang, and Nancy Cox, "A Ten-Year China-US Laboratory Collaboration: Improving Response to Influenza Threats in China and the World, 2004–2014," BMC Public Health, Vol. 19, No. 520, 2019.

engaging in joint research on the virus. The Chinese efforts to manage the outbreak of H7N9 were widely praised by governments and scientists around the world.[13] In the United States, the CDC partially activated its Emergency Operations Center to conduct epidemiological and vaccine research, provide assistance to the Chinese, and develop and distribute test kits capable of detecting the virus worldwide.[14]

HIV/AIDS: 2003–2014

Besides preparing for and responding to influenza epidemics, the United States also helped China in its campaign against HIV/AIDs. In 2002, the U.S. National Institutes of Health (NIH) gave the Chinese CDC a five-year, $14.8 million grant to develop infrastructure to improve research and better monitor the spread of the disease in the country. Beijing also partnered with the U.S. CDC to establish the CDC's Global AIDS Program (GAP) in China in early 2003. GAP quickly developed and implemented a comprehensive HIV prevention and mitigation plan across 15 Chinese provinces to promote increased surveillance of high-risk populations. The CDC, in partnership with China's National Center for AIDS/STD Control and Prevention, has assisted with capacity-building, including the improvement of the quality and geographical reach of laboratory testing capabilities, the development of an epidemiological surveillance system, and the expansion of treatment options. The U.S. CDC has assisted Chinese health authorities with the establishment of three HIV/AIDS clinical training centers in rural areas, which have educated more than 300 graduates who are now providing antiretroviral therapy for 50,000 patients in 16 provinces.[15]

2013–2019: The Years Leading Up to the 2019 Coronavirus

Ebola

In 2014, the Chinese government launched an unprecedented response to the Ebola epidemic in West Africa in 2014.[16] China's State Council dispatched one of its largest medical teams of about 1,200 clinicians, public health experts, and military medical

---

[13] Carina Perkins, "OIE Meeting Congratulates China on Bird Flu Response," GlobalMeatNews, June 4, 2013; Mara Hvistendahl, "A Decade After SARS, China's Flu Response Wins Cautious Praise," *Science*, Vol. 340, No. 6129, April 12, 2013, p. 130; Dobri Genchev, "H7N9 Response Discussed During World Health Assembly," news release, World Health Organization, November 9, 2018.

[14] Centers for Disease Control and Prevention, "Asian Lineage Asian Influenza A(H7N9) Virus" December 7, 2018. As of February 3, 2020: https://www.cdc.gov/flu/avianflu/h7n9-virus.htm

[15] Bulterys M. (2020) The US CDC Global AIDS Program in China. In: Wu Z., Wang Y., Detels R., Bulterys M., McGoogan J. (eds) HIV/AIDS in China. Springer, Singapore.

[16] Yanzhong Huang, "China's Response to the 2014 Ebola Outbreak in West Africa," *Global Challenges*, Vol. 1, No. 2, February 27, 2017.

officers after the WHO declared a Public Health Emergency of International Concern (PHEIC). The Chinese team opened a 100-bed treatment unit and established three field demonstration sites in Sierra Leone while providing free treatment. Within six months, China also built a biosafety level 3 laboratory, transporting all construction materials into the laboratory in only 87 days.[17]

The United States took similar actions but on a larger scale, with aid exceeding $1 billion. In some cases, U.S. and Chinese teams collaborated on the ground in Africa. On the international stage, the United States and China worked together at the UN Security Council, jointly declaring the Ebola outbreak a "threat to international peace and security," and called on governments around the world to respond to the crisis.[18] In June 2015, at the U.S.-China Symposium on Ebola, Research, and Global Health Security hosted by the NIH, both countries renewed their commitment to building systems to detect, prevent, and respond to global health threats.

Indeed, these collaborations between U.S. and Chinese public health agencies are the ones that the 2016 U.S.-China Strategic and Economic Dialogue highlighted as venues for deeper cooperation moving forward: "The United States and China are committed to strengthening cooperation to improve global health security," both sides agreed. They pledged to further "strengthen their partnership to build capacity to prevent, detect and respond to infectious disease threats including but not limited to influenza, malaria, laboratory capacity, and antimicrobial resistance."[19]

However, a big change in the U.S.-China relationship was on the way. Afraid of western influences, China enacted new legislative restrictions on foreign nongovernmental organization (NGO) activity on January 1, 2017; the law requires foreign-based researchers in China to have a government partner who will report their activities to central and local security agencies. Then, in 2018, due to a U.S.-China trade war, such diplomacy dialogues as the strategic and Economic Dialogue and bilateral diplomatic and security dialogues halted. Subsequently, the United States closed the National Science Foundation office in Beijing in 2018 (along with its offices in Tokyo and Brussels) and the GAP program. Currently NIH and the CDC both reduced their staff in the Beijing office.

In summary, in the 18 years since SARS, with help from the international community and through the commitment of the Chinese government, China has invested in a nationwide network of its own centers for disease control at the national, provincial, prefecture, and county levels; they are connected by a real-time, web-based reporting system for emerging public health events. The workforce for China's CDCs is large,

---

[17] Kun Tang, Zhihui Li, Wenkai Li, and Lincoln Chen, "China's Silk Road and Global Health," *The Lancet*, Vol. 390, No. 10112, December 2017, pp. 2595–2601.

[18] "Ebola 'Threat to World Security'-UN Security Council," BBC News, September 19, 2014. As of February 3, 2020: http://www.bbc.com/news/world-africa-29262968.

[19] U.S. Department of State, Office of the Spokesperson, "U.S.-China Strategic & Economic Dialogue Outcomes of the Strategic Track," Washington, D.C.: June 7, 2016. As of February 3, 2020: https://2009-2017.state.gov/r/pa/prs/ps/2016/06/258146.htm.

relative to the 15,000 employees at the U.S. CDC, consisting of 3,481 units and 877,000 public health professional positions at all levels of government. China also has a world-class National Influenza Center. However, the question on the minds of global health organizations around the world is, is China truly ready for the next pandemic?

A report in late 2018 from China's CDC casts some doubts.[20] The challenges, as the authors highlighted, are multifaceted. First, the growing public health needs (and the voids after the departure of international funders) have stretched still-limited investments in China's public health and its preparedness and response. In the past decade, many Chinese agencies have prioritized innovation in technology, including biomedical research. They have also invested in restructuring the health system for the population of 1.4 billion. Public health, in comparison, was relatively underfunded due to these competing priorities. At the local level, local CDCs are supported by provincial governments. In places where the local government's resources are less robust or declining, local public health resources, including personnel, can also suffer from insufficient funding. Low salaries are a significant barrier to the recruitment and retention of high-quality professionals, and local Chinese CDC staffing has declined at all levels. Secondly, suboptimal multisector coordination, such as inadequate communication and inconsistent data sharing between health and veterinarian sectors, between clinicians and public health professionals, can delay early detection of emerging diseases. Insufficient health care surge capacity was also identified as a potential barrier for providing sufficient response to pandemics, as well as the lack of an official technical framework to communicate an epidemic's intensity, severity, and risks to public.

These underlying issues with the Chinese CDC—especially its dwindling funding and lack of effective communication with public and other sectors—may explain the different fate of the two main surveillance systems in China for detecting and monitoring emerging pathogens. One is China's national sentinel surveillance system for influenza-like illness (ILI), as mentioned earlier, anchored by more than 500 sentinel hospitals in 31 provinces.[21] The other is the national pneumonia surveillance system, which was built and has been maintained by China's CDC since 2004. The latter is designed to monitor pneumonia of unknown etiology (PUE) and facilitate timely detection of novel respiratory pathogens, such as SARS or the 2019 coronavirus. The ILI system is able to use the hospital information system for case recording and outpatient monitoring since the network is hospital-based. The PUE surveillance system, on the other hand, belongs to the CDC system, and has not been used consistently. One study found that 29 percent of community-acquired pneumonia cases that met the PUE criteria were not reported to

[20] One hundred years of Influenza since the 1918 Pandemic -Is China prepared today? CCDC weekly; 2018:1 (4) 56-61.

[21] Dennis KM Ip, Qiaohong Liao, Peng Wu, Zhancheng Gao, Bin Cao, Luzhao Feng, Xiaoling Xu, Hui Jiang, Ming Li, Jing Bao, Jiandong Zheng, Qian Zhang, Zhaorui Chang, Yu Li, Jianxing Yu, Fengfeng Liu, Michael Y. Ni, Joseph T. Wu, Benjamin J. Cowling, Weizhong Yang, Gabriel M. Leung, and Honjie Yu, "Detection of Mild to Moderate Influenza A/H7N9 Infection by China's National Sentinel Surveillance System for Influenza-Like Illness: Case Series," *The BMJ*, Vol. 346, June 24, 2013.

the PUE system in 2009.[22] Only 1,016 PUE cases in all of China were reported during a nine-year period. A study showed that the number of cases surged when an outbreak occurred, either during the SARS outbreak or during A(H5N1) outbreaks. This surge may reflect enhanced administrative requirements from health authorities or enhanced clinician awareness of respiratory viruses.[23] This illustrated that the hospital system (a system paralleled to the CDC system) is in better fiscal condition to maintain a surveillance system compared with the CDC system, which is underused and not sensitive unless it is triggered by an established outbreak.

But a more fundamental question is, what role will China's CDC take in an outbreak response? From what I have witnessed in SARS and 2019-nCoV, the CDC's role is mostly that of consultation rather than decisionmaking.

2019–2020: Is 2019-nCoV Another SARS?

As millions of Chinese prepared to celebrate the 2020 Chinese New Year, the country was seized by anxiety over the emergence of a rapidly evolving epidemic of pneumonia associated with a new coronavirus, 2019-nCoV. At the time of this writing, more than 17,000 confirmed cases and more than 20,000 probable cases have spread throughout China and 23 other countries, causing more than 360 deaths. After person-to-person transmission was reported in four of the 23 countries known to be experiencing cases of the virus, the WHO declared a Public Health Emergency for International Concerns (PHEIC) on January 29, signaling global consensus on deeming the 2019-nCoV outbreak as an extraordinary public health risk. Therefore, to address the question, "Is this another SARS?" I will provide my thoughts from two angles: (1) Will the 2019-nCoV epidemic be similar to that of SARS? (2) What can we learn from comparing China's current response with that of SARS 18 years ago?

Agent, Host, Environment, and Transmission

2019-nCoV is the latest member of the coronavirus family. This type of virus is commonly found in humans and other mammals, such as bats, civet cats, and camels. In

[22] Nijuan Xiang, Fiona Havers, Tao Chen, Ying Song, Wenxiao Tu, Leilei Li, Yang Cao, Bo Liu, Lei Zhou, Ling Meng, Zhiheng Hong, Rui Wang, Yan Niu, Jianyi Yao, Kaiju Liao, Lianmei Jin, Yanping Zhang, Qun Li, Marc- Alain Widdowson, and Zijian Feng, "Use of National Pneumonia Surveillance to Describe Influenza A(H7N9) Virus Epidemiology, China, 2004-2013," *Emerging Infectious Diseases*, Vol. 19, No. 11, 2013, pp. 1784–1790.

[23] Xiaorong Guo, Dong Yang, Ruchun Liu, Yaman Li, Qingqing Hu, Xinrui Ma, Yelan Li, Heng Zhang, Xixing Zhang, Benhua Zhao, and Tianmu Chen, "Detecting Influenza and Emerging Avian Influenza Virus by Influenza and Pneumonia Surveillance Systems in a Large City in China, 2005 to 2016," *BMC Infectious Diseases*, Vol. 19, No. 825, September 18, 2019.

humans, coronavirus has four strains that cause mild clinical symptoms, usually referred as the common cold. Two other strains are more lethal: SARS and MERS. Currently, I do not know whether the new virus will cause clinical symptoms similar to the strains that cause the common cold or to the two strains of coronavirus that caused large-scale epidemics and fatalities. We do know that it shares a high degree of genomic similarity to coronavirus in bats, and to SARS-CoV in humans.[24] It is as contagious as SARS, but so far, the reported statistics indicate a lower proportion of case fatalities (around 2–3 percent) compared with SARS (10–14 percent) and MERS (35 percent).[25] The severe symptoms and fatalities seem to be associated with individuals with medical complications. These estimates can change if the virus continues to mutate or the data are, in reality, different from what we know. For now, the moderately high infectivity, mild clinical symptoms, and wide-ranging incubation period may mean that the novel virus is less harmful to individuals but may coexist with humans and become endemic. In this sense, 2019- nCoV has the potential to cause a pandemic.

The physical and social environments of 2020 are also very different from those in 2002.

China is wealthier and more globalized today. Today, there are 739 international air travel routes originating from China—three times the number of routes (233) available in 2002. On average, 51 million people travel between China and another country per year, a number many times higher than the 3 million back in 2002. The epicenter of the outbreak, Wuhan, is a major transportation hub in central China, sometimes known as "Chicago of China." On an average day, 30,000 people fly out of the city, and many more use the bullet trains from three railway stations in the city. The outbreak began right before the Chinese New Year, a time during which more than three billion trips typically occur under normal circumstances. January is also the time when students from overseas colleges to return to school after the winter break and students from Chinese universities start the winter break. The environmental difference between the 2019- nCoV epidemic and SARS is the scale of mobility, which makes the global spreading of the disease much easier than that for SARS.

Prevention and treatment methods are similar between SARS and 2019-nCoV. In both cases, vaccine development takes months to a year and can hardly be helpful in stopping the outbreak. Quarantines, travel bans, and case-tracing can slow down the disease transmission and buy precious time for countries to plan their responses, but they

---

[24] Peng Zhou, Xing-Lou Yang, Xian-Guang Wang, Ben Hu, Lei Zhang, Wei Zhang, Hao-Rui Si, Yan Zhu, Bei Li, Chao-Lin Huang, Hui-Dong Chen, Jing Chen, Yun Luo, Hua Guo, Ren-Di Jiang, Mei-Qin Liu, Ying Chen, Zu-Rui Shen, Xi Wang, Xiao-Shuang Zheng, Kai Zhao, Quan-Jiao Chen, Fei Deng, Lin-Lin Liu, Bing Yan, Fa-Xian Zhan, Yan-Yi Wang, Gengfu Xiao, and Zheng-Li Shi, "Discovery of a Novel Coronavirus Associated with the Recent Pneumonia Outbreak in Humans and Its Potential Bat Origin," bioRxiv, January 23, 2020.

[25] Chen Wang, Peter W. Horby, Frederick G. Hayden, and George F. Gao, "A Novel Coronavirus Outbreak of Global Health Concern," The Lancet, January 24, 2020.

are not perfect prevention methods.[26] Quarantine will only be effective if it can guarantee stopping people's mobility, which is hard to do for a city of 11 million people. Early detection is conducted using proper reverse transcription polymerase chain reaction (RT-PCR) testing kits, thanks to the Chinese scientists who have isolated the novel virus, conducted genomic sequencing, and shared the data with the world in an astonishingly short amount of time. This has helped to identify the virus and has enabled China and other countries to develop effective testing kits for early detection. The treatment of 2019- nCoV mostly focuses on supportive therapy, but a few antiviral medicines are being used experimentally.

The Chinese Government's Response to 2019-nCoV

The Chinese government's response to 2019-nCoV has followed a similar pattern to that of the SARS outbreak and is characterized by three common features: (1) delaying public acknowledgement of a public threat, (2) downplaying the severity of the outbreak in its early days, and (3) relying on quarantine, social control, and large-scale health care system mobilization to stop the outbreak. The current response also has a few major differences, including the use of social media, better research, and technology, which have helped mitigate some of the negative effects.

The first common feature response of SARS and 2019-nCoV is the delay in acknowledging the initial case cluster to be a public health threat. If we recognize that stability is what the Chinese political system values most, and an acute public health threat, such as an epidemic, is precisely the "black swan" that can threaten such stability, then it is not too difficult to understand the Chinese government's reluctance toward acknowledging an epidemic. China's law prohibits anyone from talking about a public health threat before an official government announcement. For the government to make an announcement on an epidemic, a full process of upward reporting and verifying at every political level has to be accomplished. Once the verified report reaches the Ministry level, a special expert group is often sent to investigate. Following such a process, a timely acknowledgement of an epidemic to the public is almost impossible. The exception has been when social stability itself is being threatened. For example, we saw Guangdong government officials breaking the silence three months after the first SARS case only when the public panicked after seeing phone messages regarding a deadly flu in February 2003. We also saw Wuhan health officials announcing the 27 cases of 2019-nCoV on December 31, 2019 after a few doctors in Wuhan sent WeChat messages warning their acquaintances about a "SARS-like" pneumonia. (The informants were later publicly reprimanded by the government.) In this case, wide use of social media, no

[26] Jennifer B. Nuzzo, "Past Epidemics Prove Fighting Coronavirus with Travel Bans Is a Mistake," *Washington Post*, February 2, 2020.

matter how closely monitored, helped the local officials significantly shorten the waiting period that is usually required for an official announcement.

The second characteristic of the government's response is the downplaying of the severity of the threat at the beginning of an epidemic. For SARS, the results from the first investigation did not alarm the Ministry—and therefore, there was no public announcement—in January 2003. For the next two months, the government continued downplaying the severity of SARS to the public until the Minister of Health was fired in April. In this recent response to 2019-nCoV, the first expert team went to Wuhan in January 2020 and concluded that there was no person-to-person transmission and the outbreak was well controlled after the closing of the seafood market where many cases (not all) were identified. For days, the local health officials assured the public that there were no new cases in Wuhan and no cases outside Wuhan. This inaccurate portrayal of the disease may have allowed sufficient time for the virus to be spread widely in Wuhan, to other cities in China, and to the world. It was not until the 2019-nCoV cases were confirmed in Thailand and Japan in patients who had had no exposure to the seafood market that the MOH sent a second expert group to Wuhan on January 19. This time, person-to-person transmission was immediately confirmed, and the national case reporting system was triggered on January 20. Although the downplaying of the severity of the epidemic did occur, this time it only lasted 20 days, compared with the 2.5 months during the SARS outbreak. This was due to better biomedical and research capacity of the Chinese researchers in 2019. Chinese scientists were able to quickly culture the virus and share the genomic sequencing data with international researchers by January 11. The genetic sequencing data helped many countries quickly develop testing kits for early detection of the disease. When cases showed up in Thailand and Japan, international genomic researchers were able to quickly identify the matching genomic patterns and confirm the presence of 2019-nCoV. This success helped provide the evidence for understanding the greater geographic spread of the epidemic and the role of person-to-person transmission. During the SARS epidemic, however, because of the lack of virus identification, China's pneumonia outbreaks were not linked to those in Hong Kong and Vietnam until four months after the index case happened.

Finally, during SARS, once the government finally geared up to stop the outbreak, they swiftly initiated a quarantine policy. With 2019-nCoV, the decision on quarantine was made three days after the government accepted the fact that the outbreak was fueled by person-to- person transmission. This time, the scale of the quarantine was unprecedented. The mayor of Wuhan announced that the government would shut down all public transportation, including airports and railways, in Wuhan—a city of 11 million people—on January 23, two days before the Chinese New Year. The national government also employed social policing to enforce self- quarantine, canceled public events, and prohibited crowd gatherings across the country.

Without a vaccine, a quarantine is one of the few effective ways to prevent disease transmission. China's decision on a city lockdown has been praised by the WHO and probably buys precious time for many other countries to activate their public health responses. However, there are debates on the effectiveness of the lockdown over such a large area. First, some would argue that by issuing a lockdown only two days before the Chinese New Year, the government missed many people who had left earlier, since new year travel usually starts a week before the new year. The lockdown also took effect a day after the announcement, and many people from Wuhan rushed to get out of Wuhan before it started. As the mayor of Wuhan mentioned in a news conference on January 27, about five million people had left Wuhan by then.[27] Second, the lockdown of a city of 11 million people made it harder to implement the typical door-to-door or community-by-community screening, assessment, and provision of supportive care that usually happens after a quarantine is established. Quarantine may also bring heightened fear and stigma among the affected population, accelerate the shortage of medical supplies and health care resources, and provide a false picture that the epidemic is under control. In addition, the economic impact of the quarantine can be large.

SARS cost the world 40 billion USD and China 1 percent of its GDP in 2003. China may suffer more economic loss this year due to the 2019-nCoV, given that quarantine was initiated before the Chinese new year and at a relatively early stage of the epidemic. (Quarantine may last longer than two months.) In 2003, the industries hurt most were tourism, retail, and entertainment, which was 43 percent of China's GDP. Today, these industries account for 54 percent of the GDP.[28] China now contributes 17 percent of world's economy, compared with 4.3 percent in 2003, when the SARS epidemic was unfolding. China's current stature in the world economy means that the impact of 2019-nCoV outbreak is likely to substantially exceed that of SARS.

Currently, the national case report system is in use, and the case numbers have surged in the last weeks. However, given that many hospitals in China are overwhelmed by the large volume of people with cold-like symptoms coming for testing and treatment because of the fear of the epidemic, patients are often being turned away, and delayed diagnosis and deaths that are not counted (when infected people die before the diagnosis or at home) are both possible. The two new 1,000-bed hospitals that China built in two weeks may help relieve the severe shortage of hospital beds and improve health care for many infected people. It may also help improve the accuracy of the epidemic's statistics.

In summary, the 2019-nCoV is the third of its type, after SARS and MERS, to cause a global outbreak. The Chinese government's response to 2019-nCoV has been similar to that of SARS; however, the initial delay and the "downplay" time were much shorter this

---

[27] Gerry Shih, "Coronavirus Prompts CDC to Expand Travel Warning to All of China; Top U.S. Health Official Urges Beijing to Admit Disease Experts," *Washington Post*, January 27, 2020.

[28] Bloomberg News, "Coronavirus Is More Dangerous for the Global Economy than SARS," January 31, 2020. As of February 3, 2020: https://www.bloomberg.com/news/articles/2020-01-31/the-coronavirus-is-more-dangerous-for-the-economy-than- sars.

time due to the widespread use of social media and the much-improved local research capacity. The unfolding battle against this new pandemic, meanwhile, highlights the importance of transparency and open collaboration among scientists globally. It is a reminder that all nations should prioritize and protect global health research, capacity building, and cooperation.

RECOMMENDATIONS

Given that my fellow panelists both have more experience on leading pandemic preparedness programs in the United States, I will focus my recommendations on the China-related issues. I have short-term, medium-term, and long-term suggestions.

Short Term

First, China is on the front line of a full-fledged battle with the new coronavirus. Health care workers are exhausted, and testing kits and personal protection, such as face masks, goggles, and gloves, are all in short supply and have been rationed.[29] At this time when many Chinese people are suffering from illness, anxiety, and uncertainty, it is important and opportune for U.S. public health and health care professionals to reach out to China and provide humanitarian and technical aid. Such support will boost the morale of their Chinese colleagues, serve as an international witness to the health care professionals' work at the front line of the epidemic, and help provide technical support on trials of the latest antiviral medicines. I am quite encouraged to hear that the U.S. CDC office in Beijing will be hosting a medical team in the near term.

Secondly, any efforts by the U.S. government to reduce stigma and unfriendly gestures toward people from China and Wuhan at this tense and sensitive moment will increase the soft power of the United States and bring more goodwill from Chinese people toward the United States. Conversely, stigma, prejudice, and any punitive remarks will preclude any sense of goodwill and will also more likely undermine the level of transparency the Chinese government is willing to allow now.

Finally, given that the WHO has declared 2019-nCoV a PHEIC, there are concerns regarding developing countries that do not have a health care system capable of stopping the spread of the virus. In the worst-case scenario, the epidemic may affect more people in these countries when the epidemic subsides in China and the United States. The U.S. CDC may consider working with China's CDC and the China International Development

[29] Rosie Perper, "As the Wuhan Virus Spreads, Doctors in the City Say They Face a 'Flooding' of Patients and Not Enough Protective Gear," Business Insider, January 24, 2020. As of February 3, 2020: https://www.businessinsider.com/wuhan-coronavirus-doctors-wuhan-patients-protective-gear-2020-1.

Cooperation Agency (CIDCA) to map out potential collaborations to help these countries in distress.

Medium Term

Once the epidemic is under control, studies on the country response systems and global pandemic management will begin. It might be valuable for the United States to help lead the evaluations with government officials and scholars from China and other countries. There will be several questions for China to contemplate: What can China do in the future to improve communication about new public health threats? What can be done to increase the transparency about the occurrences and the severity of the outbreak? To what extent are quarantines effective, and how should they be implemented? How can China make its CDC more sustainable and improve multi-sector communications? The lessons learned will benefit not only China, but also other countries that encounter similar issues.

To take such a leadership role, I hope the U.S. government can build a realistic and consistent policy about future U.S.-China collaboration on global health and seek consensus with China on what data to share and what rules to follow.

Long Term

As I mentioned earlier in my testimony, during most of the years between SARS and 2019- nCoV, the United States and China were working side by side to confront the challenges of epidemics. In doing so, both countries have benefited from capacity building for their current and future public health workforces. In our current situation, as the first phase of the trade war is resolved, this could be an opportune time to restart the U.S.-China dialogues on economy, diplomacy, and security. I hope U.S.-China collaboration on global health and pandemic preparedness will benefit from these future talks between the two countries.

In: Coronavirus …
Editor: Roger F. Martin
ISBN: 978-1-53617-939-2

Chapter 16

LESSONS FROM THE WEST AFRICAN EBOLA RESPONSE: HOW TO SAVE LIVES AND PROTECT OUR NATION DURING THE NOVEL CORONAVIRUS EPIDEMIC OF 2020*

Ronald A. Klain

Chairman Bera, Ranking Member Yoho, other members of the Subcommittee:

Thank you for inviting me to participate in this hearing today. I want to commend the Subcommittee for moving quickly to gather information and educate the public about the novel coronavirus epidemic that originated in Wuhan, China, and has now spread to countries around the world, including our own. It is a privilege to be able to present my perspective on this, and to answer your questions about the emerging US response.

Before I begin my substantive presentation, I want to make two preliminary points.

First, as frustrating as it may be, it is important to understand that what we know about this epidemic and the virus that causes it remains uncertain and preliminary. We know much less about coronavirus today than we did about Ebola in 2014. Scientists in the US and around the world are working at unprecedented speed to improve our understanding about the virus and its spread; new papers are being published every day, literally. Nonetheless, there are critical questions about the virus, how quickly it spreads, how infectious it might be, how lethal it will be – and others –for which we still do not know the answers, and that (once learned) will have huge impacts on our response. Part of this is due to a lack of full transparency and cooperation by the Chinese government,

* This is an edited, reformatted and augmented version of Testimony before the Asia, Pacific and Non-Proliferation Subcommittee of the House Committee on Foreign Affairs, dated February 5, 2020.

which hopefully will improve. But part of this is simply due to the fact that it takes time for science to learn key facts about a novel virus. As someone who has coordinated the policymaking and implementation of a response to an epidemic, I know that these information gaps are vexing: many decisions cannot wait, and have to be made on the best information available. But it is important that we understand this limitation, understand that policy choices will have to change as our fact base changes, and that we be careful not to make definitive or declarative pronouncements when the science does not justify such statements.

Simply put, at present, we do not know how serious this epidemic will become, how many people – in China, in the US, and elsewhere – will contract the virus, how many will die, and how grave the threat is to our own country. Such a lack of knowledge does not counsel a lack of action, indeed, perhaps it counsels just the opposite. But it does advise modesty in the forcefulness of our conclusions, and awareness of the need to make changes in policy choices as we gain more information.

Second, a point about partisanship and the response. I am an outspoken political partisan – that is well known. But I come here today in the same way that I approached my tenure as White House Ebola Response Coordinator: putting partisanship and politics aside. The coronavirus will not ask any person's partisan affiliation before infecting them. There is no Democratic or Republican approach to fighting infectious disease; only sound and unsound measures.

To reinforce this point: what we did during the Obama administration's Ebola response relied heavily on lessons learned and expertise acquired during the Bush administration's efforts to fight AIDS and malaria in Africa. Key players in the Ebola response were veterans of both Democratic and Republican administrations. President Obama's emergency funding package passed this House with strong, bipartisan support; our implementation of it domestically involved work with state and local officials from both parties, and the input of Members of Congress of all political and ideological camps. Saving lives, abroad and at home, turns on putting politics aside and allowing science, expertise, and sound decision making to govern our actions.

With these two preliminary points made, I want to move on to the subject of my testimony today: how the lessons we learned during the Ebola response in 2014-15 should shape how our government – in the Executive and Legislative branches – approaches the threat now posed by the novel coronavirus.

To be clear, the Ebola response was not without its own problems and mistakes. Particularly early on, the danger to Africa and the world was underestimated; early signs of progress in containing the disease in the Spring of 2014 led to a false sense of security. The fact that no Ebola outbreak prior to 2014 had ever involved more than 500 cases of the disease also led to a false confidence that a large-scale epidemic was unlikely. Early initiatives in West Africa lacked a full understanding of the complexities of implementation there and cultural and religious barriers to some aspects of the response.

And confusion and a lack of preparation led to missteps when the first case of Ebola arrived in Dallas, Texas, in late September, 2014.

But ultimately, the US got the response organized; quickly adapted and improved its approach; and made adjustments to what responders were doing in Africa and here at home. President Obama mustered an all-of-government response to the challenge, authorized the first-ever deployment of US troops to combat an epidemic ("Operation United Assistance"), appointed me to lead a team of dedicated and talented professionals at the White House to coordinate this effort, implemented novel and innovative policies on travel screening and monitoring, and worked with Congress to enact a $5.4 billion emergency package to fight the disease abroad and improve our preparedness at home and around the world for future such epidemic threats.

In the end, the epidemic in West Africa was tragic: an official death toll of over 11,000, with the real count likely higher. But the backdrop for this loss of life must be considered. In September of 2014, experts forecast that the death toll could be over 1 million people; thus, the response succeeded in helping to reduce the projected loss of life by as much as 98%. America's actions – as part of a global response, with Africans playing the largest part, deserving the greatest credit, and suffering the harshest losses to its health care workers – saved hundreds of thousands of lives. It was a great humanitarian achievement.

Here at home, after the initial missteps in Dallas, no one contracted Ebola on US soil, and Americans evacuated for medical care in the US were successfully treated and released, with only a lone fatality. Once implemented, our monitoring system successfully insured no domestic transmission of the disease, routed suspected cases to prepared medical facilities before those patients could be infectious, and enabled ample time for successful testing and response.

The ongoing legacy of this response is likewise enormous. With Congress' support, we implemented a national four-tiered network of hospitals and medical facilities that remain prepared to this day to identify and isolate cases of dangerous infectious disease, and to provide treatment to those who are infected – nothing like this existed in 2014 when the Ebola epidemic began, as many earlier investments made after the anthrax attacks in 2001 had been allowed to dissipate. The capacity to test for and promptly identify diseases like Ebola grew from three laboratories in the US in September 2014 to almost 100 by the end of that year. We developed rapid diagnostics that ended the risky practice of having patients wait days to learn if they were sick and/or infectious. Vaccines against Ebola were tested and developed, and as a result of that work, an effective vaccine now exists and is being used in the field. New therapeutics were developed that helped reduce the mortality rate of Ebola dramatically.

It is no wonder that this effort – without in any way minimizing the devastation in West Africa – is seen today as a huge success. Tom Friedman wrote last year that that West African Ebola response was:

> "[President Obama's] most significant foreign policy achievement, for which he got little credit precisely because it worked — demonstrat[ing] that without America as quarterback, important things that save lives and advance freedom at reasonable costs often don't happen."

From mid-October 2014 to mid-February 2015, I was proud to lead the team at the White House that coordinated this response. We saw the weekly new case count in West Africa drop from about 1,000 a week to fewer than five a week, at which point the President announced the end of Operation United Assistance and began the withdrawal of US troops serving in that mission.

This was a truly global response, with tremendous contributions by government officials, NGOs, and volunteers from around the world, with a particularly close partnership with our allies in the United Kingdom and France. With regard to the US part of this global effort, special thanks should go to the men and women on the frontlines. This includes members of the 101st Airborne (who constituted the bulk of Operation United Assistance), and also, civilian responders -- via US AID DART teams and CDC employees deployed to the region, and contractors who supported them. It includes the men and women of the US Public Health Service who staffed the Monrovia Medical Unit in Liberia. It includes career Ambassadors and other diplomats who served in all three effected countries with skill and played such a large role in the response. It includes the doctors, nurses and other health care workers – many of them volunteers -- who served in Ebola treatment units, hospitals, and other facilities – treating the sick under extreme conditions. It includes the scientists of the NIH and the CDC who pioneered new diagnostics, therapeutics, and vaccines. The US response put over 10,000 people – soldiers and civilians, government workers and NGO teams, contractors and volunteers – on the ground in West Africa in 2014-2015. It was a gargantuan undertaking, and a story in which all Americans should take pride.

To make that effort effective, and to match it with preparation and protection here at home, it took talented teams in Washington, in Atlanta at the CDC, and in government agencies and private health care facilities around the country. Public servants of all ranks and all levels worked around the clock. And as I mentioned before, Congress acted swiftly and on a bipartisan basis to approve most of the Obama administration's request for $6 billion in aid, less than five weeks after it was sent to Capitol Hill.

I would be remiss if I did not say that, of course, President Obama, too, deserves credit for this success. He weathered sharp criticism for his actions during the Ebola response, and had to ignore pressures to put aside the advice he was getting from top scientists and medical experts. He made difficult decisions about the actions we took abroad and at home. He communicated openly and directly with the American people, and chaired repeated meetings of the National Security Council as the response took shape. He used every tool at his disposal – from his bully- pulpit (to destigmatize survivors by publicly hugging Ebola patient Nina Pham in the Oval Office after her discharge from the hospital), to authorizing the massive deployment to West Africa, to personally engaging numerous world leaders to activate their resources and support for the response, to urging Congressional leaders to approve his emergency spending package, and much more: he did so much to achieve these results.

The challenge we face from the novel coronavirus that began in China late last year contains many similarities, but also, many differences from the challenge posed by the Ebola epidemic in West Africa in 2014-15. It would be a mistake to simply repeat what we did at that time, given those many differences. But likewise, it would also be a mistake to ignore the lessons that can be learned from that response, given the similarities. And hence, I am grateful for the opportunity to talk about the lessons I think are most applicable from this experience, to be applied in the current circumstance.

Among the many possible lessons that should be employed now, there are seven in particular that I would like to call out today. I will do so briefly, but I am happy to go into more depth on any of them in response to your questions or any subsequent follow-up from the Subcommittee.

First, in a complex, rapidly evolving scenario like the one we are seeing, there is no substitute for White House coordination and leadership. There should be a single official inside the National Security Council at the White House, supported by an appropriate team, working on this full-time, overseeing our response.

This does NOT mean that we need a "Coronavirus Czar" to serve the same role that I played during the Ebola epidemic. At the end of my tenure as Ebola Response Coordinator, I said, in fact, there should never be another specific "Disease Czar" at the White House. Instead, I recommended to President Obama that he create a permanent "Pandemic Preparedness and Response Directorate" inside the NSC, led by a Deputy National Security Adviser-level appointee with direct access to the President as needed, to oversee ongoing work to prepare for future infectious disease threats, and to coordinate a response when such threats arrive.

President Obama accepted this recommendation, and set up such a unit in 2015. President Trump continued with the structure, and named Admiral Tim Ziemer – a respected long-time public servant – to fill this post. If Admiral Ziemer were still in place, I believe that America would be much better positioned to respond to the coronavirus threat today.

But unfortunately, in July of 2018, when John Bolton took over as head of the NSC, he disbanded this unit, and Admiral Ziemer was reassigned to US AID. As a result, there has been no special unit at the NSC to oversee preparedness for epidemics, or the current response. In addition, the Trump administration has dismantled the Homeland Security Advisor structure that Presidents Bush and Obama used to deal with complex transnational threats, further undermining our preparedness for events like these.

The administration's recent decision to create a "Task Force" to oversee the response, led by Secretary Alex Azar, is a valuable step, but an insufficient one. This is not a criticism of Sec. Azar, who I believe is playing a critical role in the response, and brings great experience and judgment to this effort. But a response to a challenge like this one requires action from a number of federal agencies outside of Sec. Azar's authority: Homeland Security, State, US AID, Transportation, DOD – and probably also Labor, Commerce and Justice. Given the nature of Cabinet government, the fundamentals of bureaucratic behavior, and the realities of competing demands on a Cabinet secretary's time, no single Cabinet agency head can lead such a response. There are global implications as well: in dealing with other nations as the world shapes and implements the response, a single point of coordination inside the White House both emphasizes the response's importance to the President, and facilitates high-level government-to-government cooperation.

For these reasons, and many more, an effective response to a challenge like coronavirus should be led by a full-time, high-level appointee at the White House. Ideally that decision would be made by the Executive Branch, but another avenue to achieve this structure would be for Congress to move ahead on the Global Health Security Act (HR 2166), introduced by Reps.

Connolly and Chabot, as that bill would create much of this apparatus by statute.

Second, the US must "lean forward" to fight this epidemic overseas, using all of the tools and leverage that it can commit to the effort. Unlike West Africa in 2014, China in 2020 probably does not need, and would not accept, thousands of US responders on the ground treating patients, testing new approaches, conducting research, providing infrastructure, and helping bring the disease under control. This is a huge difference.

But that should not get us off our toes, or have us sitting back and believing that our only sphere of action is the homeland. Dr. Tony Fauci of NIH has publicly urged the deployment of medical researchers and investigators to China, and key administration leaders – at State and the White House – should apply pressure to encourage the most open access possible. Nations less advanced or well-resourced than China may experience significant coronavirus outbreaks and require more direct forms of US assistance, akin to what we provided during the 2014 Ebola epidemic, albeit on a smaller scale. We should send CDC experts wherever they would be helpful, and task US AID to determine where DART teams and other assistance could be usefully deployed. Likewise, we should bolster preparedness in low-income countries now – before the disease spreads further – to avoid spread in places where local containment efforts might fail.

Our diplomats should be empowered and engaged around the globe, and our government must press WHO – with stronger leadership today under Dr. Tedros Adhanom Ghebreyesu than it had during the 2014 Ebola epidemic – to do the right thing.

This is a global challenge, and America must provide global leadership. There is no room for isolationism or withdrawal. The best way to keep Americans safe is to contain and combat the virus overseas. We should do this not only because it is generous or humanitarian – though it would be generous and humanitarian, both great American traits – but because it will make America safer and reduce the risk of a larger outbreak here.

Third, the administration must ensure that science and expertise guide our actions, not fear or politics. One of the first casualties in an epidemic is rational thinking, replaced by fear, bias and poor decision-making. We saw this in 2014 with calls for needless travel bans and baseless quarantine restrictions; President Obama was right to reject these misguided calls, and to implement travel and monitoring policies based on the scientific advice he got from the nation's leading experts.

Travel warnings and advisories make sense in the face of the coronavirus; telling people not to take trips to China right now, except in special or compelling cases, is wise. That is quite different from banning people – including, for example, Americans in China, or family members of Americans – from coming back home, or going for essential purposes. Congress should press the administration for the science behind recently announced quarantines and exclusions of non-US persons from travel to the US; also, it should inquire as to the effectiveness of the measures being implemented. Banning travel to or from China altogether would impede the flow of medical assistance, expert investigation, or other key response functions; in addition, key supplies – including supplies critical to our own health care system – come from China.

More generally, there will be many policy decisions to be made in the days and weeks ahead. Science, medicine and expertise should guide them. The American people are lucky to have the world's leading experts on infectious disease working in their government, led by men and women like Tony Fauci at NIH and Anne Schuchat at CDC. They have served Democratic and Republican administrations, and helped Presidents with a wide variety of political perspectives save lives and protect our nation. This expertise should be paramount in decision making at all levels of government.

Fourth, the administration should quickly assemble, and transmit to Congress, an emergency funding package to ensure that there are no delays in responding to the coronavirus challenge. Fighting the coronavirus overseas and at home will cost money. HHS (and its units like ASPR, BARDA, NIH and CDC), US AID, DHS, and other agencies will have costs. State and local governments will feel a pinch from monitoring contacts of those who have the virus, and tracking and monitoring individuals who have been in effected countries. Hospitals treating patients with the virus may need assistance. Research and deployment of new therapeutics and vaccines needs government support, and funding for private-public partnerships. The list of needs goes on.

While Congress responded quickly to a funding request from the Obama administration for Ebola, even that short delay had some impact on our response. The delay of months in approving funding for the Zika response was quite consequential. Most importantly, Congress is unlikely to even begin considering these funding needs until the administration makes a request.

The Trump Administration has tools that we lacked in 2014, most importantly – and to the Congress' credit – it has a new Emergency Fund on which the Administration can (and has) drawn. But I expect that this will not be adequate, and it would be wise for the administration to begin putting together a Supplemental Funding request immediately.

Fifth, Congress must do its own work in dealing with the novel coronavirus. The burden of action does not rest entirely with the Executive Branch; Congress too must do its part.

This starts with the point I made above: once the administration makes an emergency funding request, Congress should act on it without delay. Of course, Congress should not rubberstamp the request: any proposal to use public funds should get scrutiny and review. But prompt action must drive this process, and divisions between parties or chambers should not result in delay. Indeed, Congress might want to begin now – given the expertise of many in this body – preparing for such a request even before it is made, and contemplating the likely funding needs.

But Congress' role does not end with acting on the emergency funding question; there are a number of other elements of the response that demand Congressional attention. Hearings like today's are important, to help ascertain how the response is going and where it needs to be improved. Congress wisely funded the Public Health Emergency Fund last year – but did so only on a limited basis. Adding to that funding, and funding an additional emergency fund specific to the development of therapeutics and vaccines via public-private partnerships, should be considered.

Additionally, as I wrote in the Post with Dr. Syra Madad in December – before the coronavirus hit -- Congress is overdue to renew the funding for the network of "Ebola and Special Pathogens Hospitals." This network was created during the Ebola epidemic in 2014, and funding for it expires in May of 2020. Pending legislation would fund only the 10 most advanced such facilities, and would end federal funding for the 60 other hospitals that screen, test, and provide initial treatment for these cases. Allowing this funding to expire in May would be a huge mistake; funding for these specialized facilities should be renewed, and the network should be strengthened with greater help for frontline facilities, EMS responders, and other touch points in our medical system that are least prepared and most exposed.

Sixth, both the Executive Branch and the Congress should take this as a wake-up call to finish the work we need to do on pandemic preparedness and readiness. Recently, America marked the 100th anniversary of the single largest mortality event in our history: the Spanish Flu epidemic of 1918-19. More Americans died from this epidemic than from World War I, World War II, the Korean War, and the Vietnam War - -combined. While, on the one hand, science has made great strides since 1918, on the other hand, increased global travel, human incursion on animal habitats, and the stresses of climate change have raised the risk that we will face such a "great pandemic" once again.

At present, it seems very unlikely that the coronavirus poses such a threat to the United States – but we cannot know for certain. Moreover, even if this current epidemic is not "the big one" that is coming, it is a reminder that this danger lurks, and our preparedness for it is lacking. As Dr. Ashish Jha of the Harvard Global Health Institute often says, "Of all the things that can kill millions of Americans quickly and unexpectedly, an epidemic is probably the most likely ... and the one in which we invest the least to prevent."

The Global Health Security Agenda, legislation such as HR 2166, Blue Ribbon Commission reports, table top exercises, proposals from members of this Subcommittee – and my own extensive writing over the past five years – have set forth detailed agendas of what we need to do to prepared for this event. These bipartisan calls for action have largely been ignored. The current public focus on infectious disease generated by the coronavirus should spur us into action. The time to act on this agenda is now. If we wait until the catastrophic pandemic arrives, it will be too late.

Seventh, we need to be on the watch for discrimination against people in our country of Chinese origin and ancestry, and speak out strongly against any such fear-driven racism. The coronavirus strikes humans – not people of any particular ethnicity or race. Chinese-Americans or Chinese people in America are no more likely to get the disease, carry the disease, or transmit the disease, than any other group of people.

Yet we have already seen signs that such people are the targets of discriminatory fear – with some already being hassled, threatened with expulsion from schools and other mistreatment. As fears of the coronavirus accelerate, so too will these incidents. This kind of discrimination not only is wrong, but also makes it harder to combat the disease. If some members of the Chinese-American community feel that they are likely to face hostility, they are less likely to work closely with authorities, and less likely to heed advice of public health experts.

It is incumbent on every person in authority in this nation to speak out against such racism, and to ensure that this does not become part of our civic life during the coronavirus epidemic.

Americans need to pull together to fight a disease, not pull apart to fight one another.

In closing, I want to thank, again, the Subcommittee for holding this hearing, and for inviting me to participate. I stand ready to answer your questions about any of these points, or any other aspects of the response.

America has the tools, the talent, and the expertise to combat the coronavirus, both abroad and at home. The question now is whether our leaders, in the Executive Branch and the Congress, will deploy them effectively; act promptly and wisely; rely on expertise – not bias and fear; organize and implement our response appropriately; and allow science and medicine tobe our touchstone. For the sake of people around the world, and for the sake of the American people, let us work to see that it is so.

In: Coronavirus …
Editor: Roger F. Martin
ISBN: 978-1-53617-939-2

Chapter 17

THE STATE OF U.S. PUBLIC HEALTH BIO-PREPAREDNESS: RESPONDING TO BIOLOGICAL ATTACKS, PANDEMICS, AND EMERGING INFECTIOUS DISEASE OUTBREAKS*

Subcommittee on Oversight and Investigations

Friday, June 15, 2018
House of Representatives, Committee on Energy and Commerce,
Washington, DC

The subcommittee met, pursuant to call, at 9:01 a.m., in room 2123, Rayburn House Office Building, Hon. Gregg Harper (chairman of the subcommittee) presiding.

Present: Representatives Harper, Griffith, Burgess, Brooks, Collins, Walberg, Walters, Costello, Carter, Walden (ex officio), Degette, Schakowsky, Castor, Ruiz, and Pallone (ex officio).

Also Present: Representative Eshoo.

Staff Present: Jennifer Barblan, Chief Counsel, Oversight and Investigations; Adam Fromm, Director of Outreach and Coalitions; Ali Fulling, Legislative Clerk, Oversight and Investigations, Digital Commerce and Consumer Protection; Christopher Santini, Counsel, Oversight and Investigations; Jennifer Sherman, Press Secretary; Alan Slobodin, Chief Investigative Counsel, Oversight and Investigations; Austin Stonebraker, Press Assistant; Christina Calce, Minority Counsel; Jeff Carroll, Minority Staff Director;

* This is an edited, reformatted and augmented version of Hearing before the Subcommittee on Oversight and Investigations, of the Committee on Energy and Commerce, House of Representatives, One Hundred Fifteenth Congress, Second Session, Serial No. 115–140, dated June 15, 2018.

Chris Knauer, Minority Oversight Staff Director; Miles Lichtman, Minority Policy Analyst; C.J. Young, Minority Press Secretary; and Perry Lusk, Minority GAO Detailee.

OPENING STATEMENT OF HON. GREGG HARPER, A REPRESENTATIVE IN CONGRESS FROM THE STATE OF MISSISSIPPI

Mr. HARPER. Good morning. Today, the subcommittee continues its longstanding oversight of the U.S. public health system's preparedness to respond to biological threats and emerging infectious diseases that endanger the public health. The purpose of today's hearing is to hear from top public health experts on the good work being done at their agencies to protect the public and to explore where improvements need to be made.

The biological threats facing the United States in today's global society are varied, ever-evolving and, in some cases, intensifying. The CDC just reported that the seasonal influenza claimed the lives of 172 children during the most recent flu season, making it the deadliest seasonal flu season for children on record.

In recent years, the U.S. has also seen an increase in the number of antibiotic-resistant bacteria. Around the world, viruses are emerging, adapting and, in some cases, reemerging. Currently, there is an Ebola outbreak in West Africa and a Nipah virus outbreak in India that has killed at least 17.

In recent years, we have also seen humans in China contract the H7N9 strain of influenza which has been confined to birds. The H7N9 influenza strain is rated by the CDC's influenza risk assessment tool as posing the greatest risk to cause a public pandemic.

The 2013 ricin mailings addressed to President Obama and Senator Roger Wicker that originated in my home State of Mississippi, as well as the 2001 anthrax mailings and foreign terrorist threats, is a reminder of the risk of intentional biological attacks.

Today's hearing is especially timely, given that the committee is considering bipartisan legislation sponsored by Mrs. Brooks and Ms. Eshoo to reauthorize the Pandemic and All Hazards Preparedness Act, PAHPA, which is set to expire at the end of September. Passage of PAHPA's reauthorization would not only provide critical certainty for public health agencies and industry partners, it would also bring about some much needed reforms. One such reform proposed in the legislation is transferring control of the Strategic National Stockpile from the CDC to HHS' Office of the Assistant Secretary for Preparedness and Response, to improve management of the stockpile.

A year ago, HHS' Office of Inspector General reported systemic issues with security and inventory management of the stockpile, risking CDC's ability to deploy the stockpile during a public health emergency. These issues need to be addressed, as does improving the training of State and local stakeholders on deployment of medical countermeasures.

Administrative reforms are also of interest. For example, are there ways to improve the timeliness of the decisionmaking process on threat assessments and appropriate countermeasures? Effective threat detection has been a subject of committee oversight. In 2016, the committee questioned the CDC about the effectiveness of its Laboratory Response Network, or LRN, which is responsible for developing assays for public health labs to test for the presence of Federal select agents.

In a May 2017 letter to the committee, the CDC reported that the LRN had only developed three assays approved by the FDA to detect specific Federal select agents. While the LRN has also had those cleared by the FDA under emergency use authorization, after nearly 20 years of this program, with about $135 million in funding over the last decade, could the LRN have cleared a significantly higher number of assays through the most rigorous FDA 510(k) process?

Finally, maintaining public confidence in critical Federal biopreparedness research is essential. In response to safety lapses in 2014 and to an expert panel's recommendations, the CDC and FDA each formed new offices in 2015 to centralize and elevate oversight of laboratory safety, with the directors of those offices reporting directly to the agency head.

These changes sent a strong message that lab safety was a top priority, backed by the clout of direct backing from the agency head. Unfortunately, both agencies seem to be backtracking from this good direction.

In the FDA's case, less than a year after this administration approved the direct report organization—or reorganization, the sudden change is curious and would seem to be a step in the wrong direction. So we need to hear more details about the basis for this new direction.

I would like to thank the distinguished members of our panel for being here today and for your service to our country.

I now recognize the ranking member of the subcommittee from Colorado, Ms. DeGette, for 5 minutes.

[The prepared statement of Mr. Harper follows:]

PREPARED STATEMENT OF HON. GREGG HARPER

Good morning, today the Subcommittee continues its long-standing oversight of the U.S. public health system's preparedness to respond to biological threats and emerging infectious diseases that endanger the public health. The purpose of today's hearing is to hear from top public health experts on the good work being done at their agencies to protect the public, and to explore where improvements in biopreparedness may still be needed.

The biological threats facing the United States in today's global society are varied, ever-evolving, and in some cases, intensifying. The CDC just reported that the seasonal influenza claimed the lives of 172 children during the most recent flu season, making it the deadliest seasonal flu season for children on record. In recent years the U.S. has also seen an increase in the number of antibiotic resistant bacteria.

Around the world, viruses are emerging, adapting, and in some cases, re-emerging. Currently, there is an Ebola outbreak in West Africa and a Nipah (*pronounced Knee – Pah*) virus outbreak in India, that has killed at least 17 people.

In recent years, we have also seen humans in China contract the H7N9 strain of influenza, which had been confined to birds. The H7N9 influenza strain is rated by the CDC's Influenza Risk Assessment Tool as posing the greatest risk to cause a possible pandemic.

The 2013 ricin mailings addressed to President Obama and Senator Roger Wicker that originated in my home state of Mississippi, as well as the 2001 anthrax mailings and foreign terrorist threats, is a reminder of the risk of intentional biological attacks.

Today's hearing is especially timely given that the Committee is considering bipartisan legislation, sponsored by Ms. Brooks and Ms. Eshoo, to reauthorize the Pandemic and All-Hazards Preparedness Act (PAHPA), which is set to expire at the end of September. Passage of PAHPA's (*pronounced Pah – Pah*) reauthorization would not only provide critical certainty for public health agencies and industry partners, it would also bring about some much-needed reforms.

One such reform, proposed in the legislation, is transferring control of the Strategic National Stockpile from the CDC to HHS' Office of the Assistant Secretary for Preparedness and Response to improve management of the Stockpile. A year ago, HHS's Office of Inspector General reported systemic issues with security and inventory management of the Stockpile, risking CDC's ability to deploy the stockpile during a public health emergency. These issues need to be addressed, as does improving the training of state and local stakeholders on deployment of medical countermeasures.

Administrative reforms are also of interest. For example, are there ways to improve the timeliness of the decision-making process on threat assessments and appropriate countermeasures?

Effective threat detection has been a subject of Committee oversight. In 2016, the Committee questioned the CDC about the effectiveness of its Laboratory Response Network (LRN), or LRN, which is responsible for developing assays for public health labs to test for the presence of federal select agents. In a May 2017 letter to the Committee, the CDC reported that the LRN had only developed three assays approved by FDA to detect specific federal select agents. While the LRN has also had assays cleared by the FDA under Emergency Use Authorization, after nearly 20 years of this program with about $135 million in funding over the last decade, could the LRN have cleared a significantly higher number of assays through the more rigorous FDA 510(k) process?

Finally, maintaining public confidence in critical federal biopreparedness research is essential. In response to safety lapses in 2014 and to an expert panel's recommendations, the CDC and FDA each formed new offices in 2015 to centralize and elevate oversight of laboratory safety, with the directors of those offices reporting directly to the agency head. These changes sent a strong message that lab safety was a top priority backed by the clout of direct backing from the agency head. Unfortunately, both agencies seem to be backtracking from this good direction, in the FDA's case less than a year after this Administration approved the direct-report reorganization. The sudden change is curious, and would seem to be a step in the wrong direction. We need to hear more details about the basis for this new direction.

I would like to thank the distinguished members of our panel for being here today and for your service to our country. I now recognize the Ranking Member of the Subcommittee from Colorado, Ms. DeGette, for five minutes.

Opening Statement of Hon. Diana DeGette, A Representative in Congress from the State of Colorado

Ms. DEGETTE. Thank you, Mr. Chairman.

I know we agree that preparing this country for a bioincident is of critical importance. The threat, as you said, is real and it's growing.

In April, the CDC reported that in 2017, Colorado saw 25 cases of an antibiotic-resistant bacteria known descriptively as the nightmare bacteria, because 50 percent of those infected by it die. Thankfully, those cases were isolated, but the same CDC study noted that it's possible for these germs to "spread like wildfire." If that happens, we need to know that we're able to respond.

We've looked at this issue in this subcommittee many times over the years, as our panel well knows. It's a regular appearance, and I want to thank you for coming again. And again and again, we've found that the Federal Government has to scramble to address biosafety incidents.

Those of us who were here during the fall of 2001 vividly recall the chaos that a few small envelopes of anthrax caused on Capitol Hill. Offices were closed. Buildings were fumigated. Some congressional business was suspended, and thousands of staffers and other personnel lined up for days to get tested for exposure. Far worse, some of the workers in our Postal Service were infected and died.

In 2009, we again had to scramble to produce sufficient doses of the H1N1 swine flu vaccine to protect against this new strain of the disease.

In 2014, hospitals and healthcare providers were not adequately prepared to deal with the arrival of Ebola patients in America. In one case, a hospital in Dallas failed to diagnose Ebola in a patient who had traveled to West Africa and discharged him. The virus was later transmitted from that patient to two healthcare workers. In the days and weeks that followed, important questions were raised about how this event was handled and were we adequately prepared for the larger event.

And then, of course, in 2015, the Zika outbreak underscored the need for the U.S. Government to focus on disease preparedness every day. And I know our panel here today does just that.

I'd like to know today, though, what lessons we've learned from these incidents, and I want to know how the agencies are using what we've learned to better prepare for the next crisis, because there will be one.

For example, do we have adequate medical countermeasures in place to respond quickly when an outbreak occurs or a toxin is released? Do we have the capacity to quickly deliver these counter-measures to the doctors and nurses who will actually use them? And do the healthcare workers understand how to deploy the coun-termeasures?

Similarly, research into emerging pathogens and existing pathogens that have mutated is key to helping us quickly respond to new and expanding outbreaks. How is this research informing our surveillance and detection methodologies? Are we prioritizing research into threats of greatest concern? And are we dedicating adequate resources to the threats?

I also want to hear more about how all of our agencies—CDC, ASPR, NIAID and FDA—coordinate their research, surveillance, and response efforts. Because while each one of these agencies today has a specific valuable role to play in ensuring preparedness, nobody can operate effectively alone.

In fact, one major finding of the Blue Ribbon Panel's 2015 report on biodefense preparedness was these agencies must ensure they're equipped to work together to respond to pandemics. The Blue Ribbon report also found that the Federal Government must dramatically increase the support provided to local jurisdictions to help them build and sustain their biodefense capabilities.

Local providers like hospitals and healthcare workers will be on the front lines in a public health emergency. I want to ensure that we're adequately supporting these providers, as well as State and local Health Departments, so they are equipped to detect incidents when they happen and respond appropriately.

Mr. Chairman, I'm really hoping we'll hear today that we've made tangible, measurable progress in this area, but, again, I urge us to revisit the work of the Blue Ribbon Panel and some of its findings to determine what more we need to do to better prepare the Nation for the threats that we will be discussing today.

I just can't thank our panel today enough for the tireless work that they put in to keeping America safe. We always have a great opportunity to hear from you, and we know that you're working hard. We think by having you come up here and take the time, it really helps us represent our constituents, and it helps all of us be better prepared for the next emergency that faces us.

Thank you, and I yield back.

Mr. HARPER. The gentlewoman yields back.

The chair now recognizes the chairman of the full committee, the gentleman from Oregon, Mr. Walden, for 5 minutes.

OPENING STATEMENT OF HON. GREG WALDEN, A REPRESENTATIVE IN CONGRESS FROM THE STATE OF OREGON

Mr. WALDEN. Thank you very much, Mr. Chairman. To all our committee members, thanks for your work on this. And to our panelists, thank you, not only for your guidance on this issue, but also what we tap into you for along the way. And so we appreciate your professionalism and your assistance in our policy debates.

The topic of biopreparedness really hits home for me. I think I was the first Member of Congress to be diagnosed with H1N1 years ago. Not a distinction I was glad to get, but one apparently I had.

But more than that, 30 years ago, a religious group called the Rajneeshees moved to Oregon. You may have seen the documentary on Netflix called Wild Country. And if you read Judith Miller's book Germs, you'll find it was the largest bioterror attack in the Nation's history, but it took the Federal Government a year, I think she wrote, to admit that that's really what it was. They grew their own salmonella and then sprinkled it over salad bars in Dalles, Oregon, and sickened 751 people, many of whom I know.

Deliberate biological attacks are just one risk. With more global travel, there's, of course, increased risk of spread of infectious diseases. As we've seen with influenza, our vaccines must be constantly updated to keep up with the latest strains. Meanwhile, other pathogens can develop antibiotic resistance, and our ability to quickly recognize evolving diseases and respond to new outbreaks is reliant on the testing and treatment and capabilities in the men and women who do the work that you all oversee.

Lack of preparation is not an option. A mock pandemic exercise hosted last month by Johns Hopkins Center for Health Security with a group of current and former government officials, including our own colleague Susan Brooks, I'm told was quite eye-opening. The exercise resulted in a failure to develop a vaccine within 20 months, and that led in this exercise to 150 million deaths globally. So obviously, we've got to do more to be prepared for these types of outbreaks.

So that's where the reauthorization of the Pandemic and All Hazards Preparedness Act comes in. PAHPA originally was adopted in 2006. It's set to expire at the end of September. We intend to move forward with legislation prior to that.

Our Health Subcommittee met just last week to consider a bipartisan discussion draft to reauthorize this law and continues to fine-tune it. It's critically important Congress reauthorizes this law in time and to make sure that all levels of government are well-equipped to handle, not just current and emerging biothreats, but also chemical attacks, radiological emergencies, cybersecurity incidents, and mass casualty events.

Through letters, hearings, and investigations, the Committee has raised numerous issues regarding biological threats to the U.S. and our nation's ability to respond to infectious disease outbreaks. For example, the Committee has examined concerns about the CDC's management and the security of the Strategic National Stockpile and the capabilities of CDC Laboratory Response Network. The Trump administration is set to transfer management of the stock-pile from the CDC to the Assistant Secretary for Preparedness and Response, known as ASPR. And we look forward to hearing more details about how this transfer will work.

Another area of interest to the Committee is the improvement of our biosurveillance capabilities. Innovation in this field could bolster our public health response in the event of an attack or epidemic. So I'll be interested in learning more about that as well.

One thing we do know, the Federal Government needs to act faster to identify and determine material threats. The Department of Homeland Security in March 2018 made a material threat determination for pharmaceutical-based agents such as Fentanyl. It took 2 years for the DHS to make this designation, yet carfentanil, a highly potent form of Fentanyl, was used in a terrorist attack more than 15 years ago. So it's only after that designation is made that the Public Health Emergency Medical Countermeasures Enterprise can approve countermeasure development and acquisition. If we knew about it 15 years ago and it took 2 years to get that designation, we can do better.

Maintaining public support for critical biopreparedness research relies on Federal scientists and researchers working with these diseases and dangerous pathogens in a safe and secure manner. Following several safety lapses at CDC and FDA labs in 2014, both FDA and CDC created new offices to oversee and prioritize lab safety. These are positive steps. The recent proposals at these agencies to lower the status of their lab safety offices raises concerns with this committee.

So I thank you for being here today.

And I'd like to yield the balance of my time to Dr. Burgess and hopefully to Mrs. Brooks.

[The prepared statement of Chairman Walden follows:]

PREPARED STATEMENT OF HON. GREG WALDEN

Mr. Chairman, thank you for holding this hearing. The topic ofbiopreparedness hits home for me. Some of you may recall that in 2009 I was diagnosed with H1N1—the swine flu. It was reported at the time that I was the first Member of Congress to contract swine flu—a distinction I'm not particularly proud of. But that's not all. The first and single largest bioterrorism attack in the U.S. occurred in my district. More than 30 years ago, a group of Rajneeshee cult members used salmonella to contaminate at least 10 restaurant salad bars in The Dalles, Oregon, causing at least 751 people to get ill.

Deliberate biological attacks are just one risk. With more global travel, there is increased risk of the spread of infectious diseases.

As we've seen with influenza, our vaccines must be constantly updated to keep up with the latest strain mutations. Meanwhile other pathogens can develop antibiotic resistance. Our ability to quickly recognize evolving diseases and respond to new outbreaks is reliant on our testing and treatment capabilities.

Lack of preparation is not an option. A mock pandemic exercise hosted last month by Johns Hopkins Center for Health Security with a group of current and former government officials, including our colleague Susan Brooks, was eye opening. This exercise resulted in a failure to develop a vaccine within 20 months and led to 150 million deaths globally. We must do more. We must be prepared for potential out-breaks.

That's where the reauthorization of the Pandemic and All-Hazards Preparedness Act (PAHPA) comes in. PAHPA, originally adopted in 2006, is set to expire at the end of September. Our Health Subcommittee met just last week to consider a bipartisan discussion draft to reauthorize this law and continues to fine tune it. It is critically important Congress reauthorizes this law to ensure that all levels of government are well-equipped to handle not just current and emerging biothreats, but also chemical attacks, radiological emergencies, cybersecurity incidents, and mass casualty events.

Through letters, hearings and investigations, the committee has raised numerous issues regarding biological threats to the U.S. and our nation's ability to respond to infectious disease outbreaks. For example, the committee has examined concerns about the CDC's management and security of the Strategic National Stockpile, and the capabilities of the CDC Laboratory Response Network. The Trump Administration is set to transfer management of the stockpile from the CDC to the Assistant Secretary for Preparedness and Response (ASPR), and we look forward to hearing more details about how this transfer will work.

Another area of interest to the committee is the improvement of our biosurveillance capabilities. Innovation in this field could bolster our public health response in the event of an attack or epidemic. I will be interested to learn whether more intensive research could help expedite addressing the technical challenges.

One thing we do know: The Federal Government needs to act faster to identify and determine material threats. The Department of Homeland Security (DHS) in March 2018 made a material threat determination for pharmaceutical-based agents such as fentanyl. It took 2 years for DHS to make this designation. Yet carfentanil, a highly potent form of fentanyl, was used in a terrorist attack more than 15 years ago. It's only after that designation is made that the Public Health Emergency Medical Countermeasures Enterprise can approve countermeasure development and acquisition. We must move faster.

Maintaining public support for critical biopreparedness research relies on federal scientists and researchers working with these diseases and dangerous pathogens in a safe and secure manner. Following several safety lapses at CDC and FDA labs in 2014, both CDC and FDA created new offices to oversee and prioritize lab safety. These were positive steps, but recent proposals at these agencies to lower the status of their lab safety offices raise concerns.

I'd like to thank our witnesses for being here with us today. We value the feedback and insight you provide and look forward to today's discussion.

Mr. BURGESS. Thank you, Mr. Chairman.

And this issue is one that is important and timely for this sub-committee. And last week, the Health Subcommittee had a hearing on the discussion draft of the Pandemic and All Hazards Preparedness Act authored by Representatives Brooks and Eshoo. At that hearing, we heard from witnesses with firsthand experience in combating these biological threats to our nation and received input on the draft legislation.

Certainly, our witness panel today is well-known to us and they are all experts. I look forward to hearing from our witnesses.

And I thank you, Mr. Chairman, and I will yield to Mrs. Brooks.

Mr. HARPER. Maybe with unanimous consent, due to your leadership role in this, 30 seconds.

Mrs. BROOKS. Thank you, Mr. Chairman.

And thank you to our witnesses for your work on this public health and national security issue.

Last February, our subcommittee here held a hearing examining how we best combat biological threats. And I'm pleased we're once again examining the state of our preparedness as we prepare to reauthorize PAHPA.

As everyone here knows, it is not a question of if we face a threat; it's a question of again, once again, when we face a threat. And we've been reminded by the stories that we've heard here today that these types of incidents have already happened in our country over the last decade and a half.

Created in 1999, the National Stockpile is the repository of vaccines, antibiotics, and supplies used in the event of an attack or an outbreak. But HHS OIG, in June of 2017, issued a report identifying serious systemic issues within the CDC's management of the stockpile.

I look forward to hearing from our witnesses today how we are going to ensure that our stockpile is properly managed and that we can be prepared as a country for whatever threat we are and may face.

I yield back.

Mr. HARPER. The chair now recognizes the ranking member of the full committee, the gentleman from New Jersey, Mr. Pallone, for 5 minutes.

OPENING STATEMENT OF HON. FRANK PALLONE, JR., A REPRESENTATIVE IN CONGRESS FROM THE STATE OF NEW JERSEY

Mr. PALLONE. Thank you, Mr. Chairman.

Ensuring that our nation is equipped to respond to pandemics, natural disasters, and the accidental or intentional release of toxins is a key part of protecting public health. Past work by this committee has suggested that our nation has not always been as prepared as we need to be, so I'm glad that we're having this hearing today, and I hope to hear that we have made tangible progress towards increasing our Nation's preparedness.

In 2015, the Blue Ribbon Panel on Biodefense conducted a comprehensive review of the Federal Government's biopreparedness efforts. The panel found that, "The Nation is dangerously vulnerable to a biological event." It produced an extensive report recommending 30 action items for our public health infrastructure to address.

While the Blue Ribbon Panel was the most recent high-level commission to examine our nation's biopreparedness, it was not the first. In fact, for many years, experts have warned that our ability to respond to biologic and other emerging threats must be improved.

These recommendations remain important today, because the emerging health threats this country faces continue to grow. Just this week, officials announced that a child in Idaho had contracted bubonic plague. Last year, an outbreak of this plague killed 200 people in Madagascar.

In March, we heard at a hearing that the threat of pandemic flu is among the greatest concerns in the public health world. And antibiotic resistance also poses a major threat to public health, killing 23,000 Americans every year and making everyday procedures like surgery and chemotherapy increasingly risky. In May, a study showed that warming temperatures were associated with higher levels of antibiotic resistance in common strains of bacteria.

Extreme weather events can also lead to serious public health emergencies. The hurricanes in Puerto Rico, the Virgin Islands, Texas, and Florida last year were a stark reminder of this fact. We must be prepared to address threats from all these sources.

The Blue Ribbon Panel produced many recommendations for improving our biopreparedness, and I hope our witnesses will show that we have made real progress. For example, I hope to hear that the agencies have established a plan for who will take the lead in response to a public health threat and how the efforts will be coordinated.

Along these same lines, I hope we will learn how CDC, NIH, ASPR, and FDA are working together to identify the greatest threats and to prioritize the research, surveillance, and response capabilities needed to target these threats.

We must also focus on how these agencies collaborate with State and local health departments as well as healthcare providers, such as hospitals. These entities are likely to be the first to see patients impacted by an infectious disease outbreak or other incident. In most cases, they'll be the ones to dispense countermeasures and to treat those impacted.

In 2014, for example, we witnessed the negative consequences that ensued when our healthcare infrastructure was unprepared to diagnose and treat patients with Ebola. A hospital failed to detect the disease in the patient in Dallas, and that patient later transmitted Ebola to two healthcare workers. This incident led to a serious question about whether we would be able to handle a larger scale event or incident. And we must make sure everyone on the ground has all the resources they need to respond effectively in such a crisis.

We also want to hear more about how we are conducting surveillance so that when an outbreak happens or a toxin is released, we know as soon as possible. While we cannot anticipate every possible new or mutated pathogen, if we can quickly detect when such a pathogen has emerged, we can respond much more effectively.

And along these same lines, I understand the CDC is gathering a substantial amount of data from laboratories, public health departments, and clinicians across the country every day. So we must ensure that this agency has the resources it needs to effectively use and analyze this data as it comes in.

And finally, I want to hear more about what we're doing to prioritize development of medical countermeasures to help us respond to a biosafety incident. Countermeasures include preventative measures like vaccines as well as therapeutics like antibiotics and antivirals.

BARDA, I understand that you work closely with the private sector to develop many of these products, and I hope that we will hear today about how these partnerships have produced useful, safe, and effective products that truly address the challenges we face.

So, Mr. Chairman, I'd like to thank our panel once again for being here. Preparing for these threats is certainly not easy, but I'm confident that you're up for the task as long as we do our part and provide you with all the resources that you need.

I yield back, Mr. Chairman.

Mr. HARPER. The gentleman yields back.

I ask unanimous consent that the members' written opening statements be made part of the record. Without objection, they will be so entered into the record.

And additionally, I ask unanimous consent that Energy and Commerce members not on the Subcommittee on Oversight and Investigations be permitted to participate in today's hearing. Without objection, so ordered.

I would now like to introduce our witnesses for today's hearing. First, we have Dr. Rick Bright, Director of Biomedical Advanced Research and Development Authority and Deputy Assistant Secretary at the Office of the Assistant Secretary for Preparedness and Response. Next is Dr. Anne Schuchat, Principal Deputy Director at the Centers for Disease Control and Prevention. Then we have Dr. Anthony Fauci, Director of the National Institute of Allergy and Infectious Diseases at the National Institutes of Health. Finally, we have Rear Admiral Denise Hinton, Chief Scientist at the U.S. Food and Drug Administration.

We welcome all of you.

And you are each aware that the Committee is holding an investigative hearing and when doing so has had the practice of taking testimony under oath. Do you have any objection to testifying under oath?

Let the record reflect that all of the witnesses have reflected that they do not.

The chair then advises you that under the rules of the House and the rules of the committee, you're entitled to be accompanied by counsel. Do you desire to be accompanied by counsel during your testimony today?

Let the record reflect that each of the witnesses reflected that they do not.

In that case, if you would please rise and raise your right hand, I will swear you in.

[Witnesses sworn.]

Mr. HARPER. You are now under oath and subject to the penalties set forth in title 18, section 1001 of the United States Code. You may now give a 5-minute summary of your written statement.

And I will begin with you, Dr. Bright. Welcome back.

TESTIMONY OF RICK A. BRIGHT, PHD, DIRECTOR, BIOMEDICAL ADVANCED RESEARCH AND DEVELOPMENT AUTHORITY, DEPUTY ASSISTANT SECRETARY, OFFICE OF THE ASSISTANT SECRETARY FOR PREPAREDNESS AND RESPONSE, U.S. DEPARTMENT OF HEALTH AND HUMAN SERVICES; ANNE SCHUCHAT, MD (RADM, USPHS), PRINCIPAL DEPUTY DIRECTOR, CENTERS FOR DISEASE CONTROL AND PREVENTION, U.S. DEPARTMENT OF HEALTH AND HUMAN SERVICES; ANTHONY FAUCI, M.D., DIRECTOR, NATIONAL INSTITUTE OF ALLERGY AND INFECTIOUS DISEASES, NATIONAL INSTITUTES OF HEALTH; AND DENISE HINTON (RADM, USPHS), CHIEF SCIENTIST, U.S. FOOD AND DRUG ADMINISTRATION

Mr. BRIGHT. Thank you.

Chairman Harper, Ranking Member DeGette, and distinguished members of the subcommittee, it's a pleasure to speak today on behalf of our Assistant Secretary for Preparedness Response to discuss the state of the Nation's health security preparedness.

I'm Dr. Rick Bright, the Director of the Biomedical Advanced Research and Development Authority, BARDA, and the Deputy Assistant Secretary for Preparedness and Response.

ASPR's mission is to save lives and protect Americans from 21st century health security threats. BARDA is a component of ASPR created to ensure that we have products to protect people from numerous dire threats that we face as a nation. ASPR's staff is dedicated to preparing for and responding to these threats.

We are currently coordinating HHS' response to the Ebola outbreak in the DRC and monitoring H7N9 influenza in China. In communities affected by last year's hurricanes, we're there for the long haul, helping local health officials manage recovery and build resilience.

ASPR coordinates across the Federal Government to support State and local partners in emergencies. We enhance medical search capacity through our National Disaster Medical System and Hospital Preparedness Program, and we oversee the development and procurement of medical countermeasures. We've made great progress in public health preparedness response since Congress established ASPR and BARDA in 2006.

BARDA was created to bridge government and industry to accelerate the development of life-saving medical countermeasures that would not otherwise be available. We use flexible authorities, multiyear advanced funding, public-private partnerships, and deep technical expertise to push vaccines, drugs, and diagnostics towards FDA approval. In our 12 years, BARDA has formed over 200 public-private partnerships with industry to accomplish our mission.

I want to pause for one second to acknowledge the hard work of our partners who, together with the U.S. Government, work very hard to create a more secure nation with not only products but capabilities to respond when needed. These partnerships have led to 35 FDA approvals of products that form a protective shield for our nation against a range of the most serious CBRN and pandemic and emerging infectious disease threats.

Through Project BioShield, BARDA has supported 27 vaccines, drugs, and devices to address national security threats, including smallpox, anthrax, botulinum, rad/nuc and chemical exposure. Fourteen of these are now in the Strategic National Stockpile for use in an emergency, and seven have now achieved FDA approval. These outcomes are the spirit of PAHPA: leadership, coordination, partnerships, and capabilities, working together to protect our nation.

While this effort has created life-saving products to be procured by the SNS, it has also created challenges to acquire and sustain sufficient quantities to address the requirements needed for each threat. Critically, each product also represents a company with a response capability that must be sustained to ensure we have these products available when they're needed. Project BioShield and the SNS together represent a marketplace for these products that would otherwise never exist and the products would quickly vanish without it.

PAHPA, ASPR, BARDA, and BioShield have all played valuable roles in enhancing our preparedness. However, the threats continue to evolve, and technology to modify and create new deadly threats have become simpler. We must modernize our capabilities, emphasizing an end-to-end approach, ranging from early detection through the last mile of administering vaccines and treatments to patients.

With new technologies and innovation, the time is here to apply transformative approaches to these daunting health security problems. Last week, we announced a new initiative called DRIVe, a nationwide business-friendly approach to identify, capture, and accelerate life-saving innovation. Using authorities you enacted in the 21st Century Cures Act, DRIVe brings together innovators, government, and now the investment community to create solutions for today's threats.

As you consider reauthorization of PAHPA, important changes to BARDA's authorities would sustain and enhance our capabilities. First, advanced appropriations for Project BioShield will attract more partners to support our mission. Without this consistent and guaranteed market, the companies are reluctant to work with us. Second, an authorization of appropriation for BARDA's pandemic influenza program will sustain our domestic flu vaccine production capabilities, modernize our vaccine technologies, and bring new treatments and faster diagnostics into the homes across America.

I look forward to working with members of this panel, this subcommittee, your congressional colleagues, and I'm grateful for the opportunity to present to you today and look forward to your questions.

[The prepared statement of Mr. Bright follows:]

WRITTEN TESTIMONY, HOUSE COMMITTEE ON ENERGY AND COMMERCE, SUBCOMMITTEE ON OVERSIGHT AND INVESTIGATIONS, THE STATE OF U.S. PUBLIC BIOPREPAREDNESS: RESPONDING TO BIOLOGICAL ATTACKS, PANDEMICS, AND EMERGING INFECTIOUS DISEASE OUTBREAKS

Statement of Rick Bright, PhD
Director, Biomedical Advanced Research and Development Authority
Deputy Assistant Secretary for Preparedness and Response

Good morning Chairman Harper, Ranking Member DeGette, and other distinguished Members of the Subcommittee. I am Dr. Rick Bright, the Director of the Biomedical Advanced Research and Development Authority (BARDA) and the Deputy Assistant Secretary for Preparedness and Response (ASPR) at the Department of Health and Human Services (HHS). Thank you for the opportunity to testify before you today on behalf of ASPR to discuss the state of our nation's preparedness for 21st century health security threats, including biological incidents, as the Energy and Commerce Committee prepares to consider the second reauthorization of the Pandemic and All-Hazards Preparedness Act (PAHPA).

My expertise is in developing drugs, vaccines, diagnostics and other medical countermeasures (MCMs) for health security threats. In this testimony, I will cover a broader range of ASPR programs and activities, including some background on the nature of the health security threats facing the United States, the mission and duties of ASPR and BARDA, and our vision for where these areas can be strengthened.

Readiness for 21st Century Health Security Threats: A National Security Imperative

One of the federal government's fundamental responsibilities is to provide for the common defense - to protect the American people, our homeland, and our way of life. The strength of our nation's public health and medical infrastructure, and the capabilities necessary to quickly mobilize a coordinated national response to emergencies and disasters, are foundational for the quality of life of our citizens and vital to our national security. The health security threats facing the United States during the 21st century are increasingly complex and dangerous. Therefore, improving national readiness and response capabilities for 21st century health security threats is a national security imperative.

Additionally, we have witnessed the impacts of naturally occurring outbreaks such as pandemic influenza, outbreaks of Ebola and SARS, and the emergence of antibiotic resistant bacteria. ASPR is currently engaged in coordinating HHS's response to the Ebola outbreak in the Democratic Republic of Congo and monitoring other potential emerging infectious diseases that could cause a pandemic, such as the H7N9 influenza strain circulating in China. This year marks the 100-year anniversary of the 1918 influenza pandemic, which killed more people than World War I. During that pandemic, more than 25 percent of the U.S. population became sick and 675,000 Americans, many of them young, healthy adults, died from the highly virulent influenza virus. As our healthcare delivery systems become more networked, cyber-attacks like the 2017 WannaCry incident that affected approximately 150 countries remind us that technological advancements have trade-offs in the form of new vulnerabilities and risks. Finally, we face extreme weather events, such as the recent 2017 hurricane season in which Hurricanes Harvey, Irma, and Maria caused an unprecedented amount of damage and destruction, reminding us of the awesome destructive power of nature and our vulnerability.

These are threats that most people would rather not think about. However, when natural disasters, disease outbreaks, or attacks occur, the people expect our federal government to be ready to quickly respond to save lives and decrease morbidity. Since September 11, 2001, the nation has made great progress in building our response capabilities to protect America from health security threats; however, we still have much to do.

Assistant Secretary for Preparedness and Response: Mission & Duties

ASPR's mission is to save lives and protect Americans from 21st century health security threats. On behalf of the Secretary of HHS, ASPR leads public health and medical preparedness for, response to, and recovery from, disasters and public health emergencies, in accordance with the National Response Framework (NRF) (Emergency Support Function (ESF) No. 8, Public Health and Medical Services), as well as the National Disaster Recovery Framework (Health and Social Services Recovery Support Function). ASPR also supports HHS's role in the delivery of mass care and human services in emergencies (NRF ESF No. 6, Mass Care, Emergency Assistance, Temporary Housing, and Human Services).

When ASPR was established by Congress a decade ago in PAHPA, the law's objective was to create "unity of command" by consolidating Federal nonmilitary public health and medical preparedness and response functions under the ASPR. This approach was modeled on the Goldwater-Nichols Act that created the Department of Defense (DoD) combatant commands; the impetus was the disorganized and fragmented response to Hurricane Katrina in 2005.

ASPR coordinates across HHS and the Federal interagency to support state, local, territorial, and tribal health partners in preparing for, responding to, and recovering from, emergencies and disasters. In partnership with HHS agencies, ASPR works to enhance U.S. medical surge capacity by organizing, training, equipping, and deploying HHS public health and medical personnel, such as National Disaster Medical System (NDMS) teams, and providing logistical support for HHS personnel responding to public health emergencies. ASPR supports readiness at the state and local level by coordinating federal grants and cooperative agreements, such as the Hospital Preparedness Program (HPP), by programs like the Medical Reserve Corps (MRC), and carrying out drills and operational exercises. ASPR also oversees advanced research, development, and procurement of medical countermeasures (e.g., vaccines, medicines, diagnostics, and other necessary medical supplies), and coordinates the stockpiling of such countermeasures. As such, ASPR manages BARDA, Project BioShield, and the Public Health Emergency Medical Countermeasures Enterprise.

ASPR Priorities for Improving Preparedness, Response, and Recovery

HHS and ASPR have made significant progress since PAHPA was enacted in 2006 and was reauthorized in 2013. However, we still have work to do to ensure we are ready to save lives and protect Americans. ASPR has four key priorities for building the necessary readiness and response capabilities for 21st century health security threats:

First, provide strong leadership, including clear policy direction, improved health security threat awareness, and secure adequate resources.

Second, seek the creation of a "regional disaster health response system" by better leveraging and enhancing existing programs – such as HPP and NDMS – to create a more coherent, comprehensive, and capable regional medical emergency response system integrated into daily care delivery.

Third, advocate for the sustainment of robust and reliable public health security capabilities. For ASPR to accomplish its mission, the Centers for Disease Control and Prevention (CDC) and other partners need support to quickly detect and diagnose infectious diseases and other health security threats. This is critical to rapidly and effectively dispensing medical countermeasures in an emergency.

Fourth, advance an innovative medical countermeasures enterprise by capitalizing on new authorities provided in the 21st Century Cures Act and advances in biotechnology and science. We must develop and maintain a robust supply of safe and efficacious vaccines, medicines, equipment, and other materiel to respond to 21st century health security threats, as well as the flexible response capabilities needed to handle the unexpected.

Strong Leadership

In the area of strong leadership, ASPR should continually evaluate and incorporate national health security threats by regularly coordinating with the Director of National Intelligence, the Department of Justice, and the Department of Homeland Security to assess current and future national health security threats.

Medical Countermeasures Enterprise

Congress established BARDA to speed up the availability and use of medical countermeasures (MCMs) by bridging the so-called "valley of death" in late stage development where many countermeasures for health security threats historically languished or failed. By using flexible, nimble authorities, multiyear advanced funding, strong public-private partnerships, and cutting edge expertise, BARDA has successfully pushed innovative MCMs, such as vaccines, drugs, and diagnostics, through advanced development to stockpiling and commercial availability with FDA approval or licensure.

In the last decade, BARDA's strong partnerships with biotechnology and pharmaceutical companies, the National Institutes of Health, and other HHS components have led to 35 FDA approvals for 31 unique MCMs addressing chemical, biological, radiological, and nuclear (CBRN) threats, pandemic influenza, and emerging and re-emerging infectious diseases. This is a staggering accomplishment in just 12 years.

BARDA has supported the development of 27 medical countermeasures against Department of Homeland Security (DHS)-identified national security threats through Project BioShield, including products for smallpox, anthrax, botulinum, radiologic/nuclear emergencies, and chemical events. Fourteen of these products have been placed in the Strategic National Stockpile and are ready to be used in an emergency and seven have achieved FDA approval. BARDA also has supported the development of 23 influenza vaccines, antiviral drugs, devices, and diagnostics to address the risk of pandemic influenza.

Because of these successes and progress, more medical countermeasures than ever before are eligible to be procured for the Strategic National Stockpile, thereby creating new challenges in terms of acquiring and maintaining sufficient quantities of medical countermeasures to address the requirements for identified health security threats.

Just last week, we announced an exciting new public-private engagement model – called DRIVe – which is designed to accelerate innovation, address some of the nation's most pressing health security challenges, and potentially affect major healthcare markets.

At a time when synthetic biology and personalized medicine are not just conceivable but attainable, the time is right to apply an innovative approach to some of the most daunting, far-reaching health security problems, such as sepsis and early diagnosis of infectious diseases.

By implementing the authorities you provided to us in the 21st Century Cures Act, we are opening our doors to more innovators, and most importantly investors, to catalyze advances in science and technology.

ASPR has recommended important changes to BARDA's authorization of appropriations to meet these challenges, including, most notably, additional advanced appropriations for Project BioShield, which would help incentivize private industry to dedicate resources to developing medical countermeasures to meet the government's national security requirements. Without this "guaranteed market," companies are reluctant to incur the costs required to focus development on MCMs for CBRN agents that would rely upon a limited government market that may not materialize when product development is complete. ASPR has also recommended adding a direct funding line for BARDA's pandemic influenza preparedness activities. This authorization of appropriations will help sustain domestic influenza vaccine manufacturing capacity, as well as support better, faster influenza vaccine technologies and antivirals and rapid response platform technologies.

Regional Disaster Health Response System

The 2017 hurricane season highlighted the importance of regional healthcare readiness and medical surge capacity. ASPR led the public health and medical responses to Hurricanes Harvey, Irma, and Maria under the NRF Emergency Support Function No. 8 mission. ASPR worked closely with state and territory health officials in affected areas to augment care with NDMS teams, U.S. Public Health Service Commissioned Corps Officers, Department of Veterans Affairs personnel and facility support, and DoD transportation, facilities, naval vessels with medical and surgical capability, clinicians, and support personnel. Federal personnel under the supervision of HHS treated over 36,000 patients, and evacuated nearly 800 patients. HHS deployed over 4,500 personnel, awarded over 200 contracts, and provided nearly 950 tons of equipment. Today, HHS continues to support recovery efforts in impacted communities.

Despite our progress, each event teaches us that ASPR needs to improve its internal capabilities as well as enhance our support for the healthcare infrastructure across the country. As with MCM development, the nation's healthcare delivery infrastructure is mostly a private sector enterprise. We must better leverage and enhance existing federal programs – such as HPP and NDMS – to create a more coherent, comprehensive, and capable regional medical emergency response system integrated into daily care delivery. We call this the foundation of a "regional disaster health response system."

NDMS was created during the Cold War to take care of military casualties from overseas conflicts in U.S. civilian hospitals. To modernize NDMS, strengthen capabilities, and ensure NDMS continues to provide critical support during and immediately after national public health and medical emergencies and national security special events, ASPR is implementing administrative changes and has recommended improvements to the NDMS statute to aid in ASPR's efforts to modernize this critical asset.

The Hospital Preparedness Program (HPP) was established after the September 11, 2001 terrorist attacks, with the goal of improving the capacity of local hospitals across the country to deal with disasters and a large influx of patients in an emergency. Using HPP funding, state grantees initially purchased equipment and supplies needed for emergency medical surge capacity. Over time, the program successfully evolved to support local coordinated healthcare coalitions, including hospitals, public health facilities, emergency management agencies, and emergency medical services providers. Fifteen years after it was established, HPP can be further strengthened to better utilize existing resources and enhance healthcare preparedness and response capabilities at the local level, and ASPR has recommended modifications to the HPP statute toward this end.

Conclusion

As Congress moves forward on the second reauthorization of PAHPA, we have the opportunity to build on the great progress made and further improve our national readiness and response capabilities for 21st century health security threats. On behalf of the HHS Assistant Secretary for Preparedness and Response, Dr. Bob Kadlec, I want to thank you, again, for your bipartisan commitment to this national security imperative, and we look forward to continuing to work together to enhance our nation's health security. I am happy to answer any questions you may have.

Mr. HARPER. Thank you, Dr. Bright.

The chair will now recognize Dr. Anne Schuchat for 5 minutes.

Welcome.

TESTIMONY OF ANNE SCHUCHAT, MD

Dr. SCHUCHAT. Thank you.

Chairman Harper, Ranking Member DeGette, and members of the subcommittee, thank you so much for the opportunity to testify before you today to describe CDC's role in preparing, detecting, and responding to biological attacks, pandemics, and emerging infectious disease outbreaks.

Today I'll highlight CDC's role in protecting the Nation against health threats. I'll describe our role in three areas: preparedness, detection, and response.

The three themes I'd like you to take away are, first, the work CDC does every day in public health lays the foundation for responding to emergencies. Second, the CDC's world-class scientific and medical expertise ensures we're ready to respond to any threat. And third, our longstanding connection to State and local health departments ensures that public health systems function effectively, both day-to-day and during emergency response.

Let me first address how we prepare for emergencies. CDC works every day with State and local health departments. In fact, we have 590 staff assigned to State and local health departments. We fund the Public Health Emergency Preparedness Cooperative Agreement Program and the Cities Readiness Initiative.

Public Health Emergency Preparedness grants go to every State, eight territories, and four cities. These funds support staff, enable exercises to test and validate capabilities, and pay for laboratory and communications equipment.

The Cities Readiness Initiative funds this nation's 72 largest cities, to develop and test plans to receive and dispense medical countermeasures from the Strategic National Stockpile.

CDC expertise helps assure protection of vulnerable populations against diverse threats. For example, CDC worked with the American Academy of Pediatrics, the FDA, and other stakeholders to address gaps in existing countermeasures for anthrax in children, taking advantage of the agency's scientific and clinical expertise and longstanding relationships with AAP.

Turning now to detecting threats. The CDC's lab and surveillance systems are able to detect and identify agents causing illness, ranging from infectious agents to chemical or radiation exposures. Every year, labs from all over the world send specimens to CDC, because they know we'll be able to identify pathogens that other laboratories cannot.

Rapid identification of disease permits intervention before a health threat becomes a crisis. CDC's Laboratory Response Network maintains an integrated, scaleable, and flexible system of 125 Federal, State, and local laboratories. The development of this laboratory network established in 1999 has provided a larger capacity to test and report more quickly than was previously possible. For example, during the Zika virus outbreak response, CDC and our Laboratory Response laboratories processed over 207,000 specimens just for Zika.

Now I'll turn to response. When there's a crisis, CDC responds. We're able to rapidly deploy scientific and medical experts anywhere in the world. By the end of the 21-month

Ebola response, 3,700 CDC staff had shifted from their day-to-day duties to assist with the response. 1,500 of our staff deployed to West Africa, making over 2,000 trips. Today, we're responding to a much smaller Ebola outbreak in the Democratic Republic of Congo.

During health emergencies, CDC communicates. For example, during the 2009 H1N1 response, CDC held 39 full press conferences and 21 telebriefings. During the Zika response, CDC published 51 morbidity and mortality weekly report articles to make sure the public health and healthcare professionals had the latest and best information.

Being able to prepare, detect, and respond to public health threats is a top priority for us at CDC. Our preparedness and response capabilities are built on broad and deep scientific, medical, and program expertise. Our longstanding partnerships with State and local public health authorities ensures an integrated approach wherever that approach is needed, resulting in better responses and better public health outcomes, which translate to better protection of the people we serve.

Thank you, and I'll be happy to answer questions.

[The prepared statement of Dr. Schuchat follows:]

WRITTEN TESTIMONY, HOUSE ENERGY AND COMMERCE COMMITTEE, SUBCOMMITTEE ON OVERSIGHT AND INVESTIGATIONS: THE STATE OF U.S. PUBLIC HEALTH BIOPREPAREDNESS: RESPONDING TO BIOLOGICAL ATTACKS, PANDEMICS, AND EMERGING INFECTIOUS DISEASE OUTBREAKS

Statement of RADM Anne Schuchat, MD
Principal Deputy Director,
Centers for Disease Control and Prevention
Department of Health and Human Services

Chairman Harper, Ranking Member DeGette, and other members of the subcommittee. I am Rear Admiral Anne Schuchat, Principal Deputy Director of the Centers for Disease Control and Prevention (CDC). I appreciate the opportunity to be here today to discuss CDC's biopreparedness mission.

CDC is the eyes and ears of the biopreparedness complex, advancing the health security of the nation by helping communities prepare for, detect, and respond to, public health consequences of all hazards. These hazards include chemical, biological, radiological, and nuclear (CBRN) threats, natural disasters, and emerging (and re-emerging) infectious disease. For 72 years, this has been CDC's core mission.

CDC draws on expertise from across the agency, including world-class laboratory testing, public health surveillance (for disease detection), epidemiology, guidance to healthcare providers, incident management, logistics, emergency risk communication, disease control programs, distribution of medical countermeasures, human and animal medicine, and responder health and well-being. Our multidisciplinary workforce and integrated national and international systems broaden our capacity to detect and respond to any developing situation that could affect the health of people in the United States. This ability is enhanced by our long-standing relationships and close collaboration with federal, state, territorial, tribal, local, and global partners.

Prepare

The CDC's Public Health Emergency Preparedness Cooperative Agreement Program (PHEP) (which includes the Cities Readiness Initiative (CRI)) is central to CDC's programs to prepare communities across the nation for the next public health emergency. Additionally, CDC's role in the Public Health Emergency Medical Countermeasures Enterprise (PHEMCE) is critical to national preparedness for chemical, biological, radiological, nuclear threats, and emerging infectious diseases.

Public Health Emergency Preparedness Cooperative Agreement Program

The PHEP cooperative agreement program is the largest CDC state program and provided approximately $600 million to state, local and territorial public health departments in FY 2017. The program supports these jurisdictions to develop plans for public health preparedness and response, and has been instrumental in integrating state and local health departments into their jurisdictions' emergency response structures. PHEP currently supports 62 awardees – the 50 states, eight territories and freely associated states, and four directly funded cities (New York City; Washington, D.C.; Chicago; and Los Angeles). Funding is awarded according to a base-plus population formula prescribed by statute, which ensures a minimum amount of funding to each awardee. These funds support preparedness and response staff, enable exercises to test and validate capabilities, provide training, and pay for laboratory and communications equipment essential to maintaining preparedness. In addition, CDC personnel support PHEP awardees by helping to identify and address gaps in preparedness capabilities, providing planning resources to ensure the needs of vulnerable populations are incorporated into response strategies, and improving response capabilities from experience gleaned during public health responses.

Cities Readiness Initiative (CRI)

CRI, funded through the PHEP cooperative agreement, enhances preparedness in the nation's 72 largest population centers, where nearly 60% of the U.S. population resides. These cities use CRI funds to develop, test, and maintain, plans to quickly receive medical countermeasures (MCMs) from the Strategic National Stockpile (SNS) and distribute them to local communities. This program, which relies on local boots on the ground, enables effective response to large-scale public health emergencies that require life-saving medications and medical supplies.

Public Health Emergency Medical Countermeasures Enterprise (PHEMCE)

Through participation in the ASPR-led Public Health Emergency Medical Countermeasures Enterprise (PHEMCE), CDC works with other HHS agencies and other federal partners to enhance preparedness for chemical, biological, radiological and nuclear threats, and emerging infectious disease. CDC brings together its scientific expertise and its experience in public health practice to inform the use of preventative measures and treatment during a public health emergency. Specifically, CDC subject matter experts from various CDC centers:

- Develop clinical guidance on the use of PHEMCE medical countermeasures – crucial to ensure health departments and clinicians know the safest, most effective way to use medical countermeasures.
- Inform operational details for SNS deployment – this includes informing which products should be deployed first based on epidemiology and laboratory data and clinical guidance.
- Provide technical expertise to state and local partners for the development and execution of deployment and dispensing plans for PHEMCE medical countermeasures.
- Conduct regular operational readiness reviews and exercises with state and local partners to prepare them and build their capacity to receive and dispense PHEMCE medical countermeasures. (In FY 2017, CDC supported 12 full-scale and tabletop exercises, and trained 3,758 Federal, state, territorial, and local emergency responders representing 13 different jurisdictions, on how to receive and distribute products from the Strategic National Stockpile).
- Provide regulatory science expertise to inform legal mechanisms (Emergency Use Authorizations, Emergency Use Instructions, and Investigational New Drug Protocols) and guidance on the use of MCM that have not received FDA approval or the use of FDA approved MCMs for – indications other than those included in FDA approval.

Protecting Vulnerable Populations during Emergencies

CDC has expertise and programs to promote effective support and care prior to, during, and after a public health emergency, for a wide variety of vulnerable populations. CDC's PHEP program requires states to develop emergency plans covering children, pregnant women, and other vulnerable populations such, as those isolated due to geography and individuals with disabilities. Subject matter experts within CDC's Children's Preparedness Unit champion the needs of children in public health emergencies and have supported 10 responses over the past 10 years. CDC also provides guidance to state and local health departments for dosage and administration of certain MCMs to certain populations. The Children's Preparedness Unit has recently completed a draft implementation plan for the pediatric use of Anthrax Vaccine Adsorbed (AVA) in the case of a large-scale event. AVA is the only FDA-licensed human anthrax vaccine in the U.S., but it is not currently approved for use in children. This implementation plan provides critical activities to ensure that programs are prepared to, and have the resources for, the efficient and safe administration of the vaccine to children.

Federal Select Agent Program

The nearly 300 entities in the U.S. that engage in laboratory research on biological select agents and toxins are regulated under the Federal Select Agent Program (FSAP), which is jointly managed by CDC and the Animal and Plant Health Inspection Service (USDA) to regulate the possession, use, and transfer of biological pathogens and toxins (e.g., anthrax, bubonic plague, smallpox, and ricin) that have the potential to pose a severe threat to human, animal, and/or plant health. The program aims to ensure that work with these dangerous agents is conducted in as safe and secure manner as possible, and that they are stored and transported safely and securely.

Detect

World-class scientific expertise in disease progression, epidemiology, and laboratory methods ensures CDC is ready and able to detect and develop a response to a broad range of threats, including highly hazardous and infectious diseases like Ebola, smallpox, Zika, anthrax, and H7N9 influenza.

CDC uses advanced molecular detection techniques that combine next-generation genomic sequencing, high-performance computing, and epidemiology to identify pathogens faster and more accurately. Laboratories from all over the world send specimens to CDC because they know CDC will be able to identify pathogens that other laboratories cannot.

Through Advanced Molecular Detection investments, CDC is able to detect outbreaks faster, before they have become widespread. These advances are applied in dozens of areas such as foodborne disease, influenza, antimicrobial resistance, hepatitis, pneumonia, and meningitis. Moreover, CDC shares genetic sequencing capabilities with state and local health departments, and funds them to acquire these tools that help them respond more quickly and effectively at the local level, lessening the chances that disease outbreaks will spread.

CDC also maintains unique laboratory capability to rapidly detect exposure to radionuclides and more than 150 chemical threat agents. This information about human exposure helps public health officials rapidly assess health risk, determine the most effective treatment, and reduce additional exposures.

A Strong Laboratory Response Network

Rapid identification of disease is critical to addressing public health threats before they become a crisis. This requires that high quality specialized laboratory testing be available around the country. CDC's Laboratory Response Network is an integrated system of federal, state, and local laboratories that provides early detection and characterization of biological, chemical and other public health threats. The linking of laboratories and close partnership between laboratorians, epidemiologists and clinicians at CDC, state and local health departments, and healthcare facilities ensures the most rapid detection and mitigation of health threats.

For example, in response to the MERS (Middle East Respiratory Syndrome), Ebola and Zika virus outbreaks, CDC provided Laboratory Response Network laboratories across the United States with assays authorized for Emergency Use to quickly identify cases of infection during these outbreaks.

Another important laboratory network, begun in 2016, is CDC's Antibiotic Resistance Laboratory Network, which supports nationwide laboratory capacity to rapidly detect antibiotic resistance in healthcare, food, and community settings, and inform local responses to prevent the spread of antibiotic resistant bacteria, and protect people. The Antibiotic Resistance Laboratory Network includes seven regional laboratories, the National Tuberculosis Molecular Surveillance Center, and laboratories in 50 states, five cities, and Puerto Rico.

Public Health Surveillance

Public health surveillance—the collection, analysis, and use of data to target public health prevention and intervention activities—is the foundation of public health practice at CDC, and continues to represent CDC's core work, whether as detective work in the field, or advanced analysis to understand disease transmission. CDC uses electronic data systems to monitor population health information around the clock to detect and track diseases. For example, following 9/11, CDC invested in using health-related data based on syndromic surveillance in Emergency Departments as an early warning system for a bioterrorist attack. Those investments are paying dividends, as this information technology system now allows officials to detect a wide range of health threats beyond biological attacks, from opioid overdoses to chemical exposures to disease outbreaks.

To ensure a nationwide surveillance capability, CDC supports surveillance infrastructure, including information technology systems, and practice at the state and local levels through the National Notifiable Disease Surveillance System, the National Syndromic Surveillance Program, the National Healthcare Safety Network, the Emerging Infections Program Active Bacterial Core Surveillance, and components of national influenza surveillance.

Beginning in fiscal year 2016, Congress recognized the large and growing threat of antibiotic resistance and appropriated funding for CDC to detect and respond to resistant pathogens, prevent the spread of resistant infections, and collaborate with partners to encourage innovation with respect to new prevention strategies.

CDC has multiple surveillance systems that can detect and track resistant threats across healthcare, food, and community settings.

CDC's Global Disease Detection Operations Center monitors outbreaks 24/7, assesses their potential risk to the United States and communities around the world, and improves global public health surveillance. Since 2017, CDC has tracked more than 170 unique diseases globally and identified outbreaks in more than 190 countries. CDC works with the 17 Phase 1 and the 14 Phase 2 Global Health Security Agenda partner countries to help them build the core public health capacities necessary for identifying and containing outbreaks before they become epidemics that could affect us all. The 17 Phase 1 countries receive direct financial support and technical assistance from CDC; the 14 additional countries receive only technical assistance from CDC. Our work through the Global Health Security Agenda emphasizes four critical areas: surveillance, laboratory, workforce development, and rapid response capability. In addition, CDC medical and public health officers staff United States Quarantine Stations that are located at 20 United States ports of entry and land-border crossings where the majority of international travelers arrive. These health officers are an important defense to prevent the introduction into, and spread of infectious diseases in, the United States.

Respond

CDC's number one priority during any public health emergency is to protect the health of the public. CDC subject matter experts respond regularly to events such as foodborne outbreaks, natural occurring anthrax and botulism cases, smallpox vaccine adverse event cases, and seasonal influenza. CDC's readiness activities, expertise, and infrastructure provides the foundation for all types of public health emergency responses and is scalable and can surge to respond to events such as the 2013 meningitis outbreaks. The expertise and systems used in such responses can be augmented further for larger public health emergency responses such as the 2009 H1N1 response, 2014 Ebola response, and the Zika response.

State and local public health agencies are the front lines of public health preparedness and response. CDC provides ongoing technical assistance and, where requested, on-the-ground personnel and materials to assist with response efforts. CDC's established relationships with state and local health departments ensure that day-to-day public health systems function effectively and efficiently, and that emergency response actions are appropriate to the threat. These continuous relationships, between and during emergency responses, ensure a level of trust and collaboration that cannot be overemphasized. During the stress of an emergency response, having a trusted partner you can turn to immediately can mean the difference between life and death for patients, and ensures the rapid delivery of public health services, such as vaccinations and clean water, for communities.

CDC experts lead and staff every activation of the agency's Emergency Operations Center (EOC), ensuring response activities are effective and efficient. CDC has activated its incident management system for 67 responses over the last 16 years. During a response, in coordination with and, sometimes at the direction/request of the Office of the HHS Assistant Secretary for Preparedness and Response, CDC's EOC rapidly deploys scientific experts, coordinates the delivery of supplies and equipment to the incident site, monitors response activities, provides resources to state and local public health departments, and disseminates timely and accurate information within government, to health care providers and to the public. During the agency's Ebola and Zika responses, 3,700 and 1,700 CDC staff participated in the response, respectively. During the Ebola response, CDC staff completed over 2,000 field deployments to West Africa. CDC also responds to public health events that do not require EOC support. In fiscal year 2017, CDC assisted state, local, and overseas public health authorities in 38 epidemiologic investigations of emerging infectious disease outbreaks. In addition, the Global Rapid Response Team, stood up following the 2014 Ebola outbreaks, has over 400 ready and rostered experts.

Since its inception, that team has provided nearly 9,000 person-days of support for response activities.

We are committed to continuously improving our response capability. After each activation, whether for a real event or exercise, we conduct a thorough after-action review to identify strengths to sustain and areas for improvement. Use of this information is key to improving performance for the next incident or event.

Conclusion

I want to leave the Committee with three primary points about CDC's role in biopreparedness.

1) Our responses are built on our longstanding partnerships with state, local, and international public health authorities;
2) Our detection capabilities and surveillance programs are based on our broad and deep scientific, medical, and programmatic expertise; and
3) Our response capacity ensures timely aid to state and local public health systems in times of crisis.

CDC has 72 years of experience in bringing top scientific expertise to health emergencies and remains a trusted partner in the United States and around the world. CDC stands ready to do its part to protect the health and well-being of the American public and save lives. We cannot necessarily predict the next disaster, but we know that being prepared protects health, saves lives, and prevents economic losses.

Thank you for the opportunity to testify.

Mr. HARPER. Thank you, Dr. Schuchat.

The chair will now recognize Dr. Fauci for 5 minutes for your opening statement.

TESTIMONY OF ANTHONY FAUCI, MD

Dr. FAUCI. Thank you very much, Mr. Chairman.

Chairman Harper, Ranking Minority DeGette, members of the committee, thank you very much for giving me the opportunity today to present to you the role of the National Institute of Allergy and Infectious Diseases in addressing biodefense and emerging infectious diseases.

Our role in this really dates back many years, but was really solidified following the attacks of 9/11 with the anthrax attacks, which prompted us, together with our colleagues at HHS, to develop a strategic plan and a research agenda. For our role in that, as you know, the NIH for years, with regard to any emerging infectious disease, is involved in having a number of approaches, stemming from basic and clinical research, research resources for both industry and academic communities, with the ultimate goal of developing vaccines, therapeutics, and diagnostics.

We have been in a very strong partnership with BARDA in developing the concepts for interventions, which were then handed over to them for advanced development.

This slide just shows a representative example of some key achievements directed specifically at the category A agents that were in our strategic plan. Very briefly, for example, a better smallpox vaccine, next-generation vaccines for anthrax, antitoxins for botulism, antibiotics for plague, and, interestingly, the development of an Ebola vaccine, which long antedated the outbreak that we experienced in West Africa in 2014.

Having said that, it is important to point out, as we have in the past and as shown in this interesting article from Newsday of 2001, the worst bioterrorist may actually be nature itself.

It is interesting to point out, Mr. Chairman, that I have been testifying before this committee for the last 33 years. The first time I did, I drew a map, and it's shown here. And the reason I drew the map is I wanted to point out that there would be emerging and reemerging infectious diseases. And the first time I testified before this committee, I put HIV on the map as shown there.

Today, the map is the same structurally, but this is what it looks like. And these are the emerging and reemerging infectious diseases. Many of them, many of them are curiosities and are not really of great public health impact, but others are really important and we've experienced them recently, such as Ebola, Zika, and the threat of a pandemic influenza.

Now, let's take one of these, Ebola. You mentioned in your opening statement, as others have, about the West Africa outbreak and the recent outbreak in the Democratic Republic of the Congo. It's important that the CDC, the NIH, and other agencies of the Public Health Service responded very rapidly there.

One thing that was proven that's important is that you can do good research in the context of an outbreak. And we developed, with others, a vaccine, which is called the VSV vaccine, which was first tried in a Phase I trial right in Bethesda at the NIH Clinical Center, and then went over to Africa in a Phase II trial. This is the vaccine that was used in the ring vaccination program that was actually involved in the West Africa outbreak.

If you then fast forward a couple of years to where we are today, with the outbreak in the Democratic Republic of the Congo, we have actually learned a lot and are applying what we learned to that. Let me give you an example. The experimental vaccine that was used in the ring vaccination program has now been deployed to the Democratic Republic of Congo, and even as we speak today, it is being used in a ring vaccination with 50 rings and 150 vaccinations per ring.

Interestingly, and as I mentioned before we came, that in 1995, there was an outbreak in Kikwit in the Democratic Republic of the Congo. To just show you the connection between clinical care and research, we brought one of the survivors of Kikwit to Bethesda, took their B cells, cloned it, made a monoclonal antibody. And now the Democratic Republic of the Congo has asked us to ship that to them for their discretion use as a countermeasure in the epidemic. So it came full circle that our collaboration with them came back with something that perhaps could help them.

I want to close in the last couple of seconds with influenza. I wrote this article just a few months ago, talking about the need for a universal flu vaccine. And, in fact, we have developed a strategic plan and a research agenda because of the threat, not only of getting a better seasonal flu vaccine, but also a threat of a pandemic. And we could only do that with a vaccine that essentially is able to protect us against all subtypes of influenza.

And I'll close on this last slide—this is not working very well, sorry—which is an article that I actually wrote 17 years ago, but it's very relevant today. And what it says is that emerging infections are a perpetual challenge. We've always had them, we have them now, and we always will have them. So if they are a perpetual challenge and a perpetual risk, we must meet them with perpetual readiness and, hopefully, we'll be able to do that.

Thank you.

[The prepared statement of Dr. Fauci follows:]

Department of Health and Human Services National Institutes of Health, National Institute of Allergy and Infectious Diseases Research Addressing Biodefense and Emerging and Re-emerging Infectious Diseases, Testimony before the House Committee on Energy and Commerce, Subcommittee on Oversight and Investigations

Anthony S. Fauci, MD
Director of the National Institute of Allergy and Infectious Diseases
June 15, 2018

Mr. Chairman, Ranking Member DeGette, and members of the Subcommittee, thank you for the opportunity to discuss the research response of the National Institutes of Health (NIH) to potential attacks with chemical and radiological/nuclear agents as well as biological threats, including emerging and re-emerging infectious diseases. I direct the National Institute of Allergy and Infectious Diseases (NIAID), the lead NIH institute for biodefense research.

The NIH conducts and supports basic and clinical research to better understand the biological effects of, and to develop medical countermeasures (MCMs) for, chemical, biological, and radiological/nuclear threats. Most of this work is conducted by the NIAID at the NIH. NIAID supports basic research on microbiology and immunology as well as applied and clinical research to evaluate candidate MCMs including diagnostics, therapeutics, and vaccines. This strategic effort includes the pursuit of foundational platform approaches that could be used to develop MCMs against multiple threats or pathogens. These platforms include molecular biological technologies for vaccines, targeted antibody therapeutics, and broad-spectrum antibiotics and antivirals.

NIH coordinates its biodefense research with partners in industry, academia, and the Federal Public Health Emergency Medical Countermeasures Enterprise (PHEMCE) to ensure that promising countermeasures for biological, chemical, and radiological public health threats can proceed to advanced development. Since fiscal year 2012, NIH has supported the early development of more than 20 candidate MCMs for high-priority threats, and ultimately transitioned support for those candidate MCMs to the Biomedical Advanced Research and Development Authority (BARDA) for advanced development, with the goal of Food and Drug Administration (FDA) approval, licensure, clearance, or authorization, and for potential inclusion in the Strategic National Stockpile. NIH funding for emerging infectious disease, including biodefense, research was approximately $2.6 billion in FY 2017.

NIH Medical Countermeasure Development

Innovative technologies and approaches supported by NIH are enabling the development of new medical countermeasures (MCMs) at an unprecedented pace. High-throughput sequencing and platform-based technologies are facilitating the development and manufacture of MCM candidates to expedite their clinical evaluation. For example, during the Zika virus outbreak in the Americas, NIAID scientists used Zika virus genetic sequence information to develop a vaccine candidate that moved from concept to first-in-human trial in less than four months – likely the shortest development period ever for such a vaccine. The vaccine was developed with a readily deployable DNA vaccine platform that is a form of gene-based immunization previously employed by NIAID to develop a candidate vaccine for West Nile virus. These types of genetic platforms could be used to respond similarly to multiple emerging and re-emerging infectious disease threats.

Other broad-spectrum approaches are being used to advance the development of therapeutics that could be used against multiple pathogens. For example, NIAID has supported development of broad-spectrum antiviral agents such as BCX4430 (galidesivir), which has demonstrated activity against Ebola and other RNA viruses, and broad-spectrum antibacterial products, including a compound with activity against the two different bacteria that cause tularemia and plague.

NIAID continues to explore other inventive approaches to treat or prevent bioterrorism threats. Monoclonal antibodies, which precisely bind to a single target, have been used to treat certain cancers, infectious diseases, and autoimmune diseases. Monoclonal antibodies also have the potential to treat emerging and re-emerging infectious diseases, and as a first line intervention to prevent or slow the progress of infectious disease outbreaks as vaccines are being developed. A notable example is ZMappTM, a cocktail of three monoclonal antibodies targeting Ebola virus. ZMappTM showed promise as a treatment for Ebola virus disease in an NIAID-supported clinical trial during the 2014-2016 outbreak in West Africa. Another innovative approach specific to vaccine development is the use of adjuvants. Adjuvants are valuable tools that can boost immune responses to otherwise modestly effective vaccines, and potentially can expedite development of vaccines for emerging pandemic threats. NIAID supports programs for discovery and development of adjuvants that have led to 50 novel adjuvants and 18 vaccine clinical trials.

NIAID also has invested in critical infrastructure and research resources to encourage the development and testing of biodefense MCMs. NIAID supports research capacity at high-containment laboratories where dangerous pathogens can be studied safely. In addition, NIAID provides qualified scientists with research resources, including microorganisms, research reagents, and preclinical development services that can fill knowledge gaps. These programs lower the financial risk for potential commercial partners and expedite the development of MCMs.

These NIH-supported activities are advancing a robust pipeline of candidate MCMs needed to ensure the development of safe and effective products to protect the public health. Notable successes are outlined below.

Ebola

NIAID partnered with the government of Liberia to establish the Partnership for Research on Ebola Virus in Liberia (PREVAIL). This clinical research partnership enabled a series of clinical trials, including studies testing several Ebola virus therapeutic and vaccine candidates, among them ZMappTM and the cAd3-EBOZ vaccine developed by the NIAID Vaccine Research Center (VRC) in partnership with industry. Several Ebola countermeasure candidates developed by NIAID have transitioned to BARDA for advanced development, including a novel vaccine approach using two candidate vaccines in a prime-boost regimen.

NIAID currently is utilizing its expertise in Ebola research to respond to the ongoing Ebola outbreak in the Democratic Republic of the Congo (DRC). NIAID is providing technical assistance to the DRC-World Health Organization (WHO) effort to plan and implement a research response to the outbreak, including vaccine, therapeutics, and diagnostic research. NIAID also has developed as a therapeutic candidate mAb114, a monoclonal antibody active against Ebola. The antibody, which has shown promise in animal testing, was originally isolated from a survivor of the 1995 Ebola outbreak in Kikwit, DRC, through a research partnership between the NIAID VRC and the DRC's Institut National de Recherche Biomédicale. At the request of the Minister of Health of the DRC, NIAID is providing courses of mAb114 for treatment of Ebola Virus Disease, with specific research protocol design to be determined.

NIAID also has deployed a team to the National Public Health Laboratory in nearby Brazzaville, Republic of the Congo, to establish additional Ebola diagnostic and sequencing capacity in case the epidemic spreads to that country.

Nipah

NIAID conducts and supports research on countermeasures for Nipah, a deadly virus with case fatality rates of 40 to 75 percent. NIAID researchers have developed a candidate Nipah vaccine that was shown to protect against infection in a monkey model. NIAID-funded researchers, in collaboration with NIH scientists, discovered a potential monoclonal antibody treatment for Nipah virus. This treatment candidate, m102.4, effectively protected ferrets and non-human primates after exposure to Nipah virus. Based on this research, NIAID is assisting with the research response to the ongoing Nipah virus outbreak in India. At the request of the WHO, NIAID researchers have been working with scientists and clinicians from India to develop a clinical trial protocol to test the experimental monoclonal antibody m102.4 against Nipah virus. NIAID researchers also have evaluated an antiviral treatment for Nipah virus in collaboration with CDC and industry. This candidate, GS-5734, has been shown to protect against Nipah virus disease in monkeys.

Smallpox

NIAID supported the early-stage development of a novel smallpox vaccine, IMVAMUNE®, and a therapeutic, TPOXX® (tecovirimat), prior to their transition to BARDA for advanced development. IMVAMUNE® was shown to produce a superior immune response compared to the currently licensed smallpox vaccine. TPOXX® currently is under consideration for FDA approval pursuant to the Animal Rule, using pivotal animal model data supported by NIAID.

Anthrax

NIAID supported the preclinical and clinical development of the anthrax countermeasure ANTHIM® (obiltoxaximab), prior to its transition to BARDA for advanced development. ANTHIM® was approved by the FDA in 2016 for the treatment and prevention of inhalational anthrax, the deadliest form of the disease. NIAID also has supported the development of AV7909, a third-generation anthrax vaccine with a dry formulation that is easy to store and has increased shelf life. AV7909 has been transitioned to BARDA for further development.

Pneumonic Plague

NIAID supported critical animal model studies of ciprofloxacin and levofloxacin for FDA approval, pursuant to the Animal Rule, as treatments for pneumonic plague. In addition, NIAID scientists conduct foundational research on the bacteria that cause plague, and the fleas that transmit them, to understand plague biology and to aid in the design of new MCMs.

Pandemic Influenza

NIAID is partnering with BARDA to support the development of vaccine candidates for influenza strains with the potential to cause a pandemic, including H7N9 avian influenza. NIAID also is working to develop broadly protective, or "universal," influenza vaccines that could protect against multiple strains of seasonal and pandemic influenza. NIAID recently developed a Strategic Plan to guide research efforts focused on the design and development of universal influenza vaccines.

Radiological/Nuclear Threats

NIH investment in radiation/nuclear research revitalized physician training and infrastructure for studying radiation injury and developing effective medical countermeasures. Since 2005, NIAID has transitioned 29 radiation/nuclear countermeasure candidates to BARDA for advanced development. Recent successes include FDA approval of NEUPOGEN® (filgrastim) and Neulasta® (pegfilgrastim) to treat radiological or nuclear injuries. In addition, NIAID is funding animal studies of Nplate® (romiplostim) for acute radiation syndrome for consideration for FDA approval under the Animal Rule.

Chemical Threats

NIAID administers a trans-NIH chemical countermeasures program that supports research and development of therapeutics for people exposed to dangerous chemicals, including nerve agents such as Sarin and VX; metabolic poisons such as cyanide; chemicals affecting the skin, eyes, and mucous membranes such as sulfur mustard; chemicals affecting the respiratory tract such as chlorine; and toxic industrial chemicals. NIH recently transitioned several candidate therapeutics to BARDA for advanced development, including those for nerve agent poisoning (midazolam and galantamine), sulfur mustard exposure (tissue plasminogen activator), and inhalation chlorine exposure (R-107 and GSK2798745).

Conclusion

NIAID has moved strategically toward a MCM research paradigm that features broader, more flexible platform technologies. This effort is yielding significant scientific advances that help protect against multiple emerging public health threats, whether man-made or naturally occurring. Together with academia, industry, and PHEMCE partners, NIAID remains committed to meeting public health emergency needs by advancing high-priority research toward development of MCMs for radiological/nuclear, chemical, and biological threats, including emerging and re-emerging infectious diseases.

Mr. HARPER. Thank you very much.

We now have the privilege of hearing from Rear Admiral Denise Hinton.

Admiral Hinton, you are recognized for 5 minutes.

TESTIMONY OF REAR ADMIRAL DENISE HINTON

Admiral HINTON. Thank you.

Chairman Harper, Ranking Member DeGette, and members of the committee, thank you for the opportunity to appear today to discuss the state of biopreparedness.

Medical and public health preparedness and response is critically important to the health and security of our nation. And I am pleased to be here today to discuss how FDA is working towards the shared goal of making sure that we have the medical products necessary to protect our nation from a range of public health threats, whether naturally occurring, accidental, or deliberate.

The outbreak of Ebola virus disease in the Democratic Republic of the Congo serves as a reminder that biological threats can and often do emerge with little to no warning and can rapidly become global challenges. I can assure you that FDA is dedicated to helping end this outbreak as quickly as possible, as we are actively engaged in supporting international response efforts.

FDA plays a critical role in facilitating preparedness for and response to biological threats. Our role focuses largely on facilitating the development and availability of medical countermeasures, or MCMs, such as vaccines, therapeutics, and diagnostic tests to protect against and respond to these threats.

Toward that end, we work closely with our HHS partners testifying here with me today as well as other U.S. Government partners, product developers, and nongovernmental organizations to facilitate the development and availability of MCMs. FDA also works closely with the Department of Defense to facilitate the development and availability of MCMs to support the needs of our nation's military personnel.

Prior to joining FDA and the U.S. Public Health Service Commissioned Corps, I proudly served as an officer in the United States Air Force. So these efforts are near and dear to me, and we are fully committed to closely working with our colleagues at the DOD to support the unique needs of the U.S. military personnel.

At FDA, we have made it a priority to utilize our authorities to proactively work with our private sector and government partners to help facilitate the translation of discoveries in science and technology into safe and effective MCMs as part of advancing public health and strengthening our national security.

We share Congress' goal of having safe and effective MCMs available in the event that they are needed, and we have made significant progress toward this important goal. For example, since 2012, FDA has approved, licensed, or cleared more than 120 MCMs, including supplemental changes to already approved products and modifications to diagnostic devices for a diverse array of threats, including anthrax, botulinum toxin, plague, smallpox, and pandemic influenza.

We have also issued more than 60 emergency use authorizations since 2005 to enable access to products to respond to threats, including for Zika virus, Ebola virus, H7N9 influenza virus, and the Middle East Respiratory Syndrome Coronavirus.

While the close collaboration and coordination among the agencies represented here today has achieved many successes in the development of MCMs, I would emphasize that developing MCMs is highly complex and there remain regulatory science gaps that can challenge development programs, such as a lack of models and biomarkers to enable the extrapolation of data generated in animal models to humans. Without such tools, it is difficult to generate the data necessary to support regulatory decisionmaking.

Addressing these regulatory science gaps remains a high priority for the FDA, and we have established a broad and robust portfolio of cutting-edge research under our MCMs Initiative regulatory science program to develop these tools and to promote innovation in the development of MCMs.

FDA is acutely aware that biothreats can emerge from an accidental release or exposure to threat agents during the course of conducting research. As such, we are working to ensure that our laboratories and workplaces are operated in a safe and secure manner to protect employees, the surrounding communities, and the environment. As the FDA's chief scientist, I can assure you that the laboratory safety is a high priority for me and the agency.

FDA remains deeply committed to working closely with its partners and fully using the authorities Congress provides to help facilitate and accelerate the development and availability of safe and effective medical countermeasures. While we have made significant progress, we know that more work remains to be done. We look forward to partnering with Congress and stakeholders as we work together to further enhance biopreparedness.

Thank you for inviting me to testify today. I look forward to answering any questions you may have.

[The prepared statement of Admiral Hinton follows:]

TESTIMONY OF REAR ADMIRAL DENISE HINTON CHIEF SCIENTIST, FOOD AND DRUG ADMINISTRATION, DEPARTMENT OF HEALTH AND HUMAN SERVICES, BEFORE THE COMMITTEE ON ENERGY AND COMMERCE, SUBCOMMITTEE ON OVERSIGHT AND INVESTIGATIONS, UNITED STATES HOUSE OF REPRESENTATIVES, "THE STATE OF U.S. PUBLIC HEALTH, BIOPREPAREDNESS: RESPONDING TO BIOLOGICAL ATTACKS, PANDEMICS, AND EMERGING INFECTIOUS DISEASE OUTBREAKS," JUNE 15, 2018

Introduction

Chairman Harper, Ranking Member DeGette, and members of the committee, thank you for the opportunity to appear today to discuss the Food and Drug Administration's (FDA or the Agency) efforts to prepare our Nation to respond to biological threats, such as biological weapons and naturally-emerging infectious diseases, like pandemic influenza, Zika virus, and Ebola virus.

Biological threats—whether deliberate, naturally occurring, or accidental—can and often do emerge with little to no warning. This was the case with the anthrax attacks of 2001, the 2009 H1N1 influenza pandemic, the 2014 Ebola outbreak in West Africa, the emergence of Zika virus in 2016, and the recent Ebola outbreak in the Democratic Republic of Congo (DRC), to name just a few.

We are continually reminded that biological threats know no borders, and that biological threats can rapidly become global challenges. As such, we must remain vigilant and continue to work to optimize our preparedness and response capabilities.

FDA's Public Health Preparedness and Response Mission

FDA plays a critical role in facilitating preparedness for, and response to, biological threats (as well as chemical, radiological, and nuclear (CBRN) threats). FDA's role focuses largely on facilitating the development and availability of medical countermeasures—such as vaccines, therapeutics, and diagnostic tests—to protect against, and respond to, these threats.

FDA works closely with its HHS and other U.S. government partners through the Public Health Emergency Medical Countermeasures Enterprise (PHEMCE), as well as with regulated industry and non-governmental organizations (NGOs), to sustain and optimize the medical countermeasure framework necessary to effectively respond to public health emergencies. FDA also works closely with the Department of Defense

(DoD) to facilitate the development and availability of medical countermeasures to support the unique needs of our nation's military personnel.

FDA's operations within its medical countermeasures mission cover a broad range of activities vital to facilitating the development of, and access to, safe and effective medical countermeasures, including:

- Reviewing marketing applications for medical countermeasures and approving those that meet standards for safety and efficacy;
- Providing regulatory advice, guidance and technical assistance to sponsors developing medical countermeasures, as well as to U.S. government partners, international regulators, and international organizations such as the World Health Organization;
- Supporting efforts to establish and sustain an adequate supply of medical countermeasures, including averting supply disruptions when feasible and, in certain situations, allowing products to be used beyond their labeled expiration dates when supported by appropriate scientific evaluation;
- Enabling access to medical countermeasures that are not yet approved—when necessary— through an appropriate mechanism, including through FDA's Emergency Use Authorization (EUA) authority;
- Proactively identifying and resolving regulatory challenges associated with medical countermeasure development and ensuring that FDA regulations and policies adequately support timely medical countermeasure development and enable preparedness and response activities and capabilities;
- Fostering the professional development of FDA scientists to ensure that FDA personnel maintain the skills and abilities to support the medical countermeasure mission; and
- Supporting regulatory science to create the tools, standards, and approaches necessary to develop and assess the safety, efficacy, quality, and performance of medical countermeasures.

Fostering Medical Countermeasure Development and Availability

FDA's Medical Countermeasures Initiative (MCMi)—established in 2010—brought enhanced resources to FDA that enabled FDA to hire additional expert staff, and to become more deeply and thoroughly engaged in medical countermeasure activities. This program continues to be key to providing certainty regarding regulatory pathways for medical countermeasures, advancing medical countermeasure regulatory science to support regulatory decision-making, and advancing important policies and mechanisms to facilitate the timely development and availability of medical countermeasures.

At FDA, we fully appreciate that the development of medical countermeasures can present complex and unique challenges. FDA's increased engagement in medical countermeasure activities has helped to resolve many challenges associated with medical countermeasures development so that programs continue to move forward. For example, since 2012, FDA has approved, licensed, or cleared more than 120 medical countermeasures (including supplemental changes to already approved applications and modifications to diagnostic devices) for a diverse array of threats including anthrax, botulinum toxin, plague, smallpox and pandemic influenza. Thirteen of these medical countermeasures have been approved under the Animal Rule, which enables animal efficacy studies to substitute for efficacy trials in humans if the results can reasonably be extrapolated to the expected human use.[1] These approvals underscore the critical role the Animal Rule and animal studies can play in advancing medical countermeasures for some of the most challenging threats. And of note, through the use of regulatory science, FDA was able to approve inhalational anthrax therapeutics and a botulism antitoxin for use in children as well as adults, despite the fact that ethical concerns precluded studying pediatric patients in clinical trials.

In the area of pandemic influenza preparedness, FDA has approved several influenza diagnostic tests, which can help facilitate an effective response to an influenza pandemic by rapidly identifying infected persons and facilitating appropriate care. In addition, FDA has approved several seasonal influenza vaccines, helping increase and sustain pandemic influenza vaccine production capacity. These approvals include the first seasonal influenza vaccine produced using modern cell culture techniques licensed in the United States, and the first seasonal influenza vaccine made through recombinant deoxyribonucleic acid (DNA) technology. Both of these vaccines offer an alternative to the egg-based process and a potential for a faster manufacturing startup in the event of a pandemic. FDA also approved the first adjuvanted influenza vaccine for use in people 18 years of age and older who are at increased risk of exposure to the avian influenza H5N1 virus subtype contained in the vaccine. This vaccine is not for commercial distribution but will be part of the national stockpile in the event it is needed. Furthermore, FDA has continued to collaborate closely with the Biomedical Advanced Research and Development Authority (BARDA), the National Institute of Allergy and Infectious Diseases (NIAID), and the Centers for Disease Control and Prevention (CDC) on developing avian influenza H7N9 virus vaccine candidates.

---

[1] To date, a total of 13 medical countermeasures have been approved under the Animal Rule, including inhalational anthrax therapeutics, a botulism antitoxin, antibiotics for the treatment and prophylaxis of plague, and treatments for acute radiation syndrome, prophylaxis against the lethal effects of soman nerve agent poisoning, and treatment of known or suspected cyanide poisoning.

Additionally, FDA approved the first intravenous antiviral drug to treat acute, uncomplicated influenza infection in adults and expanded its indication to include treatment of children ages two years and older. FDA also expanded the indications for use of the influenza antiviral, oseltamivir, to treat children as young as two weeks of age.

FDA also continues to facilitate the development of products to address antimicrobial resistance, including antibacterial drugs to treat patients with antimicrobial resistant infections, vaccines that can help prevent the emergence and spread of antimicrobial resistance, and diagnostic tests that can help rapidly identify the appropriate treatment for infected individuals. For example, FDA has been implementing Title VIII (Generating Antibiotic Incentives Now (GAIN)) of the Food and Drug Administration Safety and Innovation Act (FDASIA) since it became law in July 2012. GAIN created incentives to help develop new antibacterial and antifungal drugs intended to treat serious or life-threatening infections. Those meeting requisite criteria are determined to be qualified infectious disease products (QIDPs).[2] FDA has granted 147 QIDP designations through the end of FY 2017—approximately 74 of which were for novel drugs. Since the enactment of GAIN, 12 QIDPs have been approved.

With respect to supporting the development of diagnostic tests for antimicrobial resistant threats, FDA and CDC have collaborated to develop the AR Isolate Bank, a centralized repository of microbial pathogens with well-characterized resistance profiles. The AR Isolate Bank, which currently contains three bacterial isolate panels of pathogens of national medical concern (representing more than 160 total pathogens), provides a valuable resource to biotech and diagnostic groups in researching, designing, validating and evaluating next generation clinical tests. These tests in turn may support earlier diagnosis and development of more effective treatment options that can slow antibiotic resistance. As of January 2018, the AR Isolate Bank shipped more than 2,000 isolate panels.

There are still regulatory science gaps that can challenge development programs, however, such as a lack of animal models to support medical countermeasure development or insufficient biomarkers to enable the extrapolation of data generated in animal models to humans. Without such tools, it is difficult to generate the data necessary to support regulatory decision making. Given the urgency inherent in our medical countermeasure work, addressing these regulatory science gaps remains a high priority for the Agency.

To that end, FDA has established a broad and robust portfolio of cutting-edge research under the MCMi Regulatory Science Program to help develop these tools and promote innovation in the development of medical countermeasures. A few examples of projects include: supporting the development of "organ-on-a chip" models to assess

[2] A QIDP is defined as an antibacterial or antifungal drug for human use intended to treat serious or life-threatening infections, including those caused by an antibacterial or antifungal resistant pathogen, including novel or emerging infectious pathogens.

radiation damage in lung, gut, and bone marrow, and then using these models to test candidate medical countermeasures; collaborating to establish a publicly-available genomic sequence reference database for use by developers seeking to validate candidate multiplex *in vitro* diagnostic tests that could be used to diagnose multiple pathogens simultaneously (FDA-ARGOS); developing reference materials for developers to use to validate nucleic acid-based and serological diagnostic tests for Zika virus; supporting a project to identify and correlate biomarkers of host response to Ebola virus infection in animal models and humans to support medical countermeasure development; developing methods for obtaining safety and limited efficacy data from patients who receive medical countermeasures during public health emergencies; and establishing the Animal Model Qualification Program designed to support medical countermeasure development by promoting the development of animal models for use across multiple product applications, thereby minimizing duplication of effort and resources.

FDA is acutely aware that biothreats can also emerge from accidental release or exposure to threat agents during the course of conducting research. As such, the Agency works to ensure that its laboratories and workplaces are operated in a safe and secure manner to protect employees, the surrounding communities, and the environment. This includes ensuring that FDA is in compliance with the Select Agent Regulations as well as with Federal, state, and local occupational safety and health requirements (as appropriate), and environmental regulations.

FDA also works to establish and sustain an adequate supply of medical countermeasures. For example, FDA supports the Shelf Life Extension Program (SLEP), a Federal fee-for-service program, for extending the useful shelf life of military-significant and contingency-use medical products, including medical countermeasures that are owned by components of DoD or other Federal program participants, such as the Strategic National Stockpile (SNS).[3] FDA laboratory personnel test and evaluate drugs submitted for shelf-life extension to ensure stability and quality before a shelf-life extension is approved.

In addition, FDA works to ensure that the U.S. Government is as prepared as possible to rapidly deploy medical countermeasures when necessary. For example, FDA has worked with government partners to prepare for potential EUA authorization of stockpiled medical countermeasures against a diverse array of threats including smallpox, anthrax, and pandemic influenza.[4]

---

[3] SLEP is designed to defer drug replacement costs for date-sensitive stockpiles of drugs by extending their useful shelf life beyond the manufacturer's original expiration date.

[4] To facilitate the issuance of EUAs, FDA has developed a pre-EUA submission process. FDA works with product sponsors or government agencies, such as CDC and DoD, to develop pre-EUA packages that will form the basis of an EUA request and decision, when circumstances justify. Pre-EUA packages contain data and information about the safety and efficacy of the product, its intended use under an EUA, and information about the potential emergency situation that might unfold.

There are tremendous opportunities to continue to further the development of groundbreaking, innovative medical countermeasures, and the Agency intends to fully seize, and build upon, these opportunities.

Responding to Threats

When threats emerge, FDA works proactively with U.S. government partners, medical product developers, and, as necessary, international partners (including the World Health Organization (WHO) and international regulatory counterparts) to respond. Key FDA response activities include accelerating the development of investigational medical countermeasures, when needed, by working with U.S. government agencies that support medical countermeasure development and medical product sponsors to clarify regulatory and data requirements. For example, FDA continues to work closely with U.S. government agencies, the international community, and product developers—providing regulatory advice, guidance, and technical assistance—to advance the development and availability of medical products, including vaccines and therapies, to address Ebola virus and Zika virus. These activities are essential not only for advancing the development of investigational medical countermeasures to respond to ongoing outbreak and epidemics, but also to improve response to future outbreaks and epidemics. For example, FDA worked closely with NIH in response to the 2014 Ebola epidemic in West Africa to design an innovative and robust common clinical trial protocol to evaluate the most promising investigational products for Ebola. The experience and information gained from those efforts have been instrumental in supporting a rapid response to the recent Ebola outbreak in the DRC.

FDA also works to protect the safety of the nation's blood supply and human cells, tissues, and cellular/tissue-based products for transplantation when threats emerge. For example, FDA worked closely with developers to make rapidly available two investigational tests for blood screening for Zika virus. One of those tests has since been approved.

Another key FDA response activity to emerging threats is to enable access to investigational medical countermeasures, when necessary, through an appropriate mechanism such as under an investigational new drug (IND) application, an Emergency Use Authorization (EUA), or under expanded access mechanisms when the clinical circumstances warrant. Enabling access to available medical countermeasures in response to emerging threats is a high priority for FDA and FDA uses its authorities to the fullest to help protect public health. For example, since 2013, FDA has issued nearly 40 EUAs to enable the emergency use of in-vitro diagnostic devices for H7N9 Influenza virus, Enterovirus D68 (EV-D68), Middle East Respiratory Syndrome Coronavirus (MERS-CoV), Ebola virus, and Zika virus.

FDA also works to protect consumers against fraudulent products claiming to prevent, treat or cure conditions associated with emerging threats.

Throughout these response activities, FDA works to establish and maintain good lines of communication with WHO and regulatory authorities in affected countries, as necessary, to enable technical and information exchange, and to make sure that the needs of the affected countries are understood and addressed.

Conclusion

At FDA, we have made it a priority to proactively work with our private sector and government partners to help facilitate the translation of discoveries in science and technology into safe and effective medical countermeasures. FDA takes seriously its responsibility to help drive and foster innovation as part of advancing public health and strengthening our national security.

Active FDA involvement is essential to encouraging industry engagement in medical countermeasure development. Working closely with its partners and exercising the authorities Congress provides to the fullest extent, FDA remains deeply committed to protecting and promoting public health, both domestically and abroad, in response to public health threats.

FDA appreciates Congress's support in continually optimizing its authorities, and providing resources, to enable FDA to achieve its public health emergency preparedness and response mission. FDA stands ready to work with Congress and stakeholders to enable us to better achieve this critical work in our mission to protect the American people.

Thank you for inviting me to testify today. I look forward to answering any questions you may have.

Mr. HARPER. Thank you very much.

I ask unanimous consent that the contents of the document binder be introduced into the record and to authorize staff to make any appropriate redactions. Without objection, the documents will be entered into the record with any redactions that staff determines are appropriate.

It is now time for members to have the opportunity to ask you questions, and I will recognize myself for 5 minutes.

Let me begin by saying that in my 10 years of service in Congress, I don't know if I've ever been at a committee hearing with a better lineup of witnesses. And so thank you all for being here. We look forward to your responses today.

And this is a question that will go rather quickly for all of you. And for each witness, which biological threat is of greatest concern to you and why? Let's start with Dr. Bright and then go down.

Mr. BRIGHT. That's a difficult question. As Dr. Fauci has laid out, there are so many threats. They're constantly emerging. And I wish I could take some of them off the table, but they keep coming at us. And even more concerning is technology advancing so much that they can change the biological threats that we know today into something different that we may not be prepared for.

I think our greatest threat for any of those is our response capabilities and being able to respond to anything that comes our way.

Mr. HARPER. Dr. Schuchat, is there one biological threat that is at the top of your list? I know they're all important, but is there one that gives you the greatest concern?

Dr. SCHUCHAT. I think influenza needs to be at the top of my list. It can affect everyone rapidly and is constantly changing. And with pandemics, all of the population of the world can be susceptible. So the threat of a pandemic has to be at the top of the list, because it can all happen fast.

Mr. HARPER. Dr. Fauci.

Dr. FAUCI. My number one and maybe number two and number three is influenza also. I agree, for the reasons that Dr. Schuchat has mentioned.

When you have a respiratory virus that can be spread by droplets and aerosol, and then you have the situation if there's a degree of morbidity associated with that, you can have a catastrophe. We've experienced in real world those types of things. The one that we always talk about is the 1918 pandemic which killed between 50 and 100 million people.

It is likely that it would be an influenza, but if not influenza, an influenza-like respiratory virus. We had a scare with SARS. Fortunately, public health measures were able to contain it, but influenza first or something like influenza is the one that keeps me up at night.

Mr. HARPER. Admiral Hinton.

Admiral HINTON. Thank you for the question. I would say the threat that would keep me up at night would be the unknown. If we don't know what that threat may be, we have to be able to anticipate. So with the emerging spectrum of diseases, it would be the unknown that would keep me up at night.

Mr. HARPER. Thank you.

For each witness, what area of biopreparedness is of the highest priority and why? Dr. Bright.

Mr. BRIGHT. The area of biopreparedness of the highest priority would be the ability to rapidly detect something that has entered our community or has been used as a weapon. The sooner we detect something, the sooner we can turn on the machinery and call in the capabilities to begin making vaccines and drugs.

Mr. HARPER. Dr. Schuchat.

Dr. SCHUCHAT. I would say our global health security would be at the top of my list, because, as you know, a threat anywhere is a threat everywhere. And I think our greatest vulnerabilities are in the weakest countries of the world.

We saw in Ebola how rapidly West African countries were overwhelmed, and that was an issue for us as well. So I think being able to strengthen the ability of every country to be able to prevent, detect, and respond to threats is where I'd place my focus.

Mr. HARPER. Dr. Fauci.

Dr. FAUCI. I would agree with those two. But let me add an additional one that may not necessarily be my first, is in our ability to respond, for example, with a vaccine, the modern day 21st century technologies of platform technology, where you don't have to wait 6 to 7 months to get a vaccine, where you can really get it out there within a period of a couple of months, which is doable if we put our mind and our resources to it.

Mr. HARPER. Thank you.

Admiral Hinton.

Admiral HINTON. Our continued efforts in the Ebola, and then making sure that we contain it within the specific regions and not letting it cross the borders.

Mr. HARPER. Thank you.

Dr. Bright, if I could ask you, obviously, the need to rapidly respond to a biological threat is essential. Does the public health system have the capability to deliver and administer medical countermeasures rapidly and effectively in a timely manner as you sit there today?

Mr. BRIGHT. As we sit here today, we are much better and can respond much more quickly than we were in the past 10 years. We've built a national response capability and an international capability incorporating new sciences and technologies. There is a lot of room for improvement. It still takes too long to respond to respond adequately to protect everyone in our nation.

Mr. HARPER. Thank you very much.

I will now recognize the ranking member, Ms. DeGette, for 5 minutes for her questions.

Ms. DEGETTE. Thank you very much.

Well, building on the question by the chairman just now, Dr. Bright, what changes do we need to make to make the system for developing countermeasures work more effectively and efficiently? ASPR has been a good start, but, you know, where do we need to go?

Mr. BRIGHT. Well, given the 12 years' experience with ASPR and the enterprise, working across government and working with our public-private partnerships, we've learned a lot in the past 12 years. Not everything is working as effectively or efficiently—

Ms. DEGETTE. So what do we need to do?

Mr. BRIGHT. We need to improve our communications and our transparency and how we bridge our different agencies and bridge government with industry. We need to ensure there's consistency in funding and availability so the partners that we work with can better align their business models with our government models as well. And we need to improve the efficiency at which we communicate and respond to proposals and other contractual mechanisms that we use to work with our industry partners.

Ms. DEGETTE. Are efforts underway being made to do all of those things?

Mr. BRIGHT. Yes, efforts are underway.

Ms. DEGETTE. And is there something Congress can do to help you?

Mr. BRIGHT. Congress has been very generous with the authorities to date. There are things that we can do to improve our language in our other transactional authorities to be able to work more fluidly and flexibly with our industry partners, and we would be happy to submit language to assist in that.

Ms. DEGETTE. We would be delighted to have that language. That would really help.

Dr. Fauci, none of these hearings can go without me asking you about what's going on with pandemic flu. And you had said that we are getting closer to being able to develop a universal vaccine. And you've said that before, because you've been trying to do it for a long time.

What does your timeframe look like now and what are the barriers?

Dr. FAUCI. Congresswoman DeGette, the timeframe really varies about the level that you're talking about. There's not going to be one home run universal flu vaccine. There will be various iterations.

So I would say the timeframe. And I know every time when asked about a timeframe, people back off, and I don't want to get in court to be able to say something that's not going to be able to deliver. But since we spoke last, we have put into a Phase 2 trial a universal flu vaccine with a company called BiondVax, which is a multiple peptide prime followed by a killed vaccine boost.

Being in a Phase 2 trial means that you're another step closer to getting a product that you'll be able to use.

Ms. DEGETTE. Right.

Dr. FAUCI. So I would think that if you——

Ms. DEGETTE. How long is this trial going on for?

Dr. FAUCI. The trial will probably take—it's a Phase 2 trial, so that probably is going to take at least a year to determine if this induces the kind of response that you would predict would have some broad protection.

The first iteration of a universal flu vaccine is not going to be against all flu, absolutely. What we're hoping for is that the first iteration will cover, for example, all of a particular type, like all of the H3N2s. If we get that successful, then maybe all of the H1N1s.

There are two major groups of influenzas. The ultimate perfect one would be one that covers all of them. I think that's years and years and years away, but the first iteration may be 5 or so years away.

Ms. DEGETTE. And I'll ask you the same question I asked Dr. Bright. What can Congress do to help you?

Dr. FAUCI. I think Congress has been extraordinary in their positive effect on us in helping us. For example, in the 2018 omnibus, we were given an additional $40 million to develop a universal flu vaccine, and we're getting additional money in the proposal of the House for our 2019 budget. So you've been very supportive and we really appreciate it.

Ms. DEGETTE. We think it's a high priority. I think I can speak for everybody in this room.

One more question. You're developing lots of different vaccines: smallpox, flu, anthrax, Ebola. How do you prioritize your efforts to target the pathogens and toxins that provide the greatest risk?

Dr. FAUCI. That's a very good question. We do two things, Congressman. We target specific pathogens based on the threat. If you're talking about a bioterror threat, it's the intelligence that we get. And if you're talking about the possibility of an emerging infection, it's very difficult to guess what's going to come out.

Ms. DEGETTE. Right.

Dr. FAUCI. So we know, and it was mentioned in one of the opening statements, that H7N9, for example, if you look at the CDC chart, it's way up there as a threat. So we clearly made an investment of a considerable amount of money to develop a vaccine for that.

But as I mentioned in answer to one of the other questions, it's to develop platform technologies that's applicable to any disease, as opposed to picking out all the diseases and preemptively making a vaccine. In other words, making a kind of a vaccine that you could easily apply to whatever is the outbreak.

Ms. DEGETTE. Thank you. Thank you, Mr. Chairman.

Mr. HARPER. The gentlewoman yields back.

The chair will now recognize Dr. Burgess for 5 minutes.

Mr. BURGESS. Thank you, Mr. Chairman, and thanks to our panel for being here today.

Dr. Fauci, I wasn't going to do it, but you brought it up. And you said sometimes you'll give a timeframe, and then if it doesn't work out, then people will point that out to you. A couple of years ago, I think you gave us an 18-month figure on a Zika virus vaccine. How close are we today?

Dr. FAUCI. Thank you for that question. So when you're proving that a vaccine works or not, in the classical way, you have to get what's called an efficacy signal. There has to be infections in the community to get an efficacy signal.

Right now, thankfully for the countries involved, the Zika infections have plummeted almost to very, very few. However, the Phase IIb trial that I spoke to you about some months ago is still ongoing, and it's accruing volunteers in the study. So there's an interesting possibility here.

Let's say there are not enough Zika cases to be able to get an efficacy signal. We have been in discussions, with a lot of help from the FDA, about the possibility that if we get a considerable amount, and I say thousands of volunteers with safety data, immunogenicity data, namely inducing the kind of response that you would predict would be protective, and you bridge it to the animal studies, there's a possibility that they would at least consider that there would be an accelerated approval. You never can guarantee anything, but that's at least on the table.

So my short answer to your question, Congressman Burgess, is that we are on the road to getting a Zika vaccine, and I feel pretty confident about that.

Mr. BURGESS. And from the FDA's perspective, that expedited approval that was talked about, is that something we can look for?

Dr. FAUCI. Well, I'll let the FDA speak for themselves, but you never want to anticipate what they're going to do. You can just give them the data and the information that they ask for, but——

Mr. BURGESS. I may submit that in writing, because I do want to ask you about another—on the golly gee whiz slide that you put up with all of the things that can happen to us, enterovirus D68 was included on that list.

Dr. FAUCI. Yes.

Mr. BURGESS. And CDC has put out a paper on acute flaccid myelitis and the incidence of that. And I recognize that it's low, but it does seem to peak every other August. So as we are coming up on one of those every other Augusts, do we know any more about this illness and why it has had the effect that it has?

Dr. SCHUCHAT. Yes. The outbreak of severe respiratory disease in children from the enterovirus D68 a few years ago was of concern. It was contemporary with the outbreak of acute flaccid myelitis. Very difficult to confirm that one caused the other, but there's a good probability that they did.

The family of enteroviruses are known to be able to cause neuropathic problems. And when you have a very common set of infections, it could be that that was a real rare end of the spectrum among the common ones.

So I think we do need to be ready for that. Unfortunately, there are so many different enteroviruses that it's very difficult to pick one that you would necessarily focus on for countermeasure development. There's some work on antivirals that might be promising as having a broader protection, but that's the state of it right now.

Mr. BURGESS. As you'll recall, fairly frightening when that did occur, the concern we heard from parents.

Dr. SCHUCHAT. Exactly. It was happening the same time as Ebola in Africa. When the President visited CDC, he was briefed on Ebola and on enterovirus D68.

Mr. BURGESS. Admiral Hinton, let me ask you. When Ebola was really a much more significant problem, September of 2014, the monoclonal antibody ZMapp was in trials, and then FDA put a clinical hold on it. My understanding at the time, there was a Herxheimer-type reaction that was fairly severe and so we stopped looking at it.

Is there a way—when we've got a problem of that order of magnitude going on, I guess I want some reassurance that the regulatory side is not going to interfere with the delivery of what may be a very potent tool, because several people have mentioned ZMapp. I mean, it's now a recognized tool in the toolbox. Is that correct?

Admiral HINTON. That's correct. And Dr. Fauci can please feel free to add in, but that is correct. And the FDA is not there to be a roadblock; it's to ensure that the drugs are safe and efficacious. So the reasons behind that may not be privy to us, but we do make sure that we have safe and effective available drugs on the market to treat these and in emergency situations as well.

Dr. Fauci.

Dr. FAUCI. So ZMapp was part of a randomized controlled trial that was run by the NIH. It was published in The New England Journal of Medicine. The results, because of the diminution of cases at the time, were very strongly suggestive of efficacy, but not enough to be statistically significant. So the trial is technically still on. And right now, in DRC, they could use ZMapp either on a trial or, if they want, as compassionate use. But it is available.

Mr. BURGESS. It is available. Thank you all very much. Thanks for your testimony this morning.

Mr. HARPER. The gentleman yields back, who also serves as the chair of our Health Subcommittee.

Mr. BURGESS. Mr. Chairman, I'm also going to ask unanimous consent to place into the record the report of the Independent Panel of the United States Department of Health and Human Services to the Ebola response from 2015.

Mr. HARPER. Without objection, so entered.

[The information has been retained in committee files and can be found at https://docs.house.gov/meetings/IF/IF02/20180615/108422/ HHRG-115-IF02-20180615-SD003.pdf.]

Mr. HARPER. The chair now recognizes the gentlewoman from Illinois, Ms. Schakowsky, for 5 minutes.

Ms. SCHAKOWSKY. Thank you, Mr. Chairman. I want to agree with you, Mr. Chairman, that this is an extraordinary panel.

Dr. Fauci, 33 years before this committee, that's a long time, and we appreciate you every time we see you.

I also want Dr.—I looked this up. Dr. Schuchat, it looks like you're about 28 years. Is it more than that? How many?

Dr. SCHUCHAT. It's 30 in July.

Ms. SCHAKOWSKY. OK, 30 in July. And such experience in all of you. It's just really remarkable. I thank all of you for being here today.

I'm particularly concerned about the improper and overuse of antibiotics that's driving the growth of antibiotic resistance around the world. I noticed, Dr. Fauci, in your new map with all the lines, right at the top was antibiotic resistance on the left there.

I feel an obligation to raise this issue too for my sister and colleague, the late Louise Slaughter, who was always raising this issue. In the United States, somewhere between 20 and 50 percent of all antibiotic prescriptions in hospitals are either unnecessary or inappropriate. Evidence suggests that antibiotic stewardship programs in hospitals can improve prescribing practices and help reduce the occurrence of antibiotic resistance.

So I'm interested in hearing more from our witnesses on this program. Whoever wants to go first. Dr. Schuchat.

Dr. SCHUCHAT. Yes. The problem with antimicrobial resistance is a transformational challenge for us because it obviously threatens modern medicine. CDC has been investing in efforts to improve stewardship of antibiotics, and at this point, by our latest data, two out of three hospitals had an antibiotic stewardship program, which is a big increase from before. But we think that there's much more to be done.

In addition, we have 850 hospitals around the country are reporting on their antibiotic use data to the National Healthcare Safety Network. So we're tracking data.

What we find in the healthcare system is when you track antibiotic use and feed back to clinicians how they're doing, they can improve. A lot of clinicians are test takers, and we like to do really well on those tests. And so learning that we're not doing as well as our peers in terms of the appropriateness of our prescribing can help improve that.

We're also tracking resistance. And we've really invested, thanks to the congressional support, we've been able to invest in much better timely, accurate, quality antimicrobial resistance detection around the Nation. It's where we got those nightmare bacteria reports that we came out with recently.

So I would say that behavior change in clinicians is difficult, but we're making progress. And a stewardship program in every hospital is a good start, but it takes more than the hospital to make that happen. We need the whole plans, the outpatient prescribers as well, to be part of the system.

Ms. SCHAKOWSKY. But you're saying that we do have a tracking system now for clinicians, for hospitals?

Dr. SCHUCHAT. Right. In our National Healthcare Safety Network, I'm told that 850 hospitals are already reporting to us on their antibiotic use. It includes 80 VA hospitals and 30 military hospitals. And they're having that be part of their—it's voluntary, but it's part of their ability to monitor what's going on in their own institution and then look across institutions.

Ms. SCHAKOWSKY. What percentage of hospitals does that represent, do you know?

Dr. SCHUCHAT. I don't actually have that information, but we could get that for you.

Ms. SCHAKOWSKY. OK. Has the CDC identified any obstacles to successfully implementing stewardship programs? If so, how are you addressing those?

Dr. SCHUCHAT. I would say that incorporating the outpatient facilities in the stewardship is important. We also found that rural areas, critical areas, we're challenged in being able to do all the things that we recommend in terms of antibiotic stewardship.

Our program convened a batch of the rural or critical area hospital stewardship leads, who had figured out ways to make a difference, and we're working with them to share their best practices more broadly. So I would say that large hospitals are really on the case now, and helping the smaller facilities get up to speed is important.

Ms. SCHAKOWSKY. Thank you. In the remaining seconds, does anybody else——

Dr. FAUCI. Yes. How we address antibiotic resistance is really governmentwide, and it's a program called CARB, Combating Antibiotic-Resistant Bacteria, that was established years ago, a few years ago, that involves what Dr. Schuchat had mentioned regarding the CDC. It involves the FDA research component from the NIH to develop new drugs to understand the mechanisms of resistance to harness the immune system, but also an organization called CARB-X, which BARDA has a major role in.

So maybe, Rick, you want to just mention that briefly.

Mr. BRIGHT. Very briefly. So since 2010, BARDA has invested over a billion dollars in addressing the development of new antibiotics to address antimicrobial resistance. We have, just in the last year, had the first antibiotic drug licensed in our program. We have several more in Phase 2 and Phase 3.

We also realized that the early stage pipeline was not sufficient to have a stream of new candidates going into advanced stage development. So we did launch a public-private partnership called CARB-X, in collaboration with NIAID, also sponsored by Wellcome Trust, now Bill and Melinda Gates Foundation in the U.K. Government. So we have now funded 34 different novel technologies to address new mechanisms of action for new antibiotics and vaccines.

Ms. SCHAKOWSKY. Thank you. My time is up, but I hope that in addition to development, that we're looking at prevention here as well.

Thank you for your courtesy, Mr. Chairman. Thank you.

Mr. HARPER. Thank you. The gentlewoman yields back.

The chair will now recognize the chair of the House Ethics Committee and a valuable member of this subcommittee, the gentlewoman from Indiana, Mrs. Brooks, for 5 minutes.

Mrs. BROOKS. Thank you, Mr. Chairman.

Dr. Schuchat, and if, Rear Admiral Hinton, if you could pass that binder, please, over to Dr. Schuchat. The last page of that binder has a chart that I would like to enter into the record and ask unanimous consent to enter into the record. It's PHEMCE's budget report for fiscal year 2016–2020.

Mr. HARPER. Without objection.

[The information appears at the conclusion of the hearing.]

Mrs. BROOKS. A large percentage of the CDC's Strategic National Stockpile budget appears to not go to procuring and updating medical countermeasures for the stockpile, but instead, goes to a category entitled nonprocurement costs. And in an effort to inform the discussion today, committee staff did ask CDC to provide a breakdown for what is in this nonprocurement, but we never got it.

Can you please share with us very briefly, and you might need to supplement with written response, what makes up the non-procurement spending for the Strategic National Stockpile?

Dr. SCHUCHAT. Thanks so much for your question. As you know, the Strategic National Stockpile has an inventory of about $7 billion. So the annual appropriation is just a piece of that. Most of the dollars that are in the nonprocurement go for sustaining and operating. So that would be the rental space, the security for the warehouses, the staff that work, the salaries for the staff, as well as the clinical expertise that's helping with the guidance on how to use the product.

Mrs. BROOKS. Thank you. Could we get a written breakdown of what that is?

Dr. SCHUCHAT. Absolutely.

Mrs. BROOKS. Because we could not tell what that was.

Dr. SCHUCHAT. That should be on its way to you.

Mrs. BROOKS. Thank you very much.

Dr. Bright, last year, HHS OIG issued a report after conducting five site audits at the various Strategic National Stockpile locations over a 2-year period, and they talked about systemic issues, putting that $7 billion that was just mentioned into great concern.

So, Dr. Bright, what actions does ASPR plan to take in the transfer that is anticipated October 1 to ensure the Strategic National Stockpile assets will be available in case of public health emergencies?

Mr. BRIGHT. As you probably know, we have several working groups working very closely between CDC and ASPR to evaluate various components of the stockpile transfer. So we are still——

Mrs. BROOKS. Can I interrupt one second? We just heard, in her opening testimony, Dr. Schuchat talk about all the many things CDC does relative to public health and these emergencies. And so are you going through all of those things to make sure there is coordination? And is that what the working groups are actually doing, figuring out what part CDC is going to maintain and what part ASPR will have? Is that what the working groups are doing?

Mr. BRIGHT. Absolutely. There's five different working groups. They're meeting weekly actually, and some of them have daily communications, to understand the various components, understanding how we maintain and sustain the best science and expertise that's currently in the SNS, understanding how we're building and augmenting the relationship with States and locals to ensure that that is also maintained for a robust SNS enterprise. We're also looking at the contracting and the financing. We're looking at the non-procurement cost as well.

We assure you that we are doing everything we can to make sure that those nonprocurement costs are supporting the SNS and its mission.

Mrs. BROOKS. I have a question with respect to—I understand there have been instances where BARDA—and you mentioned it— had to use Project BioShield funds to procure FDA-approved clinical countermeasures or medical countermeasures, because, for whatever reason, CDC declined to procure those countermeasures for the stockpile.

How does that uncertainty affect BARDA's ability to partner with industry, and is that being addressed in your working groups?

Mr. BRIGHT. That uncertainty is critical. As you know, it's very difficult to make these countermeasures. It's very lengthy, very risky, and the companies put aside other very profitable and successful endeavors to work with us in these areas. That marketplace assurance is absolutely essential to them working with us.

So we realize that, as we've been more successful with our partners and making additional countermeasures, it has created an additional burden on the SNS. We are working with the SNS at the CDC and our internal staff now to make sure that we are able to address those lapses or those gaps in communication or transparency to make sure that we have a successful——

Mrs. BROOKS. Thank you. I'd also like to enter into the record a letter from the Blue Ribbon Study Panel on Biodefense that was sent to Dr. Kadlec with a very detailed seven recommendations to improve our biodefense posture.

Mr. HARPER. Without objection.

[The information appears at the conclusion of the hearing.]

Mrs. BROOKS. And among those was the need to improve the coordination with State and local partners and to address problems that have existed in the past.

Can you tell us how ASPR plans to engage with State and local partners once it assumes control of the stockpile, which is of great concern to State and local partners?

Mr. BRIGHT. I agree that it is an essential part of an effective enterprise, the end-to-end approach, from early detection down to distribution. The State and local and tribal and territorial partners are the front line. They are the ones who are distributing and administering the vaccines and treatments. So we are dedicated to working with them, making sure they have a voice in the structure, in our system, to understand how they need those medical countermeasures and how they need them to be delivered most effectively.

It doesn't do us any good to make new drugs and vaccines if they're not suitable for our frontline workers at the State and local and tribal and territories to deliver and administer those.

Mrs. BROOKS. And so they know how to deliver and administer.

Mr. BRIGHT. Absolutely.

Mrs. BROOKS. Thank you. With that, I yield back. Thank you for your time.

Mr. HARPER. The gentlewoman yields back.

The chair will now recognize the gentlewoman from Florida, Ms. Castor, for 5 minutes.

Ms. CASTOR. Thank you, Mr. Chairman.

Good morning. Last year, Florida recorded 262 known cases of Zika. They were overwhelmingly travel-related cases, but of those known cases, 136 were pregnant women, and three babies were born in Florida with congenital Zika syndrome. Thankfully, those statistics are down substantially from 2015 and 2016, but the threat to young women of childbearing years and families remains very serious.

A study was just published where researchers from the CDC and the Annenberg Public Policy Center determined that most people have let their guard down now, that they're not taking the precautions that they should when it comes to Zika.

So, Dr. Schuchat, now that you have the results of that study and the threat of congenital Zika syndrome remains very serious, what do you plan to do to help keep families informed and make sure they're taking all precautions?

Dr. SCHUCHAT. Thank you. Zika was such a devastating new problem to have. For a mosquito bite to be able to cause birth defects, not something that was on any of our radars, really.

I think you know that, in May, we issued one of our monthly high-visibility reports of vital signs on mosquito and tick-borne diseases, which have really been increasing, trying to get that word out in advance of the mosquito season so people would take these threats seriously.

We have another report that's focused on Zika that will be coming out in about 2 months, really highlighting what have we learned from the, unfortunately, thousands of pregnancies that were complicated by Zika in folks who reside in the 50 States, to show what the followups have been and what has happened to the babies as they develop.

We need to make mosquito protection much easier for individuals and we need to have better tools for countering mosquitoes, in terms of environmentally safe and acceptable tools for them. We have been appreciative of the investments in strengthening our vector control so that there's better surveillance for vector-borne disease, and also better understanding of resistance patterns so we have the right products that can be used.

Ms. CASTOR. And there must be more we can do to communicate to young women and young men, especially now that—I mean, it was very strange that Zika became transferable via sex as well. So——

Dr. SCHUCHAT. Yes. The signs are still up in the airports, but people turn them off. So I think continuing to raise concerns is a challenge when people become complacent. So it's sort of our perpetual challenge in prevention.

Ms. CASTOR. Thank you.

Responding to public health emergencies requires us to have a good understanding of what is happening on the ground in real time. And doctors and nurses and others who work directly with patients are likely to be the first to interact with individuals affected in a public health emergency.

How does CDC gather data from these clinicians to detect emerging illnesses and other threats?

Dr. SCHUCHAT. We have a variety of surveillance systems to try to identify both the known threats and then the unknown or the new unusual clusters. Most important is for there to be a close connection between the clinical community, the doctors and nurses on the front line, and their local and State public health authorities.

The first cases of West Nile virus disease in New York City were detected, there were some animal losses, but it was that link between clinicians and the local health department. So part of our day-to-day everyday public health system is vital for the unknown emerging——

Ms. CASTOR. And CDC has a Laboratory Response Network that plays a vital role in biopreparedness by ensuring that we are able to quickly diagnose public health threats using rapid testing methods known as assays, but I understand that right now, there are no assay kits or rapid tests available for many dangerous pathogens and toxins.

What is going on here, and what are the barriers to developing assays targeting a wide variety of pathogens and toxins?

Dr. SCHUCHAT. Yes. What I would say is that the Laboratory Response Network, or LRN, is a group of 125 hospitals around the— or laboratories around the country that are within a 2-hour drive of 85 percent of all of the population. They are equipped to use validated, standardized assays to detect a variety of conditions.

The CDC has the ability to detect and confirm a longer list of the select agents and dangerous pathogens, and we prioritize which of the detection methods or assays need to be deployed close to where people live, which ones can be deployed and maintained centrally, because it's quite expensive to have the standards high enough to be able to reproduce the results in all of the 125 hospitals.

So while there's 45 select agents, we have assays for nearly all of them. Many of those are managed at the CDC or at Regional Centers of Excellence, while the 125 laboratories can test for the things that we think are the most likely, including things like MERS, where we rolled out an emergency use authorization for a new diagnostic test for that, Ebola, et cetera, the H1N1 initially. So we try to deploy distally the assays for the threats that are the most important to have local ability to detect rapidly.

Mr. BRIGHT. If I can add just a second on that too. That is another area of innovation that BARDA has been focusing on with our industry partners is to drive diagnostics, not only out of centralized labs to augment that centralized laboratory network, but put the diagnostics in the hands of the physicians in the physician's office at point-of-care testing. And even go further now, to drive diagnostics into the home, so people will know earlier when they've been infected with something so they can take responsible action to either get treated sooner when drugs are more effective and also to take activities to reduce the further spread or transmission of that virus. This area is ripe for innovation to augment our national laboratory support system.

Ms. CASTOR. Thank you very much.

Mr. HARPER. The gentlewoman yields back.

The chair now recognizes the gentleman from New York, Mr. Collins, for 5 minutes.

Mr. COLLINS. Thank you, Mr. Chairman.

I want to thank our witnesses and follow up a little bit more on the Laboratory Response Network, Dr. Schuchat. I understand that's been around about 9 years or thereabouts, since I think 1999?

Dr. SCHUCHAT. Yes, since 1999.

Mr. COLLINS. Actually, I've lost 10 years. Twenty years. I deliberately lost those 10 years, by the way.

So I know you mentioned 125 labs here in the country, but this is, from what I understand also, there's international labs. We all know the key to a lot of this is early detection, whether it was Ebola or some other things, SARS, which initially people thought they had the flu, even anthrax. But early detection's the key to jumping on top of this, which means the laboratories that are located outside the country. And I know this is a collaborative effort.

Are you, let's use the word "comfortable," and how is that collaboration between the United States and other countries around the world—as you mentioned, in many cases, these could be in Africa and other places—for the ability to identify these select agents?

Dr. SCHUCHAT. The Laboratory Response Network is in other countries as well, but I would say there's other means, other laboratories that we collaborate with around the world to help have that rapid detection and response. And actually, that's really what the global health security agenda is about, making sure that there are abilities to find, stop, and prevent epidemics wherever they occur, natural or not.

And the international collaboration, I think, is strengthened by the daily links we have in partnership on other threats. As you heard, we're working on Ebola in DRC right now. The Nipah virus detection in India was based on training that CDC had given to the laboratory in India years before so that India could recognize that pathogen themselves without having to take the time to ship the specimens out of the country.

Mr. COLLINS. So, following up on that, what I would call proficiency testing that we do for all of our labs, whether it's on influenza or HIV or any of the STDs, I'm assuming there's also a proficiency testing program related to our LRNs, which is always maybe a little more complicated because the 45 select agents are not nearly as prevalent as influenza. But can you speak to the proficiency program, how often these laboratories are tested, their workers, how their grades are, so that, in fact, we're comfortable that, if there is an outbreak, they're properly identifying it?

Dr. SCHUCHAT. Yes. The proficiency testing and assuring the quality of the laboratory test is vital. That's one of the reasons that we don't have assays for every one of the select agents in each of the LRN labs, because we want to certify that lab for that test and make sure that they maintain their reagents adequately and that everyone who's working on that test is doing it the right way. So we really try to prioritize which assays will be run regularly in every lab, because we do have to make sure that year in and year out, they're getting the accurate results. Otherwise, it makes no sense to run the test.

Mr. COLLINS. Is that done yearly, more than yearly? How often is that done? And does the CDC conduct the proficiency tests themselves or do you use outside agencies like CAP or someone like that?

Dr. SCHUCHAT. Let me get the details on that for the committee in followup, because I don't have all of them myself.

Mr. COLLINS. OK. Thank you. I think that's an important piece. In the remaining time, Admiral Hinton, egg-based versus cell-based vaccines, could you comment? YIs the FDA looking at—as we're moving forward certainly through our influenza season, are you making progress on the cell-based? Are you seeing positive potential there?

Admiral HINTON. Absolutely. And we actually have both. We have the egg-based versus the cell-based vaccines available, and continue to do evaluation and work in that area. But both are available, both are promising.

Mr. COLLINS. Because, there's always been some folks—if anyone else would like to comment on potential problems with the egg-based. Are we seeing positive steps in the other or——

Admiral HINTON. We are seeing positive steps in the other direction. And then as far as the egg-based, I know we run into issues with people having allergens and the like to them and not being able to have them. So having different options there to be able to provide and treat people with is promising and is available.

Mr. HARPER. Dr. Fauci.

Dr. FAUCI. There are other problems with egg-based, which is the reason why we're really trying to get away from egg-based and get more towards more advanced platform technologies.

One of the accidental mismatches that we had in 2016–2017, particularly in Australia, was that the virus was chosen for the vaccine, was put into eggs, and as it mutated in the eggs as it was growing, it mutated so that the virus that came out of the eggs was not the virus that you put into the egg. So we had an accidental mismatch.

That doesn't happen all the time by any means, but the idea of having to grow a virus in a 6-month process is something that we really need to, as I often say, graduate into the 21st century and do it a little bit better with more advanced technologies.

Mr. COLLINS. Thank you for that. Mr. Chair, I yield back.

Mr. HARPER. The chair is going to allow Dr. Bright to finish his response that he wanted to make here quickly.

Mr. BRIGHT. Thank you very much. I'd like to add just a little bit more to that as well. It's very important to understand the need for diversified vaccine production systems for influenza. Influenza's a tricky virus. Eggs have been a reliable vaccine substrate for a number of years. We are working to find ways to not only diversify and augment our cell-based and recombinant-based influenza vaccines, but also to improve egg-based vaccines. It's important not to completely discard a reliable technology without having a modernized technology to replace that. So we are working with each of the manufacturers now to identify ways to make our flu vaccines more effective now while we wait for that universal flu vaccine candidate in the future.

Mr. HARPER. The chair will now recognize the gentleman from California, Mr. Ruiz, for 5 minutes.

Mr. RUIZ. Thank you, Mr. Chairman.

Emerging infectious diseases are a major threat to the health of American citizens and to people around the world. This includes both new diseases that emerge in populations, as well as previously known diseases that re-emerge. In just the past 2 months, for example, we have seen outbreaks of Ebola in the Congo and Nipah in Northern India.

Dr. Schuchat, what steps are we taking to monitor emerging and re-emerging infectious diseases in the developing world, and how are we partnering with international players on this?

Dr. SCHUCHAT. Yes. CDC works closely with dozens of ministries of health around the world, as well as with international partners like the World Health Organization and the World Food Organization to—or the World Animal Health Organization to be able to find, stop, and prevent epidemics.

Mr. RUIZ. Give me an example of how you do that in a very underdeveloped, poor infrastructure nation.

Dr. SCHUCHAT. Right. As you know, in Liberia, they suffered from a devastating outbreak of Ebola in 2014. We have a country office in Liberia that's working closely with them focused on four key areas: strengthening laboratory systems, strengthening surveillance, strengthening emergency operation centers and rapid response, and workforce development through the disease detective program that we call the field epidemiology training program.

That means they can shorten the time to recognition of Ebola or something else and respond capably.

Mr. RUIZ. Thank you.

And in 2014, 2016, the Ebola epidemic killed more than 11,000 people in West Africa, and we know in October 2014, a physician who traveled from West Africa to Dallas in Texas died of Ebola; two others that contracted the Ebola virus survived.

What did we learn from that experience? And what are the changes that you've made because of that?

Dr. SCHUCHAT. There are three key lessons learned. One was that we need every country to have the ability to find, stop, and prevent epidemics, and that's what we call this Global Health Security Agenda.

A second thing was that we need the world organizations, the global organizations, to be able to surge rapidly when a country's capacity is overwhelmed. And that has actually happened effectively in the Democratic Republic of Congo with this Ebola outbreak recently.

And the third thing that we've learned is that infection control is essential; that an issue that is one illness or a couple illnesses can amplify into a very large-scale problem when we don't have adequate infection control. That's important in the United States for antimicrobial resistance, it's important in developing countries for TB, and it's very important for Ebola in SARS.

Mr. RUIZ. This patient and these two other healthcare workers who contracted Ebola, obviously, were in emergency departments, went to emergency departments, were treated in emergency departments. The first line of defense against any emerging infection or outbreak in the United States is going to be the emergency departments and also the first responders.

So what are you doing in terms of the CDC to coordinate to make sure that they are well-equipped? And then I'm going to ask Dr.

Bright that same question.

Dr. SCHUCHAT. Yes. We have a family of efforts to educate and keep up-to-date clinicians that include tens of thousands of clinicians regularly getting updates from us, whether it's through phone calls——

Mr. RUIZ. It's hard for very busy clinicians who work in emergency departments, seeing 20 patients at once to——

Dr. SCHUCHAT. Right. And that's——

Mr. RUIZ. How do you integrate that into their daily practice?

Dr. SCHUCHAT. Yes. The system changes are really important. When I saw a doctor at Emory last week, before I could even talk to anyone, I was asked, Have you traveled out of the country the last 3 weeks? It's actually on their phone line before you make an appointment.

So institutions instituting systemwide checks can help make sure that you don't have problems with human error.

Mr. RUIZ. Dr. Bright?

Mr. BRIGHT. Also, I'd like to highlight that ASPR has spent a lot of time with our hospital protection program and our healthcare coalitions to establish now even a national Ebola training center and education center, so we can train the hospital and first responders.

We now have 178 Ebola assessment hospitals. We have 69 State or jurisdictions designated Ebola treatment centers. We have 10 regional Ebola and other special pathogen treatment——

Mr. RUIZ. Well, I'm an emergency physician. I have to take exams like crazy just to keep my board certifications and my licensing. So I think integrating it as part of their continuing medical education and training would be very essential.

Now, the President's budget—or the administration wants to move the strategic National Stockpile under the ASPR. I'd like to ask Dr. Schuchat what are your competitive advantages and why should I think about even considering keeping it at the CDC?

Dr. SCHUCHAT. What I could say is that there's already been an administrative decision to move the stockpile, and so currently, CDC is working diligently very closely with ASPR to make that transfer as seamless as possible and to mitigate any negative consequences that may have been unintended but that may occur.

I think the critical areas that we are going to focus on are to make sure that State and local support is seamless, and that we work with State and local health departments every day on a variety of things and know them and know where our gaps are and where we need to make progress. We need to make sure that that close relationship continues in a way that doesn't jeopardize the American public.

Second area is the deep scientific expertise that we have across the agency that has contributed to maintenance of the SNS so that when we need clinical guidance for children for anthrax counter-measures, we can get that best advice incorporated. We need to make sure that that continues, but we are well on the way to executing that seamless transition.

Mr. HARPER. The gentleman yields back.

The chair will now recognize the vice chair of the subcommittee, the gentleman from Virginia, Mr. Griffith, for 5 minutes.

Mr. GRIFFITH. Thank you, Mr. Chairman.

After a series of safety lapses in 2014 involving the mishandling of anthrax and smallpox, in response to recommendations from a lab safety expert panel, both the FDA and CDC formed new offices to provide centralized oversight of laboratory safety and science.

Rear Admiral Hinton, I have several questions for you regarding the FDA's Office of Laboratory Science and Safety.

First, how many labs does the FDA have, or oversee?

Admiral HINTON. The FDA has 56 lab facilities.

Mr. GRIFFITH. And do you oversee more than that?

Admiral HINTON. No.

Mr. GRIFFITH. And are you counting everything in a single building, or is that all your labs combined?

Admiral HINTON. Those are the facilities. Within those facilities, there might be a total of 2,800 rooms, with those rooms being described as a space, an office, a closet.

Mr. GRIFFITH. Yes, ma'am.

How many safety inspections of these labs were conducted by the OLSS over the past year?

Admiral HINTON. No inspections have been conducted by OLSS in the past year. However, their labs have been inspected by other entities.

Mr. GRIFFITH. OK. Have there been any laboratory-acquired infections at FDA labs during the past year?

Admiral HINTON. There have been two noted infections within the last year. The staff that had acquired those infections have been observed and the case is closed.

Mr. GRIFFITH. All right. And can you get us the reports on those two incidences, please?

Admiral HINTON. I'll work with my staff to get that to you. Mr. GRIFFITH. Thank you very much.

Likewise, have there been any potential exposures to threat agents at FDA labs during the past year?

Admiral HINTON. Not to my knowledge. No.

Mr. GRIFFITH. All right. At tab 5 in the document binder is a September 2016 letter to the FDA sent the committee indicating its intention to hire 13 permanent full-time employees in the Office of Laboratory Science and Safety, OLSS.

The FDA told the committee this week that OLSS is staffed by only three permanent full-time employees, and three detailees.

Why doesn't the OLSS have the 13 permanent employees that were promised in a September letter of 2016?

Admiral HINTON. Sir, we have put forth the proposal, and as soon as we have the dedicated budget for OLSS, we expect for their current staff to double.

They actually have three permanent staff and three detailed working on this space.

Mr. GRIFFITH. That still only puts you at six as opposed to the 13 that was indicated in 2016.

Admiral HINTON. I agree. And we note that, and then with the approval of the upcoming budget, we will be able to double that and they will have the 13 staff.

Mr. GRIFFITH. The FDA, in the September 2016 letter, committed to this committee, and in July of 2017, published a notice in the Federal Register evaluating the OLSS so the office would directly to the FDA commissioner instead of the chief scientist.

Earlier this week, the FDA told committee staff that the FDA has decided to reorganize again, and that under the new proposal, OLSS will no longer be a direct report to the commissioner and will report to the chief scientist again, just as they did when we had the lapses back in 2014 and contrary to the expert panel's recommendations.

I just would like to know, first, is the chief scientist reporting to you now?

Admiral HINTON. I am the chief scientist. But the Director of OLSS——

Mr. GRIFFITH. Is OLSS reporting to you?

Admiral HINTON. Yes, sir.

Mr. GRIFFITH. And then you report on up the line?

Admiral HINTON. Yes. I do.

Mr. GRIFFITH. So why did FDA reverse course in less than a year and decide to have the OLSS revert back to reporting to the chief scientist?

Admiral HINTON. Well, sir, since that was announced, we have had the chance over the past year to observe and to see where it might be best fit for the alignment within the office.

Within the office of the chief scientist, which reports into the office of the commissioner and to the commissioner, we work on cross cutting cross-scientific issues to include those within laboratory science space.

So we thought that the OLSS would be best aligned there under my direct supervision on their day-to-day activities. The commissioner will be fully apprised of those activities.

Mr. GRIFFITH. Well, and I certainly mean no disrespect to you, but that was the same setup we had when there were problems being reported and we had the expert panel come in and give us recommendations, which FDA agreed to, and now you all are back-tracking.

I understand some different personnel, but it seems to me we're just creating the same problem we had before.

I see my time is up, and I have to yield back. Thank you, Mr. Chairman.

Mr. HARPER. The gentleman yields back.

The chair will now recognize the gentlewoman from California, Ms. Walters, for 5 minutes.

Ms. WALTERS. Thank you, Mr. Chairman.

Dr. Bright and Dr. Schuchat, either through stockpile procurement or through other means, how do your agencies ensure we have sufficient diagnostic test capacity to identify cases of pandemic influenza or other infectious diseases?

Mr. BRIGHT. In terms of development, so we have worked with a number of different manufacturers through the last 10 years to develop diagnostics for influenza, not only laboratory-based diagnostics, but to standardize and update the point-of-care diagnostics for influenza to make sure those are available and in the marketplace for use for pandemic and seasonal influenza detection.

Dr. SCHUCHAT. Yes. And I would say that CDC both develops assays and helps with validation.

You know, a number of years ago, there were quite a few point-of-care tests for influenza detection, and some of them didn't perform as well in the field as we had hoped. So we did quite an effort of validation comparison, shared the data with FDA, and new labeling and improvements in the tests followed from that.

So we will develop tests against pandemic or avian flu and other high-threat concerns, develop them through to emergency use authorization when appropriate, 501(k) when possible.

The 501(k) final process is very labor intensive, very expensive, and there's a limited number of our tests that we are able to put through to that level. But we do work closely with FDA and BARDA on a number of the priority ones.

Ms. WALTERS. Thank you.

Dr. Fauci, you mentioned work by the National Institute of Allergy and Infection Diseases to support research involving diagnostic testing.

From a Homeland Security and public health perspective, multiplex point-of-care technologies are beneficial because they can be used to simultaneously test for multiple infectious disease pathogens with a single blood or urine sample.

Can you tell us about the research NIAID is doing with respect to multiplex point-of-care technologies and how these technologies enhance our ability to detect material threats and infectious diseases?

Dr. FAUCI. Thank you very much for that question.

Yes. We are very heavily involved in that, both with our grantees to get concept to develop into something that's translatable, as well as contract.

There's multiplex, as you mentioned in your statement, is a very important tool of the future now for detecting outbreaks. For example, we have multiplex assays involving a whole series of particular types of viruses. For example, the flaviviruses, which are many of them that we have, particularly in the Western Hemisphere, that we are involved right now in research for the development of a multiplex that would essentially cover all of the associated flaviviruses, and we're doing that with a number of other viruses.

So there's really a very important, I believe, and aggressive ongoing research program at the NIH, mostly through our grantees and contractors.

Ms. WALTERS. OK.

Mr. BRIGHT. If I can jump in, the challenge with the beauty of multiplex assays is that they can do a lot. And the challenge with them is they're very large instruments generally in centralized laboratories in a hospital or a public health laboratory.

The innovation that we're driving today with companies that move multiplex assays to point of care into a physician's office, and even to work with those multiplex technologies to push some of those now out into the home, one of our greatest challenges with our diagnostics for any disease is how long it takes for a patient to get to that system and into the system so they can get a sample drawn and can get a result.

Too much time elapses in that. So we're trying to also use this new technology for multiplex point of care to multiplex point of need into the home to get people earlier notification to empower patients to get treated sooner.

Ms. WALTERS. OK. Thank you.

Rear Admiral Hinton, how many multiplex point-of-care diagnostic tests has the FDA approved for use?

Admiral HINTON. Thank you for your question, ma'am.

Work in this area is progressing well at FDA. We've cleared more than 25 multiplex tests that could be suitable for point-of-care tests.

Ms. WALTERS. OK. And how many others are currently under assessment by the FDA?

Admiral HINTON. I'll have to get back to you. I don't have the exact number.

Ms. WALTERS. OK. Can you describe the range of capabilities that these tests have? You know, how many diseases can one multiplex point-of-care diagnostic test detect?

Admiral HINTON. It can detect many. We can do up to 20—and more than—at one time, which is incredibly important, especially at the point of care so that we can help to easily detect in order to find the best treatment.

Ms. WALTERS. OK. Thank you, and I yield back the balance of my time.

Mr. HARPER. The gentlewoman yields back.

The chair will now recognize the gentleman from Georgia, Mr. Carter, for 5 minutes.

Mr. CARTER. Thank you, Mr. Chairman.

And, Mr. Chairman, I want to echo your comments earlier about what an outstanding panel this is. Thank you all for the very important work that you do. It is extremely important to our country, and we appreciate it very much.

Dr. Bright, I want to start with you. Being, of course, from Georgia, I am somewhat concerned, even still, about the move of the strategic National Stockpile and the management of that from the CDC to ASPR, and I just want to be assured again from you. I've met Dr. Redfield, and I think he's doing a great job. Dr. Schuchat and I have worked together, and I just can't say enough good things about the CDC and the outstanding work that they do for our country.

And I just want to make sure that they're still going to have the opportunity to stay involved and to be involved in the medical counter-measurement development and everything else that goes along with the SNS.

Mr. BRIGHT. Sir, you have my complete assurance. I echo your comments about the CDC and the great work they are doing. Many people don't know I got my first start in science at the CDC as an ORISE fellow coming from Emory University in Georgia.

I understand and appreciate the great scientific leadership of the CDC and their relationship with state and local and the value of that.

We plan to always include that in our assessment and our programs for the new strategic National Stockpile management.

Mr. CARTER. We talked on it earlier. One of my colleagues had mentioned about the concern particularly that the transfer is not disruptive for the state and local agencies.

What would you suggest that we do to make that as least disruptive as we can?

Mr. BRIGHT. Well, the most important thing is to recognize the value of their voice in the entire process, not just in the transition of the management of the SNS, but an entire end-to-end process of our efficient response to any emergency or public health emergency threat.

So we already have an intentional working group focusing on the state and local and tribal and territory partners and their specific needs and their specific interests to make sure those are encapsulated in our management of the SNS.

Mr. CARTER. Great.

Dr. Schuchat, would you care to comment on that as well? How can well assure that this is not disruptive to our local and state communities?

Dr. SCHUCHAT. I think that change is, by necessity, disruptive, and I think our job is to mitigate that disruption so that people aren't harmed. So I think it's on our radar. We're working really closely together. The Association of State and Territorial Health Officers Board was just at CDC yesterday talking to us about how we can make sure this all goes as well as possible.

Mr. CARTER. And let me ask you—I run the risk of being a little self-serving here—but wouldn't it make sense to look at perhaps just having ASPR colocate down to Atlanta with the CDC? I recognize you're part of HHS, but we have to get out of the mindset that not everybody's got to be in Washington, D.C. We have a big country out here. Dr. Bright, I'm looking at you.

Mr. BRIGHT. We have a big and beautiful country, sir, and I agree with you, and there is no intent to move the strategic National Stockpile from Atlanta to Washington, D.C. There might be one or two individuals who are located in our ASPR office to ensure we have smooth and efficient ongoing communication with the expert staff that is in Atlanta, Georgia.

Mr. CARTER. OK. Well, that might be a good compromise, and we appreciate that very much.

The Ebola crisis that we had, obviously we learned a lot of lessons there, but I was so proud of the public/private partnership between Emory University and the CDC, and all four patients recovered.

And I just wanted to know, will you be using that model in the future for other pandemics and other risks that we might run into? Because we're very proud of the work that was done at Emory University, and I think it's a great example of what we can do in the future.

Dr. Schuchat?

Dr. SCHUCHAT. I would say that CDC benefits tremendously from being located right next to Emory, and there's a really close working relationship. We were fortunate that they such a terrific job in the Ebola—in the care of the patients there.

There's ongoing collaboration and communication and support.

I think ASPR may have a more direct role in the hospitals and the care of such patients, and Dr. Bright might want to comment.

Mr. BRIGHT. I also want to make sure that we capitalize and not lose that expert and lessons learned from Emory University.

As you may know, we stood up a National Ebola Training and Education Center. It's based in Nebraska as collaboration with Emory University, University of Nebraska, and Bellevue. It is an example of one the finest educational centers on Ebola and other epidemic treatments in the world now.

Mr. CARTER. OK. Again, I want to thank all of you for the work that you do. Extremely important, and especially shout out to CDC and the work that they do.

Thank you, and I yield back, Mr. Chairman.

Mr. HARPER. The gentleman yields back.

The chair will now recognize the gentlewoman from California, Ms. Eshoo, for 5 minutes.

Ms. ESHOO. Thank you, Mr. Chairman, for extending the legislative courtesy to me, since I'm not a member of this subcommittee, but I have a great interest in the subject matter, since we're looking to reauthorize PAHPA and all of the listening to what's taken place in this hearing and the superb testimony from each one of you. We've made great progress since the legislation was first written in 2006.

So I'm pleased, but in America, we're never satisfied with exactly where we are. We always want to improve. And so there's been an important pathway of improvement, and I thank each one of you.

I'm very proud of the two women that are here. Rear Admiral Hinton, it's really a source of pride to me to hear you respond to the tough questions that have come your way. To Dr. Schuchat, it's always a pleasure to hear you. Dr. Bright, the partnership with BARDA has been a very important one, and I think that you're taking it to new places.

And to Dr. Fauci, I don't have any questions to ask you. I wish I could canonize you. You are such a gift to our country. You could be in the private sector probably making millions of dollars. You've devoted your entire life to the people of our country, and you make the National Institutes of—the NIH really stand for the National Institutes of Hope.

You're a leader in that, and I just revere your record, your leadership, and what you've done and what you continue to do.

To Dr. Bright, how has restoring BARDA as a contracting authority led to increases in the efficiency and the certainty that surrounds the medical countermeasures at research and development? That's my first question.

And my second one is, does your agency interpret your existing authority to allow the stockpile to invest in countermeasures other than those explicitly mentioned in the current statute?

Maybe start with the second question.

Mr. BRIGHT. Thank you very much.

Ms. ESHOO. Do you need any additional authorities?

Mr. BRIGHT. To be more effective, I believe we need to modify some of the authorities that we have to allow us to work more flexibly with our industry.

Ms. ESHOO. So you don't need additional authorities?

Mr. BRIGHT. We don't need additional authorities. I believe we need to modify the authorities that we have.

Ms. ESHOO. What does that mean, modify the authorities?

Mr. BRIGHT. Our other transactional authority, for example, does have limitations on how we can interface with our industry partners and how they might qualify for that type of partnership. So we have a draft of suggested language that might allow us that greater flexibility to do so.

Ms. ESHOO. And have you gotten that to us?

Mr. BRIGHT. If it hasn't been sent to you yet, we will make sure that it is quickly.

Ms. ESHOO. Do BARDA's existing additional authorities promote work on the, and it's been brought up, not only at this subcommittee, but at others, of the antimicrobial resistance and the antibiotic development, or does your agency need additional authorities to engage in that work?

Mr. BRIGHT. We've been working with the authorities we have since 2010 to address antimicrobial resistance.

One area of authority that is lacking, we believe, would be beneficial would be a specific authority for the appropriations for pandemic influenza, because there's a lot of critical work that needs to happen in pandemic——

Ms. ESHOO. Have you gotten that to us?

Mr. BRIGHT. I do not have that authority yet.

Ms. ESHOO. Are you going to make that request of us?

Mr. BRIGHT. I believe that request has been submitted. I hope so.

Ms. ESHOO. There was some mention earlier about how important the advanced—I think you might have raised it in your opening statement, on advanced appropriations. I believe that, because the Senate has different rules on this, that we will meet the standard that needs to be met. That's probably the tidiest way for me to say it.

But it is critical, because if you don't have the advanced appropriations at BARDA, then our partners in the private sector are not going to be able to continue the important work that they're doing.

Mr. BRIGHT. That's absolutely correct. They are business partners working in long-term cycles and forward-looking cycles, and the consistency and assurance of that advanced appropriations allows them to have that assurance that we will still be there doing our part so they can plan appropriately as well.

Ms. ESHOO. Thank you very much to each one of you for what you're doing for our country. You're all heroes of mine.

Thank you, Mr. Chairman. Yield back.

Mr. HARPER. The gentlewoman yields back.

The chair will now recognize Ranking Member DeGette for concluding remarks.

Ms. DEGETTE. Thank you very much, Mr. Chairman, for the moment of personal privilege.

I wanted to bring up another issue that I think is a real crisis right now in this country.

I know we have a lot of HHS agency representatives here, and, of course, ASPR is under the purview of HHS.

Yesterday, our ranking member, Frank Pallone, wrote a letter to Secretary Azar about the HHS Office of Refugee Resettlement. And these kids who are being taken from their parents at the border, and then being put under the auspices of this agency, we have real concerns about what's happening to these children. And we have real concerns about their long-term prospects, being taken from their parents.

And, Mr. Chairman, I just wanted to bring this up, because you're going to be getting a request from the minority to have a hearing about this, and we would hope that you would seriously consider this, because we are quite concerned about the human aspects of this situation.

Thank you, and I yield back.

Mr. HARPER. The gentlewoman yields back.

The chair will recognize Dr. Burgess for a concluding remark.

Mr. BURGESS. Well, Mr. Chairman, thank you for the recognition.

I would just point out that this committee, and this subcommittee in particular, has a significant history of oversight on the ORR. I do feel obligated to point out this is not the agency that makes the decision about whether or not a family unit is kept together, but they are obligated to take care of—whether a child arrives unaccompanied or is separated from their family at the DHS facility. But that is the responsibility of, in fact, the Health Subcommittee, and we do take that responsibility very seriously.

In fact, it was our work in July of 2014 that allowed them to acquire an actual physician to be in those facilities to assess those children as they were brought in.

And it was our committee that raised the question shouldn't we at least have some way of contacting the children after they have been placed with a family, at least on a voluntary basis.

So it was our committee that did that work, and that work will continue. I've been in contact with both Secretary Azar and with the gentleman that runs ORR, and I expect to have robust discussions with them going forward, and I yield back.

Ms. DEGETTE. If the gentleman will yield, thank you very much, and I look forward to working with you on this, because it's really a critical issue, and I'm on that subcommittee, too. Thank you.

Mr. HARPER. I want to thank each of you for being here. Great insights and expertise, and I thank you for participating in today's hearing.

I remind Members that they have 10 business days to submit questions for the record, and I ask that the witnesses agree to respond promptly to any such questions.

With that, the subcommittee's adjourned.

[Whereupon, at 10:58 a.m., the subcommittee was adjourned.]

[Material submitted for inclusion in the record follows:]

U.S. House of Representatives
Committee on Energy and Commerce

June 13, 2018

TO: Members, Subcommittee on Oversight and Investigations

FROM: Committee Majority Staff

RE: Hearing entitled "The State of U.S. Public Health Biopreparedness: Responding to Biological Attacks, Pandemics, and Emerging Disease Outbreaks."

The Subcommittee on Oversight and Investigations will hold a hearing on Friday, June 15, 2018, at 9:00 a.m. in 2123 Rayburn House Office Building. The hearing is entitled "The State of U.S. Public Health Bio-preparedness: Responding to Biological Attacks, Pandemics, and Emerging Disease Outbreaks."

The purpose of this hearing is to follow up on the past biopreparedness oversight issues examined by the Subcommittee, and to receive updates from the agencies on current assessments and strategies. This hearing will also highlight the need to reauthorize the Pandemic and All-Hazards Preparedness Act (PAHPA), which is due to expire at the end of September 2018.[5]

[5] PAHPA created and expanded programs to enhance the public health system's capacity to monitor and respond to public health emergencies. The act expanded programs for state and local public health emergency preparedness activities and mandates the use of evidence-based benchmarks and standards to measure levels of preparedness. Ass'n of State and Territorial Health Orgs., *ASTHO Legal Preparedness Series Emergency*

Witnesses

Rick A. Bright, PhD, Director, Biomedical Advanced Research and Development Authority; Deputy Assistant Secretary, Office of the Assistant Secretary for Preparedness and Response, U.S. Department of Health and Human Services;

- Anne Schuchat, M.D. (RADM, USPHS), Principal Deputy Director, Centers for Disease Control and Prevention, U.S. Department of Health and Human Services;
- Anthony Fauci, M.D., Director, National Institute of Allergy and Infectious Diseases, National Institutes of Health; and
- Denise Hinton (RADM, USPHS), Chief Scientist, U.S. Food and Drug Administration.

Background

This section will outline four areas of continuing oversight interest in the area of biopreparedness: biological threats; detection and diagnostics; development and stockpiling of medical countermeasures (MCMs); and science, safety and security of laboratories in the life sciences-biodefense complex.

Biological Threats

Biological threats fall into three main categories: natural infectious diseases, synthetic biology/engineered pathogens, and bioterrorism. Synthetic biology could cause harm either intentionally (e.g., an engineered pathogen used in a bioterrorist attack) or accidentally (e.g., through the accidental release of dangerous agents from a lab conducting dual use research).[6]

In this century, the nation has witnessed the impacts of naturally occurring outbreaks such as influenza, Ebola, and SARS.[7] Health authorities are currently monitoring other potential emerging infectious diseases that could cause a pandemic, such as the H7N9

Authority & Immunity Toolkit -Pandemic and All-Hazards Preparedness Act, http://www.astho.org/Programs/Preparedness/Public-Health-Emergency-Law/Emergency-Authority-and-Immunity-Toolkit/Pandemic-and-All-Hazards-Preparedness-Act-Fact-Sheet/(last visited June 11, 2018).

6 GiveWell, *A conversation with George Poste on February 12, 2014*, https://www.openphilanthropy.org/sites/default/files/Poste%202-12-14%20%28public%29.pdf (last visited June 11, 2018). George Poste, DVM, PhD., is Director, Complex Adaptive Systems Institute, Arizona State University and an ex officio member of the Blue Ribbon Study Panel on Biodefense.

7 *See Examining the Reauthorization of the Pandemic and All-Hazards Preparedness Act Before the Subcomm. on Health of the H. Comm. on Energy and Commerce*, 115th Cong. (2018) (written testimony of Hon. Robert Kadlec, M.D., Assistant Sec'y for Preparedness and Response, U.S. Dep't of Health & Human Services).

influenza strain circulating in China.[8] Further, as recently noted by Department of Health and Human Services (HHS) Assistant Secretary for Preparedness and Response (ASPR) Robert Kadlec, "[t]errorist organizations such as ISIS and al-Qaida remain determined to attack; further ISIS has demonstrated no compunction about using chemical and other unconventional weapons in attacks overseas. State actors have already threatened our homeland with nuclear weapons and have shown the means to employ both chemical and biological weapons."[9]

The Subcommittee explored the growing nature of these biological threats and the need for an elevated response at a hearing held on February 12, 2016.[10]

An attachment to this memorandum provided by the National Institute of Allergy and Infectious Diseases (NIAID) shows examples of emerging and re-emerging infectious diseases as of June 2018.

Detection and Diagnostics

Laboratory Response Network

The Centers for Disease Control and Prevention (CDC) Laboratory Response Network (LRN) is a network of 134 local, state and federal laboratories that can provide the laboratory infrastructure and capacity to quickly respond to public health emergencies, and incidents of biological and chemical terrorism. The network, established in 1999 and overseen by the CDC, enables rapid detection of and response to emerging infectious diseases such as Zika, Ebola and influenza, as well as select agents and toxins. All 50 states have at least one member laboratory and 85 percent of the U.S. population lives within a two-hour drive of an LRN lab.

The ability of the LRN to respond to quickly unfolding emergencies is essential and, as such, the network was designed to deploy rapid detection technology and laboratory tests (known as assays) to quickly test suspicious materials and detect the presence of biological or chemical agents in the event of a bioterrorism attack.

In August 2016, the Committee launched a bipartisan investigation about the current capabilities of the CDC LRN, and two additional information request letters followed on October 26, 2016, and February 28, 2017.[11] These letters requested information regarding the LRN's lab capacity, funding levels, and laboratory test development.

---

[8] *Id.*

[9] *Id.*

[10] *See Outbreaks, Attacks, and Accidents: Combating Biological Threats Before the Subcomm. on Oversight and Investigations of the H. Comm on Energy and Commerce,* 114th Cong. (2016) Serial No. 114-117.

[11] Letter from Hon. Fred Upton, Chairman, H. Comm. on Energy and Commerce, et al. to Thomas Frieden, M.D., Dir., Centers for Disease Control and Prevention (Aug. 11, 2016) *available at* https://archives-energycommerce.house.gov/sites/republicans.energycommerce. house.gov/files/documents/114/letters/20160811CD C.pdf; Letter from Hon. Fred Upton, Chairman, H. Comm. on Energy and Commerce and Hon. Tim Murphy, Chairman, H. Comm. on Energy and Commerce, Subcomm. on Oversight and Investigations to Thomas Frieden, M.D., Dir., Centers for Disease Control and Prevention (Oct 26, 2016) (On file with the Committee); Letter from Hon. Greg Walden, Chairman, H. Comm.

In response to questions about funding for the network, the CDC provided documentation indicating that spending decreased over the last decade. The LRN's expenditures have gradually decreased from $15 million in 2007 to $9 million in 2016. Expenditures for the LRN totaled $116.2 million during that 10-year period.[12] The CDC has also at times received funding from other federal agencies to help support network activities. The Department of Homeland Security's Science and Technology Directorate, Department of Defense's Defense Threat Reduction Agency and its Joint Program Executive Office, and the Department of Health and Human Services' Office of the Assistant Secretary for Preparedness and Response (ASPR) and Biomedical Research and Development Authority (BARDA) have each provided funding for LRN support over the last 10 years. Funding has varied year-to-year by agency, but the total amount the four agencies have provided to the LRN since Fiscal Year 2008 is $21.5 million.[13]

In response to questions on lab test development, the CDC provided information about the process by which it selects and develops new assays the LRN can use to detect for biological agents, toxins and emerging infectious diseases. The CDC has indicated that the Food and Drug Administration (FDA) has approved 510(k) clearances for four assays and issued emergency use authorization for another six assays.[14] Out of a total of 45 select agents affecting humans on the current select agents and toxin list,[15] the CDC LRN has assays cleared by FDA under the 510(k) process for three, after nearly 20 years of the LRN program and more than $135 million in funding during the last decade.[16]

Most recently, the CDC arranged for the evaluation and deployment of a Department of Defense Ebola Zaire assay by the LRN amid the 2014 Ebola epidemic in West Africa. After the 2015 Zika outbreak in Brazil, the CDC also began development of an LRN diagnostic for the Zika virus.[17]

Biosurveillance

Two areas of biosurveillance of interest to the Subcommittee have been BioWatch and multiplex point-of-care technologies (MPOCTs). BioWatch is an early warning system designed to detect a large-scale, covert attack that releases anthrax or other agents of bioterrorism into the air. Overseen by the Department of Homeland Security (DHS),

---

on Energy and Commerce and Hon. Tim Murphy, Chairman, H. Comm. on Energy and Commerce, Subcomm. on Oversight and Investigations to Anne Schuchat, M.D., Acting Dir., Centers for Disease Control and Prevention (Feb. 28, 2017) *available at* https://archives-energycommerce.house.gov/sites/republicans.energycommerce.house.gov/files/documents/114/letters/20170228CD C.pdf.

[12] Letter from Anne Schuchat, M.D., Acting Dir., Centers for Disease Control and Prevention, to Hon. Greg Walden, H. Comm. on Energy and Commerce. (May 23, 2017) (On file with the Committee). In the letter to the Committee, the CDC represented that there may be additional funding sources for the LRN than those it had identified.

[13] *Id.*

[14] *Id.*

[15] *See* Fed. Select Agent Program, *Select Agents and Toxins List*, https://www.selectagents.gov/selectagentsandtoxinslist.html (last visited June 11, 2018).

[16] Schuchat, *supra* note 8.

[17] *Id.*

the BioWatch program involves a system of aerosol collectors deployed in more than 30 cities, as well as laboratory facilities and personnel to analyze samples from these collectors. This program relies heavily on CDC, and the state and local public health laboratories that are members of the CDC LRN. The program aims to reduce the time required to recognize and characterize potentially catastrophic aerosolized attacks by monitoring for the presence of certain biological agents considered to pose high risk for an aerosolized attack. A committee investigation and a U.S. Government Accountability Office (GAO) report found that DHS lacked reliable information about BioWatch's technical capabilities to detect a biological attack and therefore lacks the basis for informed cost-benefit decisions about upgrades to the system.[18] DHS continues to work on ways to upgrade the BioWatch system.

MPOCTs are technologies that can simultaneously test for more than one type of human infectious disease pathogen from a single patient sample (such as blood, urine, or sputum) in one run at or near the site of a patient. MPOCTs can enable rapid testing while the patient is at the doctor's office, clinic, or other testing location, including the home. From a homeland security and public health perspective, MPOCTs are of interest as an early detection tool, and can help assess the potential spread and effect of the disease in the case of dangerous pathogens. At the Committee's request, the GAO conducted a technical assessment of MPOCTs.[19] The GAO found that MPOCTs have a range of performance characteristics that describe, among other things, the ability of the technology to correctly identify the presence or absence of a pathogen. Developers identified several technical challenges to developing multiplex assays that can slow MPOCT development and raise costs. GAO also identified potential benefits of MPOCTs included improved patient health care and management, more appropriate use of antibiotics, improved ability to limit the spread of disease, and health care cost savings.

Development and Stockpiling of Medical Countermeasures

Public Health Emergency Medical Countermeasures Enterprise

In 2006, HHS established the Public Health Emergency Medical Countermeasures Enterprise (PHEMCE) to coordinate federal efforts to prepare for, and respond to, public health emergencies from a MCM perspective.[20]

---

[18] *See Continuing Concerns Over BioWatch and the Surveillance of Bioterrorism Before the Subcom. on Oversight and Investigations of the H. Comm. on Energy and Commerce* 113th Cong. (2013) Serial No. 113-56; U.S. Gov't Accountability Office, *Biosurveillance: DHS Should Not Pursue BioWatch Upgrades or Enhancements Until System Capabilities Are Established*, GAO-16-99 (Oct. 2015) *available at* https://www.gao.gov/assets/680/673309.pdf.

[19] U.S. Gov't Accountability Office, *Medical Devices: Capabilities and challenges of technologies to enable rapid diagnoses of infectious diseases*, GAO-17-347 (Aug. 2017) *available at* https://www.gao.gov/products/GAO-17-347.

[20] *See* 71 C.F.R. § 129 (2006) and U.S. Dep't of Health & Human Services, Assistant Sec'y for Preparedness and Response, *Public Health Emergency Medical Countermeasures Enterprise*, https://www.phe.gov/Preparedness/mcm/phemce/Pages/default.aspx (last visited June 11, 2018).

Pursuant to the 2013 Pandemic and All-Hazards Preparedness Reauthorization Act, the PHEMCE is led by the ASPR and is comprised of senior leadership from the CDC, the NIAID at the National Institutes of Health (NIH), the FDA, the Department of Defense (DoD), the DHS, the Department of Veteran's Affairs (VA) and the Department of Agriculture (USDA).[21]

The PHEMCE's mission components include:[22]

- Requirements Setting: The PHEMCE is responsible for establishing requirements for MCMs based on factors such as threat and risk assessments, which are principally conducted by the DHS.
- Early Stage Research: The NIH is the lead federal PHEMCE agency for conducting and facilitating research into areas of public health concerns, which could ultimately lead to the development of MCMs to diagnose, treat, and prevent a wide-range of public health threats.
- Advanced Development/Manufacturing: The Biomedical Advanced Research and Development Authority (BARDA), within HHS' ASPR, develops MCMs for emerging public health threats and partners with industry to accelerate development and increase MCM manufacturing capacity. In the past decade, BARDA's efforts, supported by industry and government partnerships, have resulted in 35 FDA approvals for 31 unique MCMs for threats to the public health.[23] BARDA has also supported the development of 27 MCMs against threats that have been identified by the DHS, through Project Bioshield, as being national security threats.[24]
- Regulatory Science Management: The PHEMCE endeavors to ensure MCMs are safe and effective, which is generally the responsibility of the FDA.
- Procurement/Inventory Management/Stockpiling: The PHEMCE oversees the procurement and management of MCMs to respond to public health threats. Currently, the CDC and BARDA are the lead PHEMCE agencies for this mission component.
- Response Planning, Policy, Guidance and Communication: The PHEMCE, led by CDC and ASPR, coordinates federal medical response and communication strategies when faced with a public health emergency.
- Deployment/Distribution/Dispensing/Administration: The CDC and ASPR engage and coordinate with state and local partners to facilitate the distribution of

---

[21] 42 U.S.C. § 300hh – 10.

[22] U.S. Dep't of Health & Human Services, Assistant Sec'y for Preparedness and Response, *PHEMCE Mission Components*, https://www.phe.gov/Preparedness/mcm/phemce/Pages/mission.aspx (last updated Feb. 27, 2015).

[23] Kadlec, *supra* note 3.

[24] *Id.*

MCMs and administration of other medical assets in times of public health emergencies.
- Monitoring/Evaluation/Assessment: The CDC and FDA are the principal PHEMCE agencies for monitoring the safety and performance of MCMs that have been deployed in response to public health emergencies response.

Concerns have been raised about the length of time it takes to classify a hazardous pathogen as a material threat and then approve the development of medical countermeasures. According to ASPR, it can take upwards of two years for the DHS to designate a pathogen as a material threat.[25] For example, carfentanil, a highly potent form of fentanyl, was known as a weapon of mass destruction after Russian forces used it in the Moscow theatre against Chechen terrorists in 2002,[26] but pharmaceutical-based agents, such as fentanyl, were only recently added as a material threat. ASPR would like to reduce the time it takes for the DHS to designate a material threat to 90-days or less.[27] After a pathogen is classified as a material threat, PHEMCE can approve the development of MCMs for a material threat. ASPR is currently considering other steps that could reduce the timeframe to approve countermeasure development while still maintaining an adequate level of input from all PHEMCE partners and experts, and hopes to devise a plan to reduce the MCM development timeframe by year's end.[28]

Strategic National Stockpile

The CDC is the primary federal agency responsible for public health surveillance, epidemiologic investigations, and public health communications. The CDC is also currently responsible for managing the Strategic National Stockpile (SNS), though the President's Fiscal Year (FY) 2019 Budget Request transfers SNS management authority from the CDC to HHS' ASPR.[29]

The SNS is a federal repository of MCMs such as vaccines, antibiotics, and other medical supplies that are to be used in public health emergencies.[30] For FY 2018, the SNS received a total of $610 million, including supplemental funding included in the omnibus spending bill passed earlier this year. Since FY 1999, the federal government has appropriated more than $9.15 billion to the SNS, with annual SNS funding levels

---

[25] Briefing by staff, U.S. Dep't of Health & Human Services, Assistant Sec'y for Preparedness and Response with staff, H.Comm. on Energy and Commerce, June 11, 2018.

[26] *See,* e.g., Erika Kinetz and Maria Danilova, *Lethal chemical now used as a drug haunts theater hostages*, Associated Press, Oct. 8, 2016, https://apnews.com/256605b7679d4a61bde9a8eac8906ea9.

[27] Assistant Sec'y for Preparedness and Response, *supra* note 21 and E-Mail from staff, Assistant Sec'y for Preparedness to staff, H. Comm on Energy and Commerce (June 12, 2018 9:13am).

[28] Assistant Sec'y for Preparedness and Response, *supra* note 21.

[29] U.S. Dep't of Health & Human Services, Centers for Disease Control and Prevention, *Fiscal Year 2019 Justification and Estimates for Appropriation Committees*, *available at* https://www.cdc.gov/budget/documents/fy2019/fy-2019-cdc-congressional-justification.pdf.

[30] 42 U.S.C. § 247d-6b.

significantly increasing in the years following the September 11, 2001, terror attacks and 2001 anthrax attacks.[31]

Through coordination with the PHEMCE, CDC's current responsibilities regarding the SNS include MCM procurement, shelf life analysis, and MCM replenishment. In addition, the CDC, through its Office of Public Health Preparedness and Response (OPHPR), is also responsible for the delivery of MCMs to areas that have been affected by public health emergencies. OPHPR also provides training to state and local medical personnel and public health officials on how to properly receive and distribute MCMs from the SNS in the case of a public health emergency. In 2017, OPHPR provided such training to more than 3,700 state and local personnel and led a total of 12 medical emergency simulation exercises.[32]

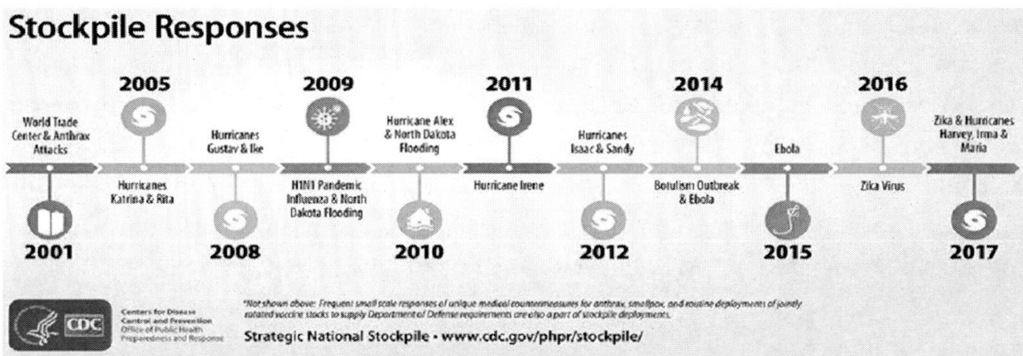

Source: Centers for Disease Control and Prevention.

Over the last few years, independent audits have raised concerns over CDC's logistical management of the SNS. In June 2017, HHS' Office of Inspector General (OIG) issued a report which called into question the readiness of the CDC to effectively deploy SNS resources during a public health emergency.[33] In its review, OIG identified "systemic issues [that] could put at risk approximately $7 billion of Stockpile inventory and negatively affect Stockpile readiness during a national emergency."[34] The OIG's conclusion was based on a review of findings from each of five SNS site audits that covered FYs 2013 and 2014, and additional information related to the value of the SNS, security, and funding.

Questions have also been raised about the SNS Division of State and Local Readiness (DSLR), which oversees expenditures of about $8.6 million. The DSLR initiatives are

[31] Source: Total tabulated from tables in Congressional Research Service e-mail to staff, H. Comm. on Energy and Commerce (June 1, 2018).

[32] Centers for Disease Control and Prevention, *Public Health Preparedness and Response 2018 National Snapshot, available at* https://www.cdc.gov/phpr/pubs-links/2018/documents/2018_Preparedness_Report.pdf.

[33] U.S. Dep't of Health & Human Services, Office of Inspector Gen., *Readiness of CDC's Strategic National Stockpile Could Be at Risk in Case of a Public Health Emergency* (A-04-16-03554) (June 2017) *available at* https://oig.hhs.gov/oas/reports/region4/41603554RIB.pdf.

[34] *Id.*

meant to ensure that local partners have the resources and training in place to distribute and properly use products from the SNS in the event they need to be deployed. ASPR, however, has identified concerns with state and local partners' current state of readiness, specifically regarding "last mile" distribution and how quickly partners are able to distribute products on the ground after receipt from SNS.[35] Among the concerns highlighted by ASPR is that state and local partners currently do not know what products are in the SNS and therefore do not know how to properly deploy the products.[36] To improve state and local readiness, ASPR intends to bolster education and training programs so local partners and first responders have familiarity with SNS products. ASPR also intends to review assessment tools used to rank state and local partners' readiness status and to design an array of distribution models that could be implemented by local entities to improve their response plans.[37]

Other issues raised regarding the CDC's management of the SNS include instances in which the CDC failed to fund the procurement of an MCM for the SNS after the MCM's development and FDA approval.[38] For example, there have been instances where BARDA has had to use Project Bioshield funding to procure MCMs that have been FDA-approved but were not ultimately purchased by the SNS. The reason for this was due to the fact that the government has to not only ensure that the specific MCMs remain available, but also must sustain a company since they are developing MCMs that do not have a traditional commercial market. Some of the MCMs that have been produced in this manner include: anthrax vaccine adsorbed; axibacumab; and obiltoxaximab.[39]

Recently, members of the Blue Ribbon Study Panel on Biodefense wrote to Dr. Robert Kadlec, HHS ASPR, with a number recommendations to enhance the United States' MCM infrastructure. Included among the Panel's recommendations were proposed SNS management reforms, which, according to the Panel, were precipitated by the CDC's inadequate management of the SNS.[40]

Pursuant to the President's FY 2019 budget, the transfer of the SNS from the CDC to the ASPR will be effective October 1, 2018.[41] According to HHS, the benefits of moving the SNS to ASPR include that: (1) a unified command for the SNS as the reorganization will vest the MCM production and stockpiling responsibilities with a single agency; (2) ASPR's mission is more targeted than that of the CDC's, enabling it to be a better

---

[35] Assistant Sec'y for Preparedness and Response, *supra* note 21.

[36] *Id.*

[37] *Id.*

[38] E-Mail from staff, Assistant Sec'y for Preparedness to staff, H. Comm on Energy and Commerce (June 12, 2018 4:02pm).

[39] *Id.*

[40] Letter from the Blue Ribbon Study Panel on Biodefense to Hon. Robert Kadlec, M.D., Assistant Sec'y for Preparedness and Response, U.S. Dep't of Health & Human Services (May 15, 2018) (on file with the Committee).

[41] U.S. Dep't of Health & Human Services, *Fiscal Year 2019 Public Health and Social Services Emergency Fund Justification of Estimates for Appropriations Committee*, *available at* https://www.hhs.gov/sites/default/files/fy-2019-phssef-cj.pdf.

advocate for the SNS; and (3) ASPR has established relationships with state/local emergency responders, who would play a critical role in a SNS deployment.[42]

National Pre-Pandemic Influenza Stockpile

In November 2005, the White House Homeland Security Council issued the *National Strategy for Pandemic Influenza*, designating HHS as the department to lead the nation's medical response to pandemic influenza.[43] According to the CDC, a pandemic influenza occurs when a new influenza A virus emerges, usually originating in animals, that is able to easily spread from person to person due to lack of effective treatments and acquired immunity.[44] The *National Strategy* also emphasized the need to ensure that the nation had an adequate MCM production capacity and stockpile to respond to potentially pandemic strains of influenza.[45] The Homeland Security Council reiterated the importance of having a pre-pandemic MCM stockpile in its *National Strategy Implementation Plan*, which was released in May 2006, categorizing the pandemic threat as a national security issue.[46]

BARDA, which was established by the Pandemic and All-Hazards Preparedness Act, is responsible for the procurement and management of the nation's pre-pandemic influenza stockpile as well as the development of influenza MCMs. BARDA is also tasked with accelerating the development and procurement of MCMs related to chemical, biological, radiological, and nuclear threats as well as threats related to emerging infectious diseases.[47]

In June 2017, and at the Committee's urging,[48] HHS issued an update to its *Pandemic Influenza Plan*, which was initially published in 2005 and had been last updated in 2009.[49] In the 2017 update, HHS stated that the national pre-pandemic influenza stockpile "satisfies requirements for vaccine and adjuvants to address influenza viruses that are assessed to be the highest risk for human infection."[50] BARDA, in collaboration with other HHS agencies, utilizes CDC's Influenza Risk Assessment Tool (IRAT) to assess pandemic risks that are associated with emerging novel influenza viruses and make

---

[42] *Id.*

[43] Executive Office of the President of the United States, Homeland Security Council, *National Strategy for Pandemic Influenza*, Nov. 2005 *available at* https://www.cdc.gov/flu/pandemic-resources/pdf/pandemic-influenza-strategy-2005.pdf.

[44] Centers for Disease Control and Prevention, *Influenza (Flu) Questions and Answers*, *available at* https://www.cdc.gov/flu/pandemic-resources/basics/faq.html (last updated May 15, 2017).

[45] Executive Office of the President, *supra* note 39.

[46] Executive Office of the President of the United States, Homeland Security Council, *National Strategy for Pandemic Influenza Implementation Plan*, May 2006 *available at* https://www.cdc.gov/flu/pandemic-resources/pdf/pandemic-influenza-implementation.pdf.

[47] 42 U.S.C. § 247d-7e.

[48] *See* Letter from the Hon. Greg Walden, Chairman, H. Comm. on Energy and Commerce, et al., to Hon. Thomas Price, M.D., Sec'y, U.S. Dep't of Health & Human Services (Apr. 20, 2017), *available at* https://archives-energycommerce.house.gov/sites/republicans.energy commerce.house.gov/files/documents/20170420HHS.pdf.

[49] U.S. Dep't of Health and Human Services, *Pandemic Influenza Plan 2017 Update* (last visited June 7, 2018) *available at* https://www.cdc.gov/flu/pandemic-resources/pdf/pan-flu-report-2017v2.pdf.

[50] *Id.*

determinations regarding a potential update to the pre-pandemic stockpile or the development of new vaccine candidates.[51]

CARB-X

CARB-X is a non-profit public-private partnership dedicated to accelerating antibacterial research to tackle the global rising three of drug-resistant bacteria.[52] With more than $500 million to invest between 2016 and 2021, CARB-X funds the research and development of new antibiotics, vaccines, rapid diagnostics and other life-saving products to tackle the global threat of drug-resistant bacteria. CARB-X was created in response to the U.S. government's 2015 Combating Antibiotic Resistant Bacteria (CARB) initiative, and the United Kingdom's government's call in 2016 for concerted global effort to address the growing drug-resistance public health crisis. Launched on July 28, 2016, CARB-X is a cooperative effort between BARDA and the NIAID. CARB-X is funded by BARDA and Wellcome Trust, the world's largest medical charity which is based in the U.K.

Science, Safety and Security of Laboratories in the Life Sciences-Biodefense Complex

Currently, there are about 1,200 high-containment laboratories in the U.S. conducting research on diagnostics and cures for highly dangerous pathogens. For more than a decade, the Subcommittee has held hearings and conducted investigations related to the Federal Select Agent Program, including on the safe handling of federal select agents and other dangerous pathogens.

Federal Select Agent Program

The Federal Select Agent Program regulates the possession, use, and transfer of biological select agents and toxins to ensure laboratory research conducted on the materials is done in a safe and secure manner. Sixty-six select agents and toxins that could potentially be used in bioterrorist attacks – including anthrax, smallpox, and plague – are currently regulated through the program. Managed jointly by HHS and the USDA, the program provides oversight of more than 275 entities that have registered through the program in order to conduct research on the hazardous pathogens.[53]

The Federal Select Agent Program was established in 1996 through the passage of the Antiterrorism and Effective Death Penalty Act. The law, passed in the aftermath of

[51] *See* Letter from Hon. Nicole Lurie, M.D., Assistant Sec'y for Preparedness and Response, U.S. Dep't of Health & Human Services to Hon. Fred Upton, Chairman, H. Comm. on Energy and Commerce (Mar. 15, 2016) *available at* https://archives-energycommerce.house.gov/sites/republicans.energycommerce.house.gov/files/documents/114/letters/20160229HHS%20Response.pdf.

[52] CARB-X, *About CARB-X*, https://carb-x.org/about/overview/ (last visited June 11, 2018).

[53] Federal Select Agent Program, *About Us*, https://www.selectagents.gov/about.html (last visited June 11, 2018).

the Oklahoma City bombing, required HHS to identify a list biological agents and toxins that could threaten public health and safety and establish regulations regarding the transfer of those agents. The September 11, 2001, terrorist attacks and the 2001 anthrax mailings led to increased concern about the threat of bioterrorism attacks, and additional restrictions which banned certain individuals from transporting or receiving select agents were included in the USA Patriot Act of 2001.[54] Congress expanded the program through the passage of the Public Health Security and Bioterrorism Preparedness and Response Act of 2002 to include regulation of the transfer and the use and possession of select agents and increased safeguards and security requirements.

Concerns raised by the mishandling of dangerous pathogens prompted the Committee to request an assessment of the select agent program by the GAO. In response to the Committee's request, the GAO reviewed oversight procedures of the select agent program and issued a report in October 2017 that highlighted deficiencies in the program's capabilities.[55] The report raised concerns about potential conflicts of interest as the select agent program is not independent from all the laboratories it oversees. The report also noted that the program has historically focused more on security and preventing thefts of select agents and toxins than on biological safety issues within the labs using the pathogens for research. The Subcommittee, which has held multiple hearings on the select agent program and safety lapses at federal labs, questioned USDA and CDC officials about the GAO report's conclusions and recommendations at a November 2, 2017, hearing.[56]

Prioritizing Lab Science and Safety

Following the 2014 incidents involving anthrax mishandling at the CDC and the smallpox discovered in storage for an FDA lab on the NIH campus, federal efforts intensified to improve the management of government labs. In particular, an external scientific working group recommended improvements to the CDC and FDA for overhauling their lab safety programs.

This included the recommendation that a program director would be a single point of accountability and would have a direct reporting relationship to the head of the agency. When Stephan S. Monroe, the CDC's Associate Director for Laboratory Science and Safety (ADLSS), testified before the Subcommittee in April 2016, he said the formation of the director position was "the most fundamental change implemented in the wake of

---

[54] *See* USA Patriot Act of 2001, Pub. L. No. 107-56, 115 Stat. 272 (2001).

[55] U.S. Gov't Accountability Office, *Coordinated Actions Needed to Enhance the Select Agent Program's Oversight of Hazardous Pathogens*, GAO-18-145 (Oct. 2017) *available at* https://www.gao.gov/assets/690/687868.pdf.

[56] *See Concerns Over Federal Select Agent Program Oversight of Dangerous Pathogens Before the Subcom. on Oversight and Investigations of the H. Comm. on Energy and Commerce* 115th Cong. (2017) *available at* https://docs.house.gov/meetings/IF/IF02/20171102/106574/HHRG-115-IF02-Transcript-20171102.pdf.

the 2014 incidents."[57] Further, Dr. Monroe noted that the fact that the ADLSS reported directly to the CDC director provided "high-level oversight and coordination of critical laboratory policies and operations" across all CDC campuses.

In response to the 2014 safety lapses,[58] the FDA's Office of Laboratory Science and Safety (OLSS) was formed in order to provide oversight and to improve security and safety across all divisions of FDA. The formation of the office was announced in 2016 as a means to consolidate oversight responsibilities and standard policies for all FDA laboratories. In 2017, the FDA issued a strategic plan outlining the goals of the new office.

According to the OLSS strategic plan, the office's mission is to:

- Ensure FDA's laboratories and workplaces are operated in a safe and secure manner to protect employees, the surrounding communities, and the environment;
- Research and disseminate innovative ideas and validated methods for safe and secure laboratory practices;
- Support high-quality (i.e., accurate, reliable, and timely) FDA laboratory results; and
- Promote a culture of shared responsibility and safety.[59]

Just as the ADLSS was organized to directly report to the CDC Director, the OLSS was also envisioned to directly report to the FDA Commissioner. A reorganization issued by the FDA in 2017 made the OLSS a direct report to the FDA Commissioner.[60] However, the FDA now plans to have the OLSS report to the Office of the Chief Scientist instead of directly to the Commissioner.[61]

In addition, the budget and staffing for the OLSS have not been consistent. In 2016, the FDA informed the Committee that the office's budget for FY 2017 was $5.2 million

[57] *Laboratory Safety at the Centers for Disease Control and Prevention Before the Subcomm. on Oversight and Investigations of the H. Comm on Energy and Commerce*, 114th Cong. (2016) (written testimony of Hon. Stephan S. Monroe, PhD., Assoc. Dir. for Laboratory Science and Safety, Centers for Disease Control and Prevention) *available at* https://docs.house.gov/meetings/IF/IF02/20160420/104823/HHRG-114-IF02-Wstate-MonroeS-20160420.pdf.

[58] Brady Dennis and Lena H. Sun, *FDA found more than smallpox vials in storage room*, WASH. POST, July 16, 2014, https://www.washingtonpost.com/national/health-science/fda-found-more-than-smallpox-vials-in-storage-room/2014/07/16/850d4b12-0d22-11e4-8341-b8072b1e7348_story.html.

[59] U.S. Food and Drug Admin., 2017-2022 Operating Model – *Office of Laboratory Science and Safety*, Updated Oct. 13, 2017, *available at* https://www.fda.gov/downloads/AboutFDA/CentersOffices/OC/OLSS/UCM583016.pdf.

[60] *See* 82 Fed. Reg. 34540 (July 25, 2017) *available at* https://www.federalregister.gov/documents/2017/07/25/2017-15564/office-of-the-commissioner-statement-of-organization-functions-and-delegations-of-authority.

[61] Briefing by staff, U.S. Dep't of Health & Human Services, U.S. Food and Drug Admin. with staff, H. Comm. on Energy and Commerce, June 11, 2018.

and that it would support 13 full time employees.[62] FDA officials subsequently told Committee staff that the FY 2017 budget for OLSS was $9 million, but that funding levels would support not just OLSS operations (including staff and contractor support) but also the Employee Safety and Environmental Management staff that were transferred to OLSS.[63] The FDA later informed the Committee that no permanent full-time employees (FTE) were hired by OLSS in FY 2017, rather the office recruited 19 individuals through temporary detail assignments and contract support.[64] In a briefing with Committee staff, the FDA confirmed that the office's FY 2018 budget is $5.6 million and the FY 2019 budget is $6 million.[65] The office currently employs three FTEs and three contractors. At this time, FDA has not reported the total number of FDA laboratories to the Committee staff. FDA has not yet reported to the Committee the number of audits that OLSS has conducted.

By contrast, the CDC's ADLSS office's FY 2016 budget was $14.5 million and supported 34 FTEs.[66] As of this month, the office had 43 FTEs with three slots vacant and oversaw audits of laboratories used by 239 teams of scientists.[67] The CDC recently reported to Committee staff that it had submitted a proposed reorganization to the Department that would eliminate the Associate Director's direct reporting relationship to the Director, and instead would report to a Deputy Director.[68]

Issues

The following issues may be examined at the hearing:

- How timely are the PHEMCE decisions regarding biological threats being made? Can the timeliness of these decisions be improved?
- How can the number of FDA-approved assays for threat agents be increased?
- Is there adequate oversight to ensure the efficacy of MCMs in the SNS and the prepandemic vaccine stockpile?

---

[62] Letter from Dayle Cristinzio, Acting Assoc. Comm'r for Legislation, U.S. Food and Drug Admin., to Hon. Fred Upton, Chairman, H. Comm. on Energy and Commerce. (Sept. 9, 2016) (On file with the Committee).

[63] E-Mail from staff, U.S. Food and Drug Admin. to staff, H.Comm. on Energy and Commerce (May 17, 2017, 3:57pm) (On file with the Committee).

[64] E-mail from staff, U.S. Food and Drug Admin. to staff, H. Comm. on Energy and Commerce (Aug. 20, 2017, 12:50pm) (On file with the Committee).

[65] U.S. Food and Drug Admin., *supra* note 57.

[66] Letter from Hon. Fred Upton, Chairman, H. Comm. on Energy and Commerce and Hon. Tim Murphy, Chairman, H. Comm. on Energy and Commerce, Subcomm. on Oversight and Investigations to Hon. Robert M. Califf, M.D. Comm'r, U.S. Food and Drug Admin. (May 18, 2016) (citing E-mail from staff, Centers for Disease Control and Prevention to staff, H. Comm. on Energy and Commerce (Apr. 15, 2016)) (On file with the Committee).

[67] Briefing by staff, U.S. Dep't of Health & Human Services, Centers for Disease Control and Prevention with staff, H. Comm. on Energy and Commerce, June 8, 2018.

[68] *Id.*

- Are U.S. public health agencies implementing recommendations to improve laboratory science and safety?

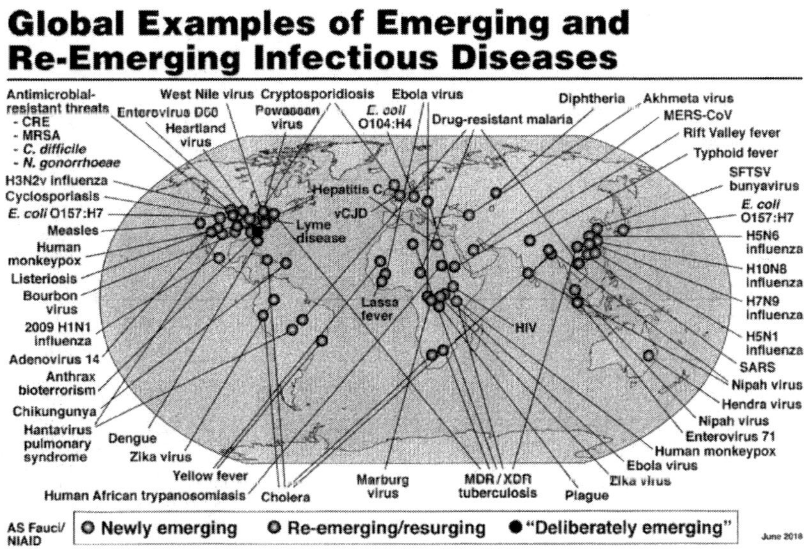

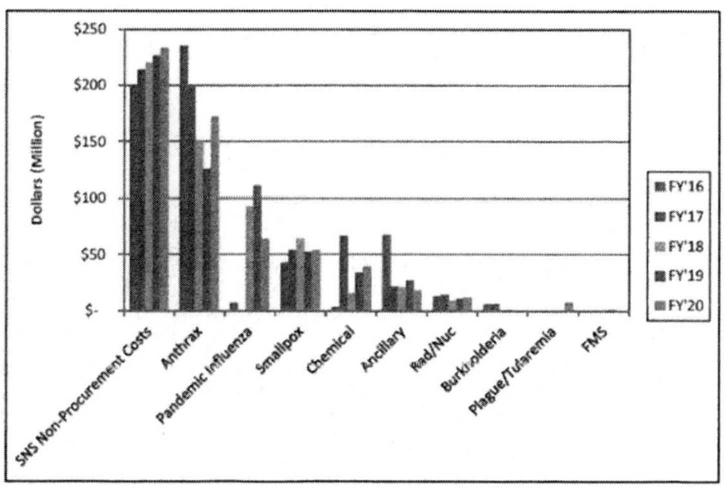

Figure 1. Estimated DSNS Spending, by Portfolio.

Blue Ribbon Study Panel on Biodefense

May 15, 2018

The Honorable Robert Kadlec
Assistant Secretary for Preparedness and Response
U.S. Department of Health and Human Services
Washington, DC

Re: Transforming medical countermeasure technology and partnerships

Dear Dr. Robert Kadlec:

The Blue Ribbon Study Panel on Biodefense recently moderated two roundtables to identify ways to overcome some of the most vexing medical countermeasure (MCM) technology, business, and policy challenges across the biological threat domain. Private sector pharmaceutical, scientific, academic, and governmental affairs representatives attended and were joined at the second meeting by federal officials from the Department of Agriculture (USDA), Department of Defense (DOD), Department of Health and Human Services (HHS), and the White House.

The MCM assets now available to civilians and to military personnel have grown substantially in the last decade. The partnerships needed to continue to build these assets to meet persistent and advancing biological threats, however, are now at considerable risk. Real and perceived under investment, unsustained investment, process uncertainty, and strategic disparity undermine what must be a vibrant enterprise. We maintain that advancing the national MCM infrastructure needed for research, development, and procurement will reduce the risk associated with biological warfare, bioterrorism, emerging infectious diseases, and biological accidents. We urge you to demonstrate your commitment to this core national security function by advancing the following recommendations.

1. Integrate animal health into the national security approach to medical countermeasures. The gross inequality between human and animal funding levels and the segregation of research between the two sectors constitute a national security liability. Many material threats. select agents, and emerging infectious diseases are human diseases with veterinary counterparts, some of which regularly cause outbreaks elsewhere in the world in livestock and wildlife. Yet conversations about the protection of human health by controlling emerging infectious diseases in animal hosts have been extremely limited, and the authority of animal health agencies to regulate has been based on animal health, not public health.
   a. *Establish a framework for combatting emerging infectious diseases.* Most emerging infectious diseases in people originate in animals. No MCM were ready when the largest Ebola outbreak the world had ever seen -likely caused by a spillover from bats to humans-occurred. In the preceding years, the government had not sufficiently determined what to fund with its limited resources. At present, HHS prioritizes efforts to address biological threat agents via Department of Homeland Security material threat determinations (MTDs), but the U.S. government has not instituted and budgeted for an analogous process for emerging infectious diseases. In accordance with Blue

Ribbon Study Panel Recommendation 7c *(A National Blueprint for Biodefense,* 2015), HHS, in coordination with DOD and USDA, should create a similar prioritization framework for emerging infectious disease threats. This framework should address pathogens and pathogen families with the potential to cause a catastrophic public health emergency and include agents known to infect wildlife and domestic animals. It should drive funding for MCM development and other areas (e.g., biosurveillance, response planning) and engage and motivate the private sector to develop and manufacture MCM. Funders must establish a vision for an emerging infectious disease MCM enterprise, define what constitutes successful emerging infectious disease MCM, and communicate this vision along with specific product requirements to industry partners.

b. *Make USDA part of the Public Health Emergency Medical Countermeasures Enterprise (PHEMCE):* BARDA was envisioned to be part of- not the entire- MCM enterprise. USDA should also participate in PHEMCE. Many diseases that could necessitate USDA MCM acquisitions are the same for DOD and HHS. USDA also has lessons to share about how it works with industry to develop effective MCM for production animals, a market in which the cost must be low and eflicacy must be high. Some veterinary companies are already using platforms to develop their animal products, and the veterinary development timeline is much shorter. This means animal health pharmaceutical companies get products to market earlier. These companies also possess extensive experience in areas like animal models and manufacturability that can help inform human MCM endeavors. These experiences are relevant and should not be ignored.

c. *Require animal disease risk assessment.* USDA should develop a risk assessment for animal diseases and work with HHS to assess the risk of diseases with zoonotic potential. USDA should assess the ability of the National Veterinary Stockpile to deploy sullicient MCM to combat high-consequence animal diseases within 24 hours of request. USDA should also use these risk assessments to prioritize the pathogens identified on the USDA *High-Consequence Foreign Animal Diseases and Pests* list. USDA should use the findings to inform its budget request; drive federal priorities for MCM innovation; and incentivize public-private partnerships to develop, transition, approve, license, and procure these products.

2. Reduce market and process uncertainty at BARDA. Variability and lack of certainty are two of the foremost hurdles to expanding industry participation in MCM advanced development and manufacturing. Indeed, these hurdles may prove so significant for some companies, even those that have successfully delivered MCM, that they may exit the market entirely. Although all

biopharmaceutical ventures carry risk, larger companies can manage this risk through a balanced portfolio of projects, the most successful of which can yield a high return on investment. Pervasive market uncertainty in the far less profitable MCM enterprise makes business endeavors unattractive and unsustainable.

a. *Create fiscal certainty.* In order to develop national security MCM, industry partners forego potential profit margins orders of magnitude higher than for commercial products. These companies need certainty in procurement to convince them and their investors that engaging in MCM development makes reasonable business sense. The annual appropriations process for advanced development and procurement, and dependency on emergency supplemental appropriations for unanticipated threats, make doing business with companies that base their operations on multi-year outlooks and planning unsustainable. In accordance with Blue Ribbon Study Panel Recommendation 28b *(A National Blueprint for Biodefense,* 2015),

Congress must reinstate the advanced appropriation for Project BioShieid for ten years at a minimum of $7.1 billion. Additionally, in accordance with Blue Ribbon Study Panel Recommendation 28c, Congress and the HHS Assistant Secretary for Preparedness and Response (ASPR) should address prioritization and the need for guaranteed, sustained funding for pandemic influenza preparedness. The appropriation levels must be tied to rigorously established MCM requirements based on risk analysis.

b. *Create process certainty:* In the last several years, the f IHS Biomedical Advanced Research and Development Authority (BARDA) noticeably shifted away from process and partnership toward product. Prioritizing products over partnerships has damaged partnerships and preparedness. The rules governing BARDA and *DOD* processes for advanced development and manufacturing should be defined with industry partners up front and with far greater clarity and commitment. Companies need to understand when and how much of their proposed product the government will procure, as the frequent moving of goalposts throughout development and procurement creates an untenable business environment For projects in which the government is not interested, federal public health security leaders need to relay that quickly (i.e., white papers should be reviewed and comment provided within 45 days). The BARDA process at this stage of review should be more like that of the Defense Advanced Research Projects Agency (DARPA), for which program managers, not contracting officers, are the central deciding figures.

3. Accelerate platform technologies. One way to create MCM quickly, safely, and effectively for unpredictable emerging infectious diseases and outbreaks is to develop a suite of platfonn technologies. Generally, platform technologies rely

upon a common manufacturing process backbone that uses a standard process to insert foreign genes. By relying upon a well-established manufacturing process and customization though standardized processes, platform technologies can reduce the risk associated with development. These production platforms may be based on, but not limited to, RNA expression systems; DNA cloning vectors; various virus, plant, or bacterial expression vectors; and viral-vectored vaccines. With targeted government and industry investments, these technologies could come to fruition within three to four years, especially for vaccines and diagnostics. To mature the technology, however, the government must mature the way it invests in the technology and ensure that partnership and business plans accompany technical plans for leveraging any platform capability. There is presently no business model in place that addresses how the government can work with industry to develop MCM platforms. At a minimum, elements of certification, expedited review, and the role of the HHS Centers for Innovation in Advanced Development and Manufacturing must be addressed.

a. *Certify platforms:* The Food and Drug Administration (FDA) approves products, not platforms. FDA, in consultation with DOD, BARDA, and other PHEMCE partners, should establish an MCM platform certification process. A regulatory construct that allows for the consideration of a company's novel platform as a basis for future MCM products would serve as an industry incentive. Its establishment would effectively reduce the risk of future product development using that platform. Determining what constitutes a platform will be difficult, but the definition should include a regularized chemistry, manufacturing, and controls (CMC) process and standardized general release criteria. The USDA Center for Veterinary Biologics policy, "Licensing Guidelines for Production Platform-Based, Non-Replicating, Nonviable Products," allows for rapid swapping of closely related immunogenic determinants, and could provide a starting point from which FDA could build a platform certification process for human products.
b. *Priority review platforms:* The platform certification process described above is likely to be extensive and should result in a thorough FDA understanding of the platform technology (e.g., CMC, clinical experience). This advanced understanding will enable subsequent review by the FDA under the expedited Priority Review process of other products based upon that certified platform. FDA commitment to the accelerated approval times associated with Priority Review for subsequent products utilizing a certified platform would provide significant incentive for industry to utilize appropriate platform technologies.
c. *Leverage CIADMs,'* The HHS CIADMs and the DOD MCM Advanced Development and Manufacturing facility (ADM) were envisioned to make

such platform-based products a reality. They could enable advanced development and manufacturing of platform technologies if aggressively integrated into the product development process. They should become places where companies want to go to advance their promising technologies. They should shrink development schedules and address significant business difficulties. At present, two major challenges prevent this: small companies are concerned about protecting their intellectual property when handed over to a privately owned ADM with its own MCM interests, and large companies are concerned about risks to their commercial business during regulatory review. The Salk Institute, a private nonprofit organization, was essentially the forenmner of what we think of as an ADM today, and BARDA should consider Salk's example as it revisits the business model for these kinds of facilities. DOD and BARDA should undertake planning for ClADM reconfiguration immediately. Planning should include industry and all federal agencies with MCM responsibility. Considerable thought must be given to contracting reform (discussed below) as the Federal Acquisition Regulation (FAR)-based, cost- reimbursable contract system in place does not work. An independent assessment (outside of DOD and HHS) of the existing CIADM model is needed to support this rcconfiguration. This planning must consider the role of the USDA and its industry partners in using the CIADMs to enable mutually beneficial technologies and to keep the facilities in use.

4. Reform FDA process to develop products faster. We can get closer to on-demand MCM in just a few years and investments to improve production cycling by days or weeks are possible. These kinds of advances, however, will not provide the same near-tenn relief that FDA could achieved on release testing. Investment in enabling technologies must go, therefore, hand in hand with reform of regulatory process. FDA needs to be part of the advanced development process early on, describing what it wants to see in a product or an investigational new drug. Advances in the speed with which products are marketed should not compromise the FDA's high safety and efficacy standards.
    a. *Standardize and clarify regulatory process.* The FDA, in collaboration with its upstream development government partners, must address development and standardization of regulatory processes that will provide needed transparency to MCM developers. The MCM industry needs to understand all elements of the process, and the government needs to mitigate the inherent risk. Several areas of regulatory reform should be considered- for example, reducing risk associated with clinical trials, and allowing companies to focus their resources on development. Through P.L. 115-92, Congress authorized DOD to request, and FDA to provide, assistance to expedite the FDA review process for MCM for military personnel. DOD and

FDA have now put a work plan in place to coordinate planning for this process. FDA and BARDA should develop a parallel plan. Expedited release testing and a plan for increased usage of emergency use authorizations (EUAs) should be addressed as part of this plan.

b. *Expedite release testing:* Even with a vaccine platfonn, the response time to produce a vaccine for the foreseeable future will be 6-12 months for mass-produced product. While maintaining safety and efficacy standards, acceptable FDA release testing during an outbreak might be different from acceptable release testing at other times. FDA should consider options. For instance, FDA might release products for use on an interim basis with final release testing to follow. FDA might identify suitable surrogates in place of full toxicology panels- or at least utilize a process to pre-identify what those surrogates would be. FDA should describe what an accelerated schedule would look like in an emergency. This will be especially important for platforms that could address multiple infectious diseases. Once in place, manufacturers could then propose specific schedules for a given MCM.

c. *Examine increased usage of Emergency Use Authorizations:* EUAs are designed for those MCM that are sufficiently well characterized to be oflikely clinical benefit in an emergency. FDA essentially certifies that a given MCM fulfills EUA requirements. FDA should detennine when more aggressive utilization ofEUAs would be appropriate.

5. Improve contracting authorities. BARDA must be empowered to make decisions in the best interest of fulfilling its mission. This means ensuring that the contracting process is as smooth, flexible, and transparent as possible. Other Transactional Authority (OTA) is most prominent among the existing contracting authorities that would incentivize MCM partnerships, yet it is utilized very rarely and limited by the statute that provided OTA authority to BARDA.

a. *Amend the OTA statute.* Congress modeled the OTA authority addressed in the *Pandemic All-Hazards Preparedness Act (PAHPA)* after DOD's OTA statute. In its reauthorization of *PAHPA,* Congress should customize OTA authority to fit BARDA's needs. Congress should also remove references to DOD and the need for approval by the senior executive for projects above $20 million (as it did previously for DOD). OTA contracts should become far more common than they are now, perhaps as common if not more than FAR-based contracts.

b. *Adopt OTAfor the CIADMs:* FAR-based contracting does not work for rapid response procurements.

Using OTA for the ADMs is critical to prevent abandonment of partnerships when rapidity is imperative, when the science does not go as planned, and when intellectual property and FAR-based requirements arise. DOD has adopted this OTA-based model for its ADM.

c. *Move contracting authority back to BARDA.* In accordance with Blue Ribbon Study Panel Recommendation 29a *(A National Blueprint for BiodO fense,* 2015), and the *21st Century Cures Act* Section 3082, contracting authority should be the exclusive responsibility of BARDA, not the office of Acquisition, Management, Contracts and Grants in the Office of the ASPR. This move must be finalized.

6. Foster innovation and new capabilities. The government often bases MCM-related plans on budgets instead of basing budgets on need. A similar mindset is seen with the government's approach to industry, often issuing solicitations to assess existing capabilities, rather than fostering new capabilities to meet national security needs. At the time of its authorization in *PAHPA,* Congress envisioned BARDA to be on the leading edge ofMCM innovation. Over the past decade, BARDA has focused on more, well-established, product development technologies and investments in technologies closer to full maturity. This approach certainly justified much of the development portfolio. Live viral vaccine platforms and therapeutics based on monoclonal antibodies may well provide near- to medium-term solutions. Yet BARDA needs to devote sufficient resources to novel and high-risk product development activities in parallel with their less risky investments.

a. *Invest in novel and high-risk products.* Meeting emerging national security threats will require BARDA to employ a high-risk, high-reward model for at least a portion of its investments. Instead of issuing solicitations to assess current industry capabilities, agencies should aggressively work with the private sector to build capabilities to meet national security needs. While investment in tried-and-true technologies will remain important, aggressively pursuing technologies that fall outside BARDA's comfort zone is imperative. The *21st Century Cures Act* authorized the Director of BARDA to engage an independent. non-profit innovation partner. BARDA should leverage this opportunity to dedicate additional resources to high-risk, high-reward outputs. It should further consider the role of the animal sector in providing needed technological advancements. The animal sector has existing markets for certain pharmaceuticals (for instance, with respect to coronavimses and influenza viruses, which happen to be the most significant viral pandemic threats to the human population) that are lacking in in the human sector. A shared interagency approach to planning for, and funding in, such areas could' lead to needed innovative breakthroughs. Precedence for interagency funding mechanisms can be found in the funding HHS provided to USDA in 2009 to conduct domestic biosurveillance for swine influenza virus, a pathogen with minimal health impacts on the animal carrier but large potential impacts on public health.

b. *Invest in rapid diagnostics,* The nation needs to invest far more in patient-side, point-of-care diagnostics.

Diagnostics can guide prioritization of MCM resources, but MCM conversations often refer only to vaccines and therapeutics, omitting diagnostics altogether. Rapid diagnostics cannot continue to be an afterthought. In accordance with Blue Ribbon Study Panel Recommendation 30a *(A National Blueprint for Biodejimse,* 2015), DOD and BARDA need to invest in rapid diagnostics as a core element of their MCM portfolios. This work should identity generalized biomarkers that would enable such technologies.

c. *Drive decision-making with early warning and predictive tools.* Leadership has yet to embrace predictive science as a core capacity that can support traditional and transformative MCM development. Advances in genomics and proteomics, risk mapping, and biosurvcillance data analytics should all be leveraged to create early warning that could both inform and spare the stockpile. Budget requests and corresponding appropriations should support these efforts and ensure that they are an integral part of the federal MCM development and procurement strategy by aligning MCM investments with the threats identified through early warning programs.

7. Establish end-to-end enterprise coordination. Although PHEMCE was envisioned as a coordinating body for the federal MCM enterprise, it has been too HI·IS-centric to do this effectively. Development of a far more forward-looking process -from idea to procurement to dispensing- is needed. As the Office of the ASPR reimagines the end-to-end nature of the enterprise, it has an opportunity to address some specific challcngcs in thc currcnt construct.

   a. *Improve interagency product transitions.*Successful research projects at the National Institutes of Health, DARPA, or other agencies, must begin competition anew for advanced development- if advanced development funding is even available or prioritized. This creates major bureaucratic hurdles to product advancement. The National Biodefense Strategy should direct the creation of more streamlined interagency transition mechanisms. A wards can be structured to assume transition from one agency to the next.

   b. *Transfer management oftlte Strategic National Stockpile under specific conditions.*In the President's Budget Request for FY 2019, the Administration moved management responsibility of the Strategic National Stockpile (SNS) from the Centers for Disease Control and Prevention (CDC) to the ASPR. CDC management of the SNS has been inadequate, resulting in industry confusion and losses when the agency suddenly decided to remove elements from the stockpile that it had previously approved. The

Administration made this move, in part, to better enable HHS leadership to direct acquisition for, and deployment of, the SNS. The move has the potential to create a more cohesive development-to- distribution structure and apply more process certainty to procurement decisions. Concems about how BARDA and the SNS will interact once the move is finalized, and whether investments made by BARDA will inadvertently or intentionally force the SNS to acquire those MCM it developed, must be addressed. Congress should authorize the transfer of management of the SNS to the ASPR only if it also requires the ASPR to fix SNS-related problems that the CDC and state, local, tribal, and territorial (SLTT) partners previously encountered or created, and to put controls in place to prevent automatic uptake ofBARDA products by the SNS just to demonstrate BARDA success. Congress should also direct the ASPR to establish a meaningful SNS training program for SLTT partners that focuses on more than just anthrax, takes SLTT ability to distribute SNS pallets upon receipt into consideration, and does not assume distribution will occur the same as in the military.

c. *Produce an MCM response framework.* In accordance with Blue Ribbon Study Panel Recommendation 22a *(A National Blueprint for Biodefense,* 2015), the Office of the ASPR, CDC, and the Federal Emergency Management Agency should, together with non-federal partners, identify requirements and capacities needed to achieve successful distribution and dispensing of MCM from the SNS as well as from local caches. The framework they develop must address unresolved issues. A progressive and innovative approach should push beyond what a given agency might devise and the bureaucratic impediments associated with a federal-only distribution system. If implementation exceeds funding available through current grant allocations, additional funding must be requested.

Sincerely,

Joseph I. Lieberman, CHair
Donna E. Shalala

James C Greenwood

Thomas J. Ridge,
Chair

Thomas A. Daschle

Kenneth L. Wainstein

Rick Bright,
CC BARDA Director

Jenn Alton

Greg Walden, Oregon
Chairman

Frank Pallone, Jr., New Jersey
Ranking Member

One Hundred Fifteenth Congress
Congress of the United States
House of Representtives
Committee on Energy and Commerce

July 12, 2018
Dr, Rick A. Bright
Director, Biomedical Advanced Research and Development Authority
Deputy Assistant Secretary,
Office of the Assistant Secretary for Preparedness and Response
U.S. Department of Health and Human Services

Dear Dr. Bright:

Thank you for appearing before the Subcommittee on Oversight and Investigations on June I 5, 2018, to testify at the hearing entitled' "The State of U.S. Public Health Biopreparedness: Responding to Biological Attacks, Pandemics, and Emerging Disease Outbreaks."

Pursuant to the Rules of the Committee on Energy and Commerce, the bearing record remains open for ten business days to permit Members to submit additional questions for the record, which are attached. To facilitate the printing of the hearing record, please respond to these questions with a transmittal letter by the close of business on Thursday, July 26, 2018. Your responses should be mailed to Ali Fulling, Legislative Clerk, Committee on Energy and Commerce, 2125 Rayburn House Office Building, Washington, DC 20515 and e-mailed in Word format to Ali.Fulling@mail.house.gov.

Thank you again for your time and eff011 preparing and delivering testimony before the Subcommittee.

Sincerely,

Gregg Harper
Chairman
Subcommittee on Oversight and Investigations

cc: The Honorable Diana DeGette, Ranking Member, Subcommittee on Oversight and Investigations
Attachment

HOUSE ENERGY AND COMMERCE COMMITTEE, SUBCOMMITTEE ON OVERSIGHT AND INVESTIGATIONS, "THE STATE OF U.S. PUBLIC HEALTH BIOPREPAREDNESS: RESPONDING TO BIOLOGICAL ATTACKS, PANDEMICS, AND EMERGING INFECTIOUS DISEASE OUTBREAKS," DR. RICK BRIGHT, DIRECTOR OF ASPR'S BIOMEDICAL ADVANCED RESEARCH AND DEVELOPMENT AUTHORITY, FRIDAY, JUNE 15, 2018

The Honorable Gregg Harper

1) In the 2017 update to HHS' Pandemic Influenza Plan, HHS provided benchmarks for manufacturing and distributing vaccines during declared influenza pandemics. HHS stated that it aims to ensure that limited vaccine distribution occurs within 12 weeks of a pandemic being declared, with distribution sufficient to meet overall public demand occurring within 16 weeks. Could you tell us why this process seemingly takes so long, and provide any recommendations for improving it? If the 12 and 16-week benchmarks are HHS's goals, what are our current capabilities?

ASPR Response

Domestic manufacturing capacity for pandemic influenza vaccine is a critical component of pandemic preparedness to ensure vaccine is available as soon as possible after emergence of a pandemic virus. ASPR/BARDA has made significant gains in pandemic influenza vaccine preparedness over the last 10 years, including supporting the licensure of faster, more flexible cell-based, recombinant and adjuvanted influenza vaccines and modernizing and expanding domestic manufacturing capabilities. These advancements have dramatically increased the domestic influenza vaccine antigen capacity increasing from 60 million doses to 600 million doses.

Building on these successes, and to ensure vaccine is available within 12 weeks of pandemic declaration, ASPRJBARDA has a multifaceted approach in place. First

ASPR/BARDA is partnering with companies to support the development of novel technologies that rely less on viral growth properties to improve the speed and robustness of vaccine production. For example, ASPRJBARDA supported the first licensed recombinant influenza vaccine (Flublok®), and ASPRJBARDA continues to fund recombinant vaccine-related efforts, moving away from the slow, inflexible production of vaccine in eggs. Second, ASPRJBARDA is supporting the sustainment of domestic production capabilities to ensure vaccines are available when necessary. Third, ASPRJBARDA is supporting further development of recombinant and cell-based vaccines through comparative efficacy clinical studies to expand use indications for a broad range of high- risk and special populations. Fourth, ASPRJBARDA is supporting the addition of currently approved adjuvanted influenza vaccines for all ages into both seasonal and pandemic vaccines, while also developing additional adjuvant options that provide safe and enhanced effectiveness to influenza vaccines that are faster to produce. Lastly, ASPRJBARDA is targeting advancements in vaccine delivery and administration to develop new approaches that would reduce reliance on needles and syringes supply chain surge capacity and allow faster and more efficient immunization with pandemic vaccine.

2) In general, what is the shelf-life for the H7N9 influenza strain vaccine that is in BARDA's pre-pandemic stockpile that will protect against the 2013 H7N9 strain? When was the last time BARDA performed a potency test on these vaccines?

ASPR Response

The pre-pandemic vaccine made in eggs against the 2013 H7N9 avian influenza virus strain is very stable, with over 80% stability as of the last potency test conducted November, 2017. The most recent potency testing for the egg based vaccine was performed in May 2018 and we are awaiting results of this testing.

3) How serious of a pandemic threat does the BARDA view the 5th wave H7N9 influenza strain, currently circulating in China? If a pandemic were to occur, how severely would it impact public health? Is BARDA currently overseeing the manufacturing of a vaccine for storage in its pre-pandemic stockpile which will match this H7N9 influenza strain?

ASPR Response

BARDA views the 5th wave H7N9 influenza outbreak as a serious concern, as reflected by the high Influenza Risk Assessment Tool (IRAT) score assigned by CDC. Since this assessment system, which assesses the threat of influenza viruses with pandemic potential, was initiated in 20 II, the 5th wave H7N9 strain has the highest Potential Impact Risk of any influenza strain evaluated.

Given the human mortality rate seen to date, if the viruses changed to allow them to spread easily between humans, the impact on public health could be catastrophic in the absence of effective medical countermeasures such as vaccines. There is also evidence that some H7N9 influenza viruses may be resistant to most available antiviral drugs.

In response, BARDA produced bulk vaccine, currently held in storage, which matches the 5th wave H7N9 strain. Additionally, the National Institutes of Health (NIH) and BARDA are conducting clinical trials to better understand optimal vaccination approaches in the event mass vaccinations are necessary.

4) How much is BARDA currently spending on CARB-X? Does the agency anticipate maintaining this level of spending over the next five years?

ASPR Response

BARDA established CARB-X in collaboration with the NIH's National Institute of Allergy and Infectious Diseases in 2016. CARB-X, an innovative public-private partnership that addresses the threat of antibiotic resistant bacteria, has received $85 million in support from BARDA over two years. CARB-X is also funded by the Wellcome Trust. In 2018 the Bill &Melinda Gates Foundation and the United Kingdom Government's Department of Health and Social Care joined as funding partners. BARDA's support for new antibiotics and diagnostics is critical to address 21st century health security threats including genetically engineered bacterial pathogens, complications of bacterial infections as a result of exposure to priority threats such as nuclear and chemical agents, and to quickly identify bacterial pathogens and their susceptibility to antibiotics. BARDA anticipates continued support based on availability of funds.

5) What is the PHEMCE's role in making a material threat determination, and how can the length of time it takes for such a determination be reduced?

ASPR Response

The Public Health and Emergency Medical Countermeasure Enterprise (PHEMCE), a Federal advisory and coordinating body led by ASPR, does have a role in advising on medical countermeasure requirements for national security material threats identified by the Department of Homeland Security (DHS). DHS's newly established Countering Weapons of Mass Destruction Office issues material threat assessments (MTAs) and the Secretary of the Department of Homeland Security (DHS) issues material threat determinations (MTDs). MTAs and MTDs are done in collaboration with other interagency departments, but the responsibility for generating these national, strategic overviews and quantification of the threat is identified by statute (section 319F-2(c)(2) of the Public Health Service Act (42 U.S.C. 247d-6b(c)(2)), added by the Project BioShield

Act of 2004") as a DHS authority and responsibility. The PHEMCE benefits from these determinations and uses them to forecast medical countermeasure requirements (type, quantity, special considerations). ASPR is currently working with other PHEMCE interagency partners to evaluate and identify opportunities to streamline and speed up these deliberative steps. We would be pleased to brief the Committee on potential process improvements after the evaluation is completed.

6) After ASPR assumes operational control of the Strategic National Stockpile on October 1, 2018, what role will CDC play in support of the stockpile's mission?

ASPR Response

ASPR recognizes and appreciates the tremendous expertise of CDC subject matter experts including on infectious diseases, other public health threats, epidemiological and laboratory surveillance, as well as understanding of the capabilities of state and local public health departments. CDC is an active partner on the PHEMCE, which is led by ASPR and provides a venue for sharing information across HHS agencies and with interagency partners with a role in medical countermeasures requirement setting, research, development, regulatory review, procurement, stockpiling, distribution and use. CDC will remain an active participant in all PHEMCE workgroups and committees.

In order to ensure a smooth transition of the Strategic National Stockpile with no degradation of operational capability, ASPR and CDC have set up several joint transition workgroups to evaluate all aspects of the program transition. Some of the details involved in the transition have not been finalized. However, we would be pleased to provide a full briefing for Committee staff at any time before the end of the fiscal year. Subsequent to this hearing, the SNS successfully transferred from CDC to ASPR on October 1, 2018.

CDC will maintain its strong working relationships with state and local public health agencies, playing a key role in distribution and dispensing of medical countermeasures. CDC will accomplish this by continuing to provide technical guidance and funding through cooperative agreements and embedding experts in state and local health departments. Coordination with state and local agencies will be enhanced by incorporating ASPR's extensive relationships with health care organizations and emergency management agencies.

Further, to continue to increase collaboration across the Department, ASPR has invited and instituted a new senior CDC liaison who is working within the ASPR Immediate Office.

7) How prepared are the nation's hospitals to respond to biological threats or infectious diseases? What are the most pressing challenges facing non- governmental health systems and what could we do to improve their response capabilities?

ASPR Response

Since the Hospital Preparedness Program (HPP) was established, investments have been made to enhance the overall preparedness of the nation's healthcare infrastructure. Initially, HPP supported the procurement of materials and supplies (e.g., generators, masks, etc.) that would be used should a community be impacted by a public health or medical event. In 2012, HPP shifted its focus from purchasing supplies to investing in health care coalitions (HCCs). HCCs are groups of health care and response organizations that collaborate to prepare for and respond to medical surge events. HCCs incentivize diverse and often competitive health care organizations to work together. During recent events, ranging from mass shootings (e.g., Las Vegas, Florida night club), hurricanes (e.g., Matthew, Harvey, Irma, and Maria), and the most recent tornados in Iowa, we have witnessed the value of the HCCs in enabling communities to quickly assess healthcare capabilities to continue to support communities without requesting assistance from the federal government.

Prior to the 2014 Ebola outbreak in West Africa, the United States did not have an organized, systematic approach to preparing for, and responding to, an outbreak of a highly infectious pathogen. CDC in collaboration with ASPR developed a tiered approach to prepare U.S. health care facilities to safely and rapidly identify, isolate, evaluate, and manage, travelers or patients who have possible or confirmed Ebola. This included providing rapid technical assistance to hospitals strategically located near airports with a large number of travelers returning from Ebola-affected countries and in communities where large numbers of persons from these West African countries reside. To support this, HPP provided awardees with approximately $214 million of Ebola emergency supplemental funding to establish a nationwide, regional treatment network for Ebola and other infectious diseases. The funding provided through HPP Ebola Preparedness and Response activities is intended to establish the foundation required for the nation's health care system to safely and successfully identify, isolate, assess, transport, and treat patients with Ebola virus disease or under investigation for Ebola (or other highly infectious diseases). Through this mechanism, ASPR awarded cooperative agreements to all 50 states, Washington D.C., all U.S. territories and freely associated states, and select metropolitan jurisdictions, over a five-year project period. Additionally, ASPR competitively awarded funding to 10 regional Ebola and other special pathogen treatment centers (i.e., one in each of the 10 HHS regions).

Additionally, to prepare for, and provide safe and successful care of patients with Ebola, HHS (in a collaboration between ASPR and CDC) awarded funding to establish a National Ebola Training and Education Center (NETEC). The NETEC provides expertise, training, technical assistance, peer review, monitoring, and recognition to state health departments, regional Ebola and other special pathogen treatment centers, state- and jurisdiction-based Ebola treatment centers, and assessment hospitals. NETEC is a consortium of three U.S. health facilities that safely and successfully treated a confirmed

Ebola patient- Emory University in Atlanta, Georgia; University of Nebraska Medical Center/Nebraska Medicine (UNMC) in Omaha, Nebraska; and the New York City Health and Hospitals Corporation/HHC Bellevue Hospital Center in New York, New York.

Going forward and leveraging the best practices from investments made with the Ebola supplemental appropriations, ASPR is developing innovative tiered regional demonstration projects that can serve as a model for building a regional disaster health response system across the country. Subsequent to this hearing, ASPR awarded two grants- Nebraska Medicine in Omaha, Nebraska and Massachusetts General Hospital in Boston, Massachusetts to conduct pilot projects that show the potential effectiveness and viability of a Regional Disaster Health Response System (RDHDS).

The Honorable Michael C. Burgess

1) Dr. Bright, in 2010, BARDA established three centers to develop and manufacture medical countermeasures, such as vaccines and therapeutics, to protect our citizens during public health emergencies. Texas A&M's Center for Innovation in Advanced Development and Manufacturing is one of these centers, and was intended to focus on surge capacity for flu vaccines. I understand that the initial contract period with the Texas facility expires at the end of this month. How does BARDA plan to utilize these centers in the future? Will BARDA maintain and grow existing partnerships that have the infrastructure to deploy capabilities in the wake of a crisis?

ASPR Response

BARDA established the Centers for Innovation in Advanced Development and Manufacturing as public private partnerships in 2012. The program has made important investments in the domestic capacity for medical countermeasure production for public health emergencies. Each of the three centers in Texas, Maryland and North Carolina were funded to establish pandemic influenza vaccine manufacturing surge capacity, core service capabilities, and workforce development programs. Program successes include: process updates that resulted in a fourfold increase in yield for the domestically-produced cell based inactivated influenza vaccine; the development of commercially run facilities in Texas and Maryland; and a well- established workforce development program at Texas A&M in College Station, Texas. BARDA recently issued a six month extension to the base period for the Texas A&M center to facilitate additional partnering opportunities.

BARDA is currently evaluating how best to sustain and strengthen the domestic medical countermeasure manufacturing capabilities needed for the nation to be optimally prepared for 21" century health security threats.

2) How do you communicate with centers such as Texas A&M about what medical countermeasures they should develop? How involved is BARDA in helping these "centers" identify additional partners with whom they can work?

ASPR Response

Each Center has a designated federal contracting officer representative and contracting officer. These officials monitor completion of contract requirements and subsequent task orders that the centers have to meet per the terms of the contract. BARDA also holds frequent site visits and regular status calls with each of the Centers and has encouraged potential partner discussions through those interactions. Lastly, the Centers are required to maintain other commercial business/partnerships to make use of established capacity, to offset costs, and be a shared resource.

The Honorable Frank Pallone, Jr.

1) With respect to the three types of threats we often hear about- natural, intentional, and accidental-to what extent do preparedness efforts for the different types of threats overlap?

ASPR Response

ASPR coordinates with states and local officials before, during, and after emergencies to test existing response capabilities. While each incident, whether naturally occurring, man-made, or accidental, has its own considerations, there are common requirements that spread across all emergencies. Common elements include supporting situational awareness and information sharing between and among all supporting officials, supporting and augmenting local healthcare entities in treating the impacted population, ensuing critical assets are available to communities in need, and supporting the recovery of the community.

Investing in technologies that have the potential to yield multiple diagnostics, vaccines or therapeutics against different pathogens ensures that capabilities are nimble and flexible to support vaccines and therapeutics for future threats. Examples of this type of investment are how BARDA is supporting development of vaccines against the Ebola Zaire virus. Currently, BARDA is supporting two candidates under Project BioShield. There is the potential that same vaccine platform used to develop the Ebola Zaire virus vaccines could be used to develop vaccines against Ebola Sudan or Marburg viruses, by replacing just one element (glycoproteins). In addition, the vaccine platform could be used to express proteins from newly identified pathogens and expedite development of a vaccine for clinical trials.

2) How can we plan long-term therapeutics and vaccines in order to respond to outbreaks that we cannot yet anticipate?

ASPR Response

It often takes 10 or more years and over $1 billion to develop a new drug or vaccine.

ASPR/BARDA utilizes many of the innovative authorities authorized by amendments made by the Pandemic and All-Hazards Preparedness Act to the Public Health Service Act to support development of medical countermeasures. Authorities like Other Transaction Authorities (OTA) mean ASPR/BARDA can enter into innovative agreements to support development and procurement. As an example, the first BARDA OTA was within the broad spectrum antimicrobial program. Currently three out of six BARDA OTAs are focused on development of antimicrobial products. BARDA has also utilized CARB-X- an innovative public-private partnership conducted under a cooperative agreement- to address the threat of antibiotic resistant bacteria. CARB-X involves seven partners in the U.S. and U.K. and is backed with half a billion dollars in funding. $85 million in BARDA CARB-X investment resulted in nearly $500 million in private equity follow on investment. The partnership has 28 different companies making novel antibacterial drugs, vaccines, and diagnostics, including eight new classes of antibiotics.

3) BARDA's CARB-X program is developing many nontraditional products at the preclinical stage. Can you briefly explain why you have supported these products, and what BARDA is doing to make sure that enough products move on to clinical trials?

ASPR Response

Under the National Action Plan for Combating Antibiotic Resistant Bacteria (CARB), published by the White House in 2015, ASPR was directed to establish a biopharmaceutical accelerator in collaboration with NIH. BARDA established CARB-X in collaboration with the NIH's National Institute of Allergy and Infectious Diseases (NIAID), in NIH, in 2016. This was two years ahead of the three year milestone to establish the partnership. CARB-X is an international consortium offunders including BARDA, NIAID, Wellcome Trust, the Bill &Melinda Gates Foundation, and the UK Government's Department of Health and Social Care.

BARDA does not support the product portfolio alone; instead it is a collaborative effort across multiple, international organizations. BARDA funds non-traditional products because antibiotics are a solution but not the only solution for antibiotic resistant bacteria. In addition, all of the candidate products supported under CARB-X can support new treatment options for genetically engineered biothreat pathogens or the secondary bacterial infections that will result from exposures to threat agents, such as ionizing radiation from a nuclear blast or burn injuries resulting from nuclear or chemical agents.

Five products under the CARB-X portfolio have advanced to phase I clinical trials with more expected in the coming years. Candidate products may move into clinical trials when clinical trial proposals and data to support investigational new drug status are submitted to the FDA and data review does not show prohibitive adverse risk-benefit concerns. BARDA, as a funder and as a member CARB-X, works closely with the cooperative agreement awardee's program team to make sure that products are meeting the scientific milestones to advance in development.

4) Can you explain what BARDA is doing to foster public-private partnerships, and why this is important?

ASPR Response

BARDA established and manages the Tech Watch Program (https://www.phe.gov/aboutlbarda/Pages/BARDA-techwatch-Mtgs.aspx). Under Tech Watch, companies can come and discuss their technologies with BARDA to determine if the product is appropriate for BARDA to consider funding in the future. If the program does not align with BARDA priorities, we will refer them to other federal agencies that may be able to assist them with development. BARDA holds 150-200 Tech Watches per year.

BARDA also holds an annual BARDA Industry Day (BID), consistent with its authorities under the Public Health Service Act. This meeting brings together BARDA and other PHEMCE partners with industry, academic, and non-government organizations. It provides an opportunity for BARDA to highlight current and future strategic plans and priorities. BID also provides companies the opportunity to discuss their programs and how they might be able to address existing or future requirements.

Lastly, BARDA attends national and international conferences to discuss our portfolio of products, potential additional candidates, and our strategic plans. Numerous stakeholders attend these conferences allowing for another venue for BARDA to meet with potential partners.

BARDA cannot develop countermeasures alone. Public-private partnerships are critical to the continued success of BARDA and all of the ongoing medical countermeasure development initiatives.

5) ASPR has a number of programs in place, including the Hospital Preparedness Program and the Medical Reserve Corps, which are designed to help ensure readiness at the state and local level. How do these programs ensure that our front- line responders are able to respond effectively in a public health emergency situation?

ASPR Response

ASPR's mission is to save lives and protect Americans from 21st century health security threats. On behalf of the Secretary of HHS, ASPR leads public health and medical preparedness for, response to, and recovery from disasters and public health emergencies.

All of ASPR's programs and capabilities work together to create "unity of command" by consolidating Federal nonmilitary public health and medical preparedness and response functions. ASPR coordinates across HHS and the Federal interagency to support state, local, territorial, and tribal health partners. ASPR works to enhance medical surge capacity by organizing, training, equipping, and deploying HHS public health and medical personnel, such as National Disaster Medical System (NOMS) teams, and providing logistical support for HHS personnel responding to public health emergencies. ASPR supports readiness at the state and local level by coordinating federal grants and cooperative agreements, such as the Hospital Preparedness Program (HPP), by programs like the Medical Reserve Corps (MRC), and carrying out drills and operational exercises. For example, HPP prepares the nation's health care system to save lives during emergencies and disasters. It is the only source of federal funding for health care system readiness. HPP prepares the health care system to save lives through the development of health care coalitions (HCCs). HCCs are groups of health care and response organizations that collaborate to prepare for and respond to medical surge events. HCCs incentivize diverse and often competitive health care organizations to work together, allowing them to plan together and respond jointly in emergencies.

Specific to how ASPR supports first responders, ASPR routinely partners with state and local governments, hospitals, and responders to conduct drills and exercises to test various aspects of medical response capabilities. Drills and exercises provide opportunities at all levels to examine plans, procedures, and capabilities and to work with all government partners to employ resources in response to a specific event or scenario. One recent example is ASPR's Tranquil Terminus Exercise that brought together four regions, seven states, eight cities and three federal departments to test the nation's ability to transport patients with a highly infectious disease. Communities and responders benefitted by having the opportunity to test and rehearse plans with all partners participating. They learned from each other as well as identified best practices for inclusion in their plans and procedures.

6. CDC recently concluded an operational readiness review to assess whether state and local governments and public health services will be able to effectively get medical countermeasures to the appropriate person at the appropriate time. How does BARDA work with CDC and health departments to ensure that we develop countermeasures with this "last mile" of delivery in mind?

ASPR Response

Through its active role in PHEMCE, CDC shares information across HHS agencies, including ASPRIBARDA, who have a role in medical countermeasures requirement setting, research, development, regulatory review, procurement, stockpiling, distribution and use. Through this channel, as well as through established direct program-to-program collaborations with BARDA, CDC provides input on how countermeasure development can better meet end user needs. This includes criteria for how products developed may be stored and packaged to improve/simplify stockpiling and distribution, improved product delivery systems, simplified dosing considerations, etc. These factors assessed by CDC, impact how products are distributed, dispensed/administrated and used.

Greg Walden, Oregon
Chairman

Frank Pallone, Jr., New Jersey
Ranking Member

One Hundred Fifteenth Congress
Congress of the United States
House of Representatives
Committee on Energy and Commerce

July 12, 2018

Dr. Anne Schuchat
Principal Deputy Director
Centers for Disease Control and Prevention

Dear Dr. Schuchat:

Thank you for appearing before the Subcommittee on Oversight and Investigations on June 15, 2018, to testify at the hearing entitled "The State of U.S. Public Health Biopreparedness: Responding to Biological Attacks, Pandemics, and Emerging Disease Outbreaks."

Pursuant to the Rules of the Committee on Energy and Commerce, the hearing record remains open tOr ten business days to permit Members to submit additional questions for the recordt which are attached. To facilitate the printing of the hearing record, please respond to these questions with a transmittal letter by the close of business on Thursday, July 26, 2018. Thank you again for your time and effort preparing and delivering testimony before the Subcommittee.

Sincerely,

Gregg Harper

Chairman, Subcommittee on Oversight and Investigations

cc: The Honorable Diana DeGette, Ranking Member, Subcommittee on Oversight and Investigations

ATTACHMENT-ADDITIONAL QUESTIONS FOR THE RECORD

The Honorable Gregg Harper

1. Have there been any laboratory-acquired infections or potential exposures to pathogens at CDC labs during this past year? If so, what was the nature of the exposure or infection, and were any hospitalizations required as a result?

2. How scrious of a pandcmic thrcat docs thc CDC vicw the 5th wave II7N9 influenza strain, currently circulating in China? If a pandemic were to occur, how severely would it impact public health?

3. What are the present challenges that are preventing the broader utilization of cell-based influenza vaccines, and what steps can be taken to become less reliant on egg-based vaccines? What are the advantages of utilizing cell-based influenza vaccines over egg- based ones?

4. Is there currently an approved anthrax vaccine that can be administered to children? If so, what are the dosing guidelines for pediatric administration? If not, are there any pediatric anthrax vaccines currently under development, and what is the status of this development?

5. Were any FY 2017 funds for the non·procurement costs of the Strategic National Stockpile (SNS) used for any CDC expenses outside of the SNS program? If so, please identify the type and amount of these expenses.

6. How many laboratories currently make up the Laboratory Response Network (LRN)?

7. How much funding is there for the LRN in FY 2018?

The Honorable Michael C. Burgess

I. Dr. Schuchat, in your written testimony you mentioned CDC's use of electronic data systems to monitor population health information. How does CDC use and disseminate this data such that it can coordinate a timely response? Is the data platform that CDC uses integrated or interoperable with other biosurveillance platforms?

The Honorable Frank Pallone, Jr.

1) How does CDC ensure that its laboratories are gathering data from as many sources as possible?
   a. Do you need additional resources to help you analyze this data more effectively?

d. Please provide an update on CDC's concerns about the growth of antibiotic resistant bacteria?

e. In the case of an emergent biological threat, how does CDC's Emergency Operations Center coordinate the response at the front lines, such as at the state and local level?

f. Please describe how CDC uses its Public Health Emergency Preparedness Cooperative Agreement Program to help states and local municipalities identify and address gaps in preparedness. Is there anything you need from Congress to make sure this program works as intended?

g. What are the biggest challenges to successfully deploying countermeasures at the state and local level? How is CDC addressing these challenges?

Greg Walden, Oregon
Chairman

Frank Pallone, Jr., New Jersey
Ranking Member

One Hundred Fifteenth Congress
Congress of the United States
House of Representatives
Committee on Energy and Commerce

July 12, 2018

Dr. Anthony S. Fauci; Director
National Institute of Allergy and Infectious Diseases
National Institutes of Health

Dear Dr. Fauci:

Thank you for appearing before the Subcommittee on Oversight and Investigations on June 15, 2018, to testify at the hearing entitled "The State of U.S. Public Health

Biopreparedness: Responding to Biological Attacks, Pandemics, and Emerging Disease Outbreaks."

Pursuant to the Rules of the Committee on Energy and Commerce, the hearing record remains open for ten business days to permit Members to submit additional questions for the record) which are attached. To facilitate the printing of the hearing record, please respond to these questions with a transmittal letter by the close of business on Thursday, July 26, 2018. Thank you again for your time and effort preparing and delivering testimony before the Subcommittee.

Sincerely,

Gregg Harper
Chairman
Subcommittee on Oversight and Investigations

cc: The Honorable Diana DeGette, Ranking Member, Subcommittee on Oversight and Investigations

HOUSE ENERGY AND COMMERCE COMMITTEE, SUBCOMMITTEE ON OVERSIGHT AND INVESTIGATIONS, "THE STATE OF U.S. PUBLIC HEALTH BIOPREPAREDNESS: RESPONDING TO BIOLOGICAL ATTACKS, PANDEMICS, AND EMERGING INFECTIOUS DISEASE OUTBREAKS," FRIDAY, JUNE 15, 2018

The Honorable Gregg Harper

1. What do we need to do as a country to be better prepared for an outbreak of pandemic influenza in the U.S.?

NIAID Response

The National Institute of Allergy and Infectious Diseases (NIAID), the lead institute for research on influenza at the National Institutes of Health (NIH), is conducting and supporting basic, translational, and clinical research that will improve our ability to prepare for and respond to potential pandemic influenza outbreaks. A particular challenge in preparing for an outbreak of seasonal or pandemic influenza is that current influenza vaccines do not provide protection that is long-lasting or effective against a large number of influenza virus strains. To address this challenge, NIAID is prioritizing the development of universal influenza vaccine candidates that could provide long-lasting protection against multiple influenza strains including those with pandemic potential.

NIAID is galvanizing research efforts to develop universal influenza vaccine candidates and convened influenza experts from the U.S. and throughout the world at a research agenda-setting workshop in 2017. Following this meeting, NIAID outlined its universal influenza vaccine research priorities in a strategic plan that focuses on three key areas: improving knowledge of the transmission and pathogenesis of influenza infection; characterizing influenza immunity and immune factors that correlate with protection against influenza; and supporting the design of universal influenza vaccines. NIAID is actively engaging federal partners, including U.S. Department of Health and Human Services agencies and other key domestic and international stakeholders involved in influenza vaccine research, to coordinate and advance activities outlined in the strategic plan. For example, NIAID continues to collaborate with the Biomedical Advanced Research and Development Authority (BARDA) to advance the development and clinical testing of promising infl uenza vaccine candidates. The additional $40 million in funding for universal influenza vaccine research provided through the Consolidated Appropriations Act, 20 I 8 (P.L. 115-141) will support targeted research investments for the development of universal influenza vaccines that could protect vaccinated individuals against seasonal or pandemic infl uenza virus strains.

In addition to pursuing universal infl uenza vaccine strategies, NIAID is working to develop novel vaccine production strategies - such as recombinant DNA manufacturing techniques -that may allow for a more rapid production of targeted vaccines in response to newly emerging or changing strains of infl uenza virus than current egg and cell-based technologies. These vaccine production techniques could help to speed the availability of vaccines that protect against new or evolving pandemic infl uenza virus strains.

While investing in research to improve infl uenza vaccines, NIAID also continues to support the development of novel diagnostics to rapidly identify infl uenza viruses, including potential pandemic strains, and antiviral drugs that could help to limit infl uenza morbidity and mortality in a pandemic. NIAID will continue to play a key leadership role in seasonal and pandemic infl uenza outbreak preparedness and response efforts by conducting and supporting the basic, translational, and clinical research needed to identify and develop effective medical countermeasures.

2. In your testimony, you mentioned that there will be several iterations of a 'universal' flu vaccine. How many universal vaccine candidates are currently being developed at, or supported by, NIAID and what strains will they target? Where does this research currently stand? How many iterations of a universal flu vaccine does NIAID ultimately envision?

NIAID Response

A truly universal influenza vaccine would represent a groundbreaking advance in the fight against influenza by providing protection against a number of seasonal and pandemic influenza virus strains. NIAJD currently is exploring at least 10 different strategies toward the development of universal infl uenza vaccine candidates. Each of these strategies may have multiple vaccine candidates in various stages of development that are being investigated by NIAID intramural researchers or NIAID-supported grantees in academia and industry. Notable highlights of NIAID universal influenza vaccine research include thc dcvclopment of a ferritin nanoparticle-based vaccine candidate by the NIAID Vaccine Research Center (VRC), Phase I clinical trials of a VRC-developed DNA vaccine candidate using a prime-boost strategy with a standard inactivated seasonal infl uenza vaccine, and the recent launch of a NIAID-sponsored Phase II clinical trial to evaluate the M-001 vaccine candidate, which contains several infl uenza fragments recognized by the immune system that are common among multiple influenza virus strains. Additionally, NIAID is sponsoring a Phase I clinical trial to evaluate the safety and immunogenicity of a prime-boost regimen using an intranasal vaccine candidate followed by a licensed, quadrivalent seasonal influenza vaccine.

We anticipate that progress toward the goal of a universal infl uenza vaccine will occur in several stages, with each intennediary stage represented by several vaccine candidates that protect against progressively greater numbers of influenza virus strains. NIAID is pursuing strategies that could protect against all strains of a single subgroup of influenza virus, such as the H3N2 strains. This could be considered a universal influenza vaccine Version 1.0. As we make progress towards more broadly protective infl uenza vaccines, a Version 2.0 could protect against two or more subgroups of influenza, such as all HINI strains and all H3N2 strains. This may lead to developing a universal infl uenza vaccine candidate that by itself could durably protect against all subgroups of influenza, thereby protecting against virtually any infl uenza strain. Each universal influenza vaccine candidate will need to be evaluated over several infl uenza seasons to detennine the level of protection that is induced, and the durability of that protcction.

Version 1.0 of a universal influenza vaccine may be available in a few years, representing an incremental improvement on currently available intlucnza vaccines. A universal infl ucnza vaccine that covers all major infl ucnza strains may be many years away, with several iterations may be likely needed to ultimately achieve a broadly protective vaccine against all or nearly all infl uenza strains.

3. What are the present challenges that are preventing the broader utilization of cell-based influenza vaccines, and what steps can be taken to become less reliant on egg-based vaccines?

NIAID Response

NIAID supports the development of flexible vaccine manufacturing processes, including the use of molecular biological techniques, to help shorten manufacturing times and increase production efficiency for current and future influenza vaccines. Barriers to the broader utilization of cell-based and recombinant technologies to produce influenza vaccines include differences in manufacturing needs, development costs, and public awareness of alternatives to egg-based influenza vaccines.

NIAID is working to address these challenges through the support of basic and translational research for the development and manufacture of novel influenza vaccine strategies. NIAID scientists have devised a new method to manufacture an experimental whole virus inactivated influenza vaccine using a cell-based system. This method would provide another alternative to currently licensed egg-based and cell-based influenza vaccines. NIAID researchers also are developing and evaluating an additional cell-based system for whole virus influenza vaccine candidates to try to determine the most efficient cell-based system to produce influenza vaccines, both in terms of manufacturing time and cost. Data from these NIAID- supported studies will help improve vaccine manufacturing processes and vaccine efficacy, leading to the design of better influenza vaccines. NIAID also has supported studies of improved vaccine strain selection and optimized high-yield vaccine strains as part of the Seasonal Influenza Vaccine Improvement (SIVI) initiative, an interagency collaboration launched in 2016.

In addition to supporting the development of innovative seasonal influenza vaccines, NIAID has made a strategic shift toward a research paradigm that features broader, more flexible vaccine platform technologies such as recombinant DNA manufacturing techniques that can be rapidly mobilized when pandemic influenza viruses emerge. NIAID continues to support the early development of candidate pandemic influenza vaccine candidates that can be transitioned to BARDA for advanced development, with the goal of Food and Drug Administration (FDA) licensure and potential inclusion in the Strategic National Stockpile. NIAID also will continue to work closely with industry partners to advance promising influenza vaccine candidates, including cell-based and recombinant vaccine strategies.

The Honorable Michael C. Burgess

1. Dr. Fauci, the National Institute of Allergy and Infectious Diseases is on the front lines of vaccine development, especially in the wake of Ebola and Zika hitting the United States. You wrote an article in the Journal of the American Medical Association in November 2017 that detailed the critical role of biomedical research in pandemic preparedness. Can you share with us some of the research approaches NIAID uses to prepare for pandemics, such as a new flu strain, that have yet to hit our shores?

NIAID Response

As outlined in the 2017 article in the Journal of the American Medical Association, *The Critical Role of Biomedical Research in Pandemic Preparedness,* comprehensive pandemic preparedness requires a multifaceted approach. A critical component is biomedical research to support the development of vaccines, diagnostics, and therapeutics that may be quickly deployed in response to an emerging or re- emerging infectious disease of pandemic potential. NIAID supports a comprehensive portfolio of basic research on microbiology and immunology to better understand the mechanisms of pathogenesis and immune responses, as well as applied and clinical research to evaluate candidate diagnostics, therapeutics, and vaccines. This strategic effort includes the pursuit of several research approaches, including: (1) research targeting specific pathogens; (2) prototype pathogen efforts, in which fundamental research to understand the disease caused by one pathogen may inform the development of countermeasures for a closely related pathogen; and (3) development of platform-based technologies and broad-spectrum products that may be easily and quickly deployed against multiple pathogens. NIAID research complements other elements of pandemic preparedness by improving understanding of infectious disease pathogenesis and by developing candidate medical countermeasures that could be used in a pandemic.

NIAID supports a broad portfolio of pathogen-specific basic, translational, and clinical research. NIAID investments in pathogen-specific research include priority pathogens of the United States Government as designated by the Centers for Disease Control and Prevention (CDC), as well as other emerging andre-emerging diseases identified as priority pathogens by NIAID. For example, NIAID supported development ofml02.4, a candidate monoclonal antibody treatment for Nipah virus infection. NIAID also is supporting the development of improved influenza vaccine candidates, including universal influenza vaccines that could provide broad protection for a range of pandemic and seasonal influenza strains. Additionally, it was an NIAID investment in basic research nearly 40 years ago that enabled the development of the novel influenza antiviral Xofluza (baloxavir marboxil), which was approved for use in Japan in early 2018 and is currently undergoing FDA priority review for use in the United States.

NIAID has built upon increased understanding of infectious disease pathogenesis to move strategically toward a medical countermeasures research paradigm that features broader, more flexible platform technologies that can be used to respond to several biological threats. High-throughput sequencing and platform-based technologies are facilitating the development and manufacture of vaccines, targeted antibody therapeutics, and broad-spectrum antibiotics and antivirals by significantly decreasing the time from identification of a public health threat of an emerging infection to clinical evaluation of candidate countermeasures. For example, in 2015-2016 when Zika virus emerged in the Americas, clusters of microcephaly and other birth defects were identified, and a Public Health Emergency of International Concern was declared by the World Health Organization. NIAID scientists rapidly used Zika virus genetic sequence information to develop a DNA-based vaccine candidate that moved from concept to a first-in-human trial in less than four months. The experimental DNA-based Zika vaccine, which currently is in Phase II/IIb clinical testing, was developed with a readily deployable DNA vaccine platform that is a form of gene-based immunization previously used by NIAID to develop a candidate vaccine for West Nile virus. The development of a broadly applicable platform technology facilitated an accelerated response to a previously unrecognized public health threat. As mentioned in the 2017 article in the Journal of the American Medical Association, NIAID is supporting development of additional vaccine platform technologies, including nanoparticle, virus-like particles, and mRNA platforms. NIAID also supports development of broad-spectrum therapeutics, including antiviral and antibacterial agents that have demonstrated activity against multiple viral or bacterial pathogens.

Together with academia, industry, and Public Health Emergency Medical Countermeasures Enterprise (PHEMCE) partners, NIAID remains committed to meeting public health emergency needs by advancing high-priority research to support development of medical countermeasures for emerging and re-emerging infectious diseases, including influenza viruses with pandemic potential. NIAID-supported research into specific pathogens, prototype pathogens, and the development of platform-based technologies will continue to play an essential role in PHEMCE pandemic preparedness and response efforts.

The Honorable Frank Pallone, Jr.

1. How can we plan long-term for therapeutics and vaccines in order to respond to outbreaks that we cannot yet anticipate?

NIAID Response

NIAID supports a comprehensive portfolio of basic research on microbiology and immunology to better understand the mechanisms of pathogenesis and immune response, as well as applied and clinical research to evaluate candidate diagnostics, therapeutics, and vaccines. This strategic effort includes the pursuit of foundational platfonn approaches that could be used to develop medical countenneasures against multiple pathogens.

NIAID is pursuing the development of platforn1 approaches including molecular biological technologies that could be rapidly mobilized to generate candidate vaccines against emerging infectious disease threats. For example, during the 2015-2016 Zika virus outbreak in the Americas, NIAID scientists developed a novel DNA-based vaccine for Zika virus using viral genetic sequence information. The candidate vaccine moved from concept to a first-in-human trial in less than four months, and currently is in a Phase II/IIb trial. In order to respond so quickly, NIAID utilized a readily deployable DNA vaccine platform that was previously used by NIAID to develop a candidate vaccine for

West Nile virus. These types of genetic platfonns could be used to respond similarly to multiple emerging and re-emerging infectious disease threats.

NIAID investments in basic, translational, and clinical research also are contributing to the development of novel broad-spectrum therapeutics that can target several pathogens. For example, NIAID has supported early-stage development of broad-spectrum antiviral agents such as BCX4430 (galidesivir), which has demonstrated activity against Ebola and other RNA viruses, and broad-spectrum antibacterial products, including a compound with activity against ilie two different bacteria that cause tularemia and plague. Such broad-spectrum therapeutics may decrease the time necessary to identify and distribute an effective treatment during an outbreak setting.

NIH, led by the Fogarty International Center and NIAID, also supports the development of research infrastructure and partnerships in foreign countries to aid in the identification, monitoring, and response to the emergence and reemergence of infectious diseases. Long-standing international investments in disease monitoring and response made by NIH were vital in the immediate response to the 2014-2016 Ebola outbreak in West Africa and provided critical in-country expertise that helped to contain the spread of the disease. In addition, the clinical research partnership between NIAID and the government of Liberia, the Partnership for Research on Ebola Virus in Liberia (PREVAIL), demonstrated the ability to do rigorous scientific research in developing countries. The PREVAIL partnership enabled in-country clinical trials testing of several Ebola virus therapeutic and vaccine candidates, among them the ZMappTM therapeutic, the Merck VSV vaccine, and the cAd3-EBOZ vaccine developed by the NIAID VRC in partnership with industry. NIAID, through a partnership with the French National Institute of Health and Medical Research (Inserm), the London School of Hygiene and Tropical Medicine, and the host country governments, has launched the Partnership for Research on Ebola VACcination (PREYAC), a Phase II clinical trial comparing three experimental Ebola vaccination strategies in Mali, Guinea, Sierra Leone, and Liberia. Medical countermeasures tested by the PREYAIL partnerships were recently deployed in the Democratic Republic of the Congo to help address an Ebola outbreak from May to July 2018, emphasizing the key contributions of this effort. NIAID-supported international research partnerships also contribute to the development of site infrastructure and sustainable research capacity in developing countries, enhancing global preparedness to respond to unanticipated outbreaks and to conduct clinical research to better understand the disease and to test candidate countermeasures during these outbreaks.

2. In your view, are there specific pathogens or diseases we should be most concerned with?

a. With so many dangerous pathogens, how do we prioritize research to try to target those posing the greatest threat?

NIAID Response

NIAID prioritizes research and early-stage development of medical countermeasures against bioterror threats and emerging and re-emerging infectious diseases of public health importance. The persistent threat of pandemic influenza and other respiratory viruses that may spread quickly and cause significant morbidity and mortality, such as severe acute respiratory syndrome coronavirns (SARS-CoV) or Middle East respiratory syndrome coronavirus (MERS-CoV) remain a particular area of concern. NIAID maximizes its efforts to develop effective medical countermeasures against these, and other potential emerging and re-emerging diseases, by prioritizing research into broad-spectrum antibiotics and antiviral drugs, as well as efficient platform technologies to more rapidly develop vaccines and diagnostics for a variety of threat pathogens.

NIAID'·s efforts to develop a broader, more flexible research paradigm is yielding scientific advances that will facilitate public health emergency preparedness and our ability to respond to emerging public health threats. NIAID is supporting the development of diagnostics platforms capable of distinguishing between several pathogens, as well as broad-spectrum therapeutics, including novel antiviral agents, effective against several pathogens. In addition, NIAID is prioritizing the development of several vaccine platforms that could be used to quickly develop vaccine candidates against newly identified threats. This includes the DNA-based platform used to develop a candidate vaccine against Zika virus that moved from concept to a first-in-human trial in less than four months. The development of these and other broad-spectrum therapeutics and platfonn technologies remains a NIAID priotity.

In addition to supporting the development of platform technologies and broad-spectrum therapeutics that may decrease response time in the event of a pandemic, NIAID also supports a targeted portfolio of basic, translational, and clinical research on priority pathogens with pandemic potential, including influenza and other respiratory viruses. This includes detailed studies of immune system responses to infection, as well as research to better understand the transmission, evolution, and pathogenesis of the viruses to inform the development of vaccines, diagnostics, and therapeutics that could be deployed during a pandemic. The NIAID Vaccine and Treatment Evaluation Units currently are conducting two Phase II clinical trials of a new vaccine candidate to protect against emerging H7N9 influenza virus strains, and NIAID intramural scientists are conducting clinical studies of prime-boost vaccine regimens for swine (H l) and avian (H7) influenza viruses.

NIAID is galvanizing research efforts to support the development of universal influenza vaccine candidates. A universal influenza vaccine that is effective against both seasonal and pandemic influenza strains would be a vital tool to prepare for future pandemics, as well as to improve our ability to prevent seasonal influenza. In addition, NIAID is supporting novel antiviral therapies for influenza, including RNA polymerase inhibitors, peptide inhibitors, and next-generation neuraminidase inhibitors. NIAID support for influenza diagnostics research has led to the development of a rapid molecular *in vitro* assay recently cleared by the FDA to accurately distinguish influenza A fi·om influenza B in nasal swab specimens.

NIAID continues to make progress against other respiratory viruses with pandemic potential. NIAID is supporting early-stage clinical trials of antibodies designed to treat people infected with MERS-CoV, as well as development of a vaccine candidate forMERS-CoV based on information from previous vaccine studies on SARS-CoV. NIAID-funded researchers also have identified a novel SARS-related virus, swine acute diarrhea syndrome coronavirus (SADS-CoV). SADS-CoV was responsible for 25,000 piglet deaths in China in 2016-17; however, no infections in humans have been identified. The identification of pathogens with zoonotic potential such as SADS-CoV that may emerge as human diseases contributes to our preparedness, as it may facilitate early identification if the pathogen becomes capable of causing disease in humans. NIAID will continue to prioritize research on pathogens with pandemic potential such as influenza and other respiratory viruses and support the development of platform-based technologies and broad-spectrum products that may be easily and quickly deployed against multiple pathogens.

3. Can you briefly explain the barriers that make it harder for scientists to discover new antibiotics?

NIAID Response

NIAID supports a comprehensive basic research portfolio on antibiotic resistance to aid in the discovery of new antibiotics. NIAID antimicrobial resistance research includes the elucidation of major mechanisms of pathogenesis, host-pathogen and drug-pathogen interactions, and the identification of new candidate antibiotics. NTAID has found that the major challenges in the development of new antibiotics are in the later stages of clinical development of these drugs. NIAID has identified three main barriers to the advanced development. of new antibacterial therapeutics: 1) the scarcity of new antibacterial drug candidates effective against Gram-negative infections; 2) the challenge of enrolling patients in clinical trials needed to show efficacy of new therapeutics, especially in the case of Gram-negative drug-resistant infections; and 3) a lack of market incentives for pharmaceutical companies to invest in the final stages of antibiotic development and licensure. NIAID is working to address these challenges in several ways, including through the support of basic, translational, and clinical research to identify and advance promising antibacterial candidates to late-stage development. NIAID estimates that more than 25 percent of the antibacterial candidates currently in clinical development previously received some form of NIAID support.

NIAID is addressing these challenges by supporting early-stage development and clinical trials of new therapeutics to help offset the investment required to successfully test these therapeutics and bring them to market. The NIAID-supported Antibacterial Resistance Leadership Group (ARLG) has supported over 35 clinical studies investigating new therapeutics, optimized treatment regimens, diagnostic devices, and projects on antimicrobial stewardship. The ARLG places a priority on research involving Gram-negative bacteria that represent a major antimicrobial resistance threat. NIAID-supportcd scientists also completed two Phase I clinical trials for a new class of antibiotics (CRS3123) to treat *Clostridium dijficile* infections, which are increasingly difficult to treat effectively. In addition, NIAID is supporting clinical trials to evaluate the efficacy of new therapeutic candidates, as well as new treatment regimens that utilize existing antibiotics in new combinations or regimens. NIAID also has solicited research for the development of tools to advance drug discovery of agents against Gram-negative pathogens through the "Partnerships for the Development of Tools to Advance Therapeutic Discovery for Select Antimicrobial-Resistant Gram-Negative Bacteria" program. NIAID is facilitating scientific discussions and partnerships to address key questions and challenges in the development of new antibiotics. NIAID and The Pew Charitable Trusts sponsored the 2017 scientific workshop entitled, "Challenges in the Discovery of Gram-negative Antibacterials: The Entry & Efflux Problem." The goal of the workshop was to identify next steps and opportunities for collaborations to determine factors that affect the entrance of antibiotics into, and accumulation within, Gram-negative bacteria to inform the identification and design of new types of antibiotics. Resolving these early-stage research qnestions will help address the growing threat of resistant Gram-negative bacteria by facilitating the later-stage development of promising new therapeutic candidates.

NIAID also addresses barriers to the advanced development of new antibacterial therapeutics by helping to de-risk antibacterial product development for researchers in industry and academia through targeted research support and services. NIAID supports the National Database of Resistant Pathogens, which contains genomic data for more than 205,000 drug-resistant microbes. This database was established by the NIH, in partnership with FDA and CDC, as a publicly available resource that scientists from all over the world can access to inform the development of novel antibacterial products. NIAID also funds the Centers of Excellence for Translational Research that have recently discovered a new class of antibiotics produced by soil-dwelling bacteria. These antibiotics, known as malacidins, have a unique mechanism of action that may make the development of resistance less likely. NIAID also supports CARB-X, a unique public-private partnership led by BARDA. CARB-X is dedicated to accelerating the development of innovative antibacterial products from target/candidate identification and characterization through Phase I clinical trials. CARB-X is currently supporting 29 therapeutic candidates, including 11 new classes of antibiotics, as well as 6 diagnostics products. To facilitate the discovery and development of promising therapeutic candidates, NIAID provides unique no-cost preclinical and clinical services that include screening tests for antimicrobial activity and access to research reagents to assist in product testing. Additionally, NIAID supported preclinical development and first-in-human Phase I clinical testing of VNRX-5133, a novel beta-lactamase inhibitor (BLI). VNRX-5133 is the first BLI in clinical development that inhibits all known classes of beta-lactamases bacterial enzymes involved in resistance to the beta- lactam class of broad-spectrum antibiotics snch as penicillin.

NIAID continues to support the development of antibacterial products in collaboration with academia, industry, and federal partners. A concerted research effort is required to combat the growing public health threat of antibiotic resistance. NJAID remains committed to facilitating the development of new antibiotics by supporting innovative research and offsetting the development costs of industry and academia.

Greg Walden, Oregon
Chairman

Frank Pallone, Jr., New Jersey
Ranking Member

One Hundred Fifteenth Congress
Congress of the United States
House of Representatives
Committee on Energy and Commerce

July12, 2018

Rear Admiral Denise Hinton
Chief Scientist
U.S. Food and Drug Administration

Dear Admiral Hinton:

Thank you for appearing before the Subcommittee on Oversight and Investigations on June 15, 2018, to testify at the hearing entitled "The State of U.S. Public Health Biopreparedness: Responding to Biological Attacks, Pandemics, and Emerging Disease Outbreaks."

Pursuant to the Rules of the Committee on Energy and Commerce, the hearing record remains open for ten business days to permit Members to submit additional questions for the record, which are attached. To facilitate the printing of the hearing record, please respond to these questions with a transmittal letter by the close of business on Thursday, July 26, 2018.

Thank you again for your time and effot1preparing and delivering testimony before the Subcommittee.

Sincerely,

Gregg Harper
Chairman
Subcommittee on Oversight and Investigations

cc: The Honorable Diana DeGette, Ranking Member, Subcommittee on Oversight and Investigations

ATTACHMENT-ADDITIONAL QUESTIONS FOR THE RECORD

The Honorable Gregg Harper

I. Medical countermeasure (MCM) development can be a costly, time-consuming venture for the private sector. It is often one of the reasons why companies are reluctant to enter the MCM product space. How could the FDA provide better guidance and get involved earlier in the development process to help reduce this burden?

The Honorable Michael C. Burgess

I. Pharmaceutical companies face economic barriers to discovering and developing urgently needed new antibiotics to address drug resistant infections. I was encouraged by Commissioner Gottlieb's announcement earlier this week that FDA is working with CMS and other agencies to develop new payment models that would incentivize antibiotic research and development and the appropriate use of new antibiotics. Can you describe how these new models may work? Does Congress need to provide additional authorities or resources?

The Honorable Frank Pallone, Jr.

I. When a crisis does occur, what can FDA do to fast-track approval of countermeasures like vaccines and therapeutics?

2. How have GAIN and ADAPT helped FDA to incentivize antibiotic development in the private sector?

In: Coronavirus …
Editor: Roger F. Martin
ISBN: 978-1-53617-939-2

Chapter 18

FACING 21ST CENTURY PUBLIC HEALTH THREATS: OUR NATION'S PREPAREDNESS AND RESPONSE CAPABILITIES, PART I*

Committee on Health, Education, Labor, and Pensions

Wednesday, January 17, 2018
U.S. Senate, Committee on Health, Education, Labor, and Pensions
Washington, DC.

The Committee met, pursuant to notice, at 10:04 a.m. in room SD–430, Dirksen Senate Office Building, Hon. Richard Burr, presiding.

Present: Senators Alexander, Burr [presiding], Isakson, Collins, Cassidy, Young, Murkowski, Murray, Casey, Bennet, Murphy, Warren, Kaine, Hassan, Smith, and Jones.

OPENING STATEMENT OF SENATOR BURR

Senator Burr [presiding]. I would like to call this hearing to order, the Senate Health, Education, Labor, and Pensions Committee.

This morning, we are holding a hearing titled, "Facing the 21st Century Public Health Threats: Our Nation's Preparedness and Response Capabilities." We will hear from Dr. Robert Kadlec, the Assistant Secretary for Preparedness and Response at the Department of Health and Human Services; Dr. Stephen Redd, Director of the Office of Public Health

* This is an edited, reformatted and augmented version of Hearing of the Committee on Health, Education, Labor, and Pensions, United States Senate, One Hundred Fifteenth Congress, Second Session, Publication No. S. HRG. 115–712, dated January 17, 2018.

Preparedness and Response at the Centers for Disease Control and Prevention; and Dr. Scott Gottlieb, Commissioner of the Food and Drug Administration.

This is the first of two hearings we plan to have on this topic. The second will be noticed for Tuesday, January 23.

Senator Murray and I each have an opening statement, then I am going to turn to Senator Alexander and Senator Casey for any opening remarks they might have. After that, we will introduce our panel of witnesses and hear their testimonies. And then each Member will have up to 5 minutes for any remarks and questions.

First, I would like to welcome the Chairman and thank him for giving me the opportunity to hold the gavel today. This hearing discusses a topic that is critical to our national security and has seen many years of bipartisan work in this Committee and in this Congress.

Together, we have developed and strengthened the framework to ensure we are prepared for chemical, biologic, radiological, and other nuclear threats with the potential to jeopardize the health of all Americans.

The Pandemic and All-Hazards Preparedness Act of 2006 created a framework which has grown and changed as we have learned from each public health experience we have been through. We should be proud of the accomplishments under PAHPA and the progress made over the last decade.

Our work has resulted in strong partnerships with our states and local counterparts, created greater certainty and accountability to bring forward medical countermeasures, and established a clear strategy with which we can combat the full range of public health threats we face today and those we may encounter in the future. Despite this progress, we are not fully prepared and more work remains to accomplish our goals. The Blue Ribbon Study Panel on Biodefense stated in their 2015 report that there are, and I quote, "Serious gaps and inadequacies that continue to leave the Nation vulnerable to threats from nature and terrorists alike."

As we move forward in revisiting this successful and bipartisan law, I want to make it very clear to my colleagues that this is a reauthorization of a national security bill, and I look forward to working with each of you on this important issue.

The threats we face continue to evolve and it is critical that we bring, with this discussion, the vigilance, urgency, and resolve this mission demands. We are in an unprecedented era of technological and biomedical innovation and advancement.

In November 2016, the President's Advisory Council on Science and Technology warned that, and I quote, "While the ongoing growth of biotechnology is a great boon for society, it also holds serious potential for destructive use by both states and technically competent individuals."

I urge the U.S. Government's past ways of thinking and organizing to meet biological threats needs to change to reflect and address this rapidly developing landscape. For this reason, it is critical that fostering and advancing innovation, particularly in the development of medical countermeasures, is top of mind and that we work through this reauthorization process to ensure CDC, FDA, ASPR, BARDA have what they need to keep pace with these rapidly changing and evolving threats.

This Committee has worked to push the Federal Government, and HHS in particular, to meet these challenges. An HHS that fosters innovation in the development of medical countermeasures and across PAHPA's framework provides the greatest hope to ensure the safety of the American people. The witnesses we have before us today will be able to provide insight into the urgency of this mission and the promise innovation holds if properly leveraged.

I look forward to hearing from each of you about the progress that we have made, and where we can continue to improve policies and programs to realize their full potential to save Americans' lives.

Now, I would like to turn to Senator Murray for any comments she might have.

STATEMENT OF SENATOR MURRAY

Senator MURRAY. Thank you very much.

And thank you, to all of you, for joining this hearing on our Nation's preparedness to combat public health threats as we look toward now reauthorizing the Pandemic and All-Hazards Preparedness Act later this year.

I especially want to thank Senator Casey and Senator Burr for their bipartisan work and leadership on this really important issue. Local Washington state papers show why today's discussion is so important to families across this country. We have headlines like, "Flu Deaths And Cases Increasing In Pierce County." And, "Flu Outbreak In Snohomish County Kills Five; 50 Hospitalized."

A bad flu season can be a nightmare for families and too often ends in horrible tragedy. Just as we must continue to improve our public health response across the board to prevent those tragedies on the local level, we have to also make sure we are vigilant against pandemics of a global scale.

A pandemic could affect half a billion people, more than the entire population of the United States; and that is not speculation. It happened 100 years ago. The 1918 influenza epidemic was a tragedy more deadly to the human race than World War I. And today, the threat of pandemic flu is joined by new threats.

What have we learned in the last century? Are we better prepared for the next catastrophe?

When we consider Ebola and how the Centers for Disease Control and Prevention, and so many partners, supported Nigeria as they instituted evidence-based policies and tracked the path of that disease, and contained it when the outbreak reached Lagos, the answer is clearly, yes.

When you consider our Strategic National Stockpile which can deliver 50 tons of emergency medical supplies anywhere in the U.S. in 12 hours, the answer is clearly, yes.

When you consider the FDA's approval of new medical counter- measures to combat anthrax, and flu, and radiation, and plague, the answer is clearly, yes.

However, our track record is far from perfect. We still can do better.

We can do better than the President's way too slow response in Puerto Rico and the U.S. Virgin Islands after Hurricane Maria. The storm left many Americans without access to clean water, and electricity, and healthcare for months.

We can do better than the Administration's response to the opioid epidemic. President Trump declared the crisis a public health emergency 83 days ago and has taken little meaningful action since.

So I am glad this Committee will continue its bipartisan work to address the opioid crisis in another hearing soon.

We can also do better than our slow response in approving funding to combat Zika in 2016. The World Health Organization declared Zika a global health emergency in February. Instead of a fast response with needed funding, the response got politicized around some Republicans who pushed to undermine women's healthcare and access to contraception, which was a key requirement to prevent the virus from causing devastating birth defects. As a result, that took Congress 9 months to pass emergency funding for a public health crisis that endangered mothers, and babies, and families across the world. That delay hurt people and it harmed families in ways they are going to carry for the rest of their lives. So we have to do better.

We are most successful at protecting our families against pandemic threats when we respond with quick, bipartisan action.

We need decisions based in science and expert medical opinion, not ideology, especially when it comes to women's health.

We need Federal, state, and local agencies to hire the people, and capacity, and have the funding they need to protect communities. Hiring freezes and funding cuts make us less prepared, not more. We need to plan for everyone. We cannot overlook the young or the elderly. We cannot forget pregnant women, or individuals with disabilities, or those fighting chronic diseases like diabetes.

We need innovative medical countermeasures to protect us from today's threats like a universal flu vaccine and antibiotics to combat resistant bacteria. And we must continue strong partnerships with industry that will allow us to rapidly respond to new threats. We need to stop fear and uncertainty before they create panic by getting families helpful and accurate information from sources that they trust. We cannot allow anyone to undermine the science of proven solutions like vaccines.

We need to respond to global health crises abroad before they travel here to home. Diseases are not stopped by borders, or walls, or bans. This is a place where the United States can, and should, lead.

We should continue to show our international partners that we are focused on these issues and will be their ally in preparing for, and addressing, public health threats.

Congress has a strong, bipartisan track record of addressing these challenges through the PAHPA, which strengthened our Nation's public health preparedness and created new roles, and programs, and authorities for public health emergency response.

Reauthorizing the Act in 2013, we built on that record and enhanced medical surge capacity. We modernized biosurveillance capabilities and increased our focus on at risk individuals.

I am hopeful we can continue that progress with legislation that focuses on the science and evidence based policies we know work to mitigate public health crises, that considers the needs of everyone, and puts families and women before politics, supports state and local public health officials, ensures communities do not spend months waiting for emergency resources, and enables us to respond to the next crisis with foresight rather than learn from the next tragedy with hindsight.

We do not know what the next public health threat will be. We do not know where, or when, or even how it will start. But we do know that being prepared starts now.

All of you here today have a critical role to play in keeping our communities healthy and safe. The Food and Drug Administration helps facilitate the development and review of medical counter-measures and grants emergency use authorizations for products that are needed on the frontlines.

The Assistant Secretary of Preparedness and Response guides our Nation's preparedness planning. They help ensure our healthcare system is ready to face any emergency. And it invests

in the medical countermeasures pipeline through biomedical advanced research and development authority.

The Centers for Disease Control and Prevention is on the frontlines supporting state and local public health departments, overseeing the Strategic National Stockpile, gathering and analyzing key data, and serving as a trusted source of information to the public.

I am interested to hear from all of you today about your work to fulfill these important roles and keep our country safe.

Mr. Chairman, I do want to say I am frustrated that Director Fitzgerald is, once again, unable to join us here today. Due to conflicts of interest presented by investments, our CDC Director still has to recuse herself on some of the important health issues that we face, including issues related to data collection and information sharing, which are very relevant to the conversation that we are having today. I am concerned that she still cannot give her full attention to all the pressing health threats we face and hope that these conflicts of interest will be resolved soon.

Thank you, Dr. Redd, for joining us in her place and I look forward to hearing from you.

Thank you, Mr. Chairman.

Senator BURR. Thanks, Senator Murray. Senator Alexander.

STATEMENT OF SENATOR ALEXANDER

The CHAIRMAN. Thank you, Senator Burr.

Senator Burr, thank you for your willingness to chair this hearing.

In March 2013, President Obama signed into law the bipartisan Pandemic and All-Hazards Preparedness Reauthorization Act. Senator Burr was the author of that reauthorization and the original legislation, which became law in 2006. He worked with many Senators on this Committee, both Democratic and Republican, and I thank them all for that. Senator Murray, Senator Casey, and others, Senator Isakson was another of those. So Senator Burr is chairing the hearing and I thank him for that.

I would also like to welcome Senator Smith from Minnesota, who is joining our Committee and replacing Senator Franken, who was a valuable Member of the Committee.

Senator Jones, from Alabama, is also a new Member of the Committee. We welcome him. He replaced Senator Whitehouse, who was a very valuable Member of the Committee, and who has taken a lesser assignment on the Finance Committee for some reason.

[Laughter.]

The CHAIRMAN. But we will miss Sheldon and his work on this Committee.

Mr. Chairman, I am going to withhold my comments, although what I would like to do is call on Senator Isakson for 1 minute, just to make some comments, and then we will go to Senator Casey.

Senator BURR. Senator Isakson.

Senator ISAKSON. Thank you, Mr. Chairman.

I just wanted to, in reference to the statements made by the ranking Member, Senator Murray, whom I have talked to about Dr. Fitzgerald. I talked with Dr. Fitzgerald yesterday.

As chairman of the Ethics Committee, I have gotten her in touch with the appropriate people to deal with the issue. She is forthrightly dealing with it to the best I can determine and I am working expeditiously to see we get it done as quickly as possible, so she will not have any conflict to testify whatsoever. And that is her desire as well.

Thank you.

Senator BURR. Senator Casey.

Statement of Senator Casey

Senator CASEY. Thank you very much, Senator Burr.

I am grateful for this hearing, and grateful to be working with you again on this reauthorization, and commend your work on this for many, many years.

I also want to thank, of course, the Chairman, Chairman Alexander and Ranking Member Murray for this bipartisan hearing on the Nation's preparedness and response capabilities in advance of the reauthorization of the Pandemic and All-Hazards Preparedness Act known as PAHPA.

I will give you one story, one brief story, but I think, instructive about how important preparation is. This is a good example of preparedness infrastructure that PAHPA supports, in this case, in the aftermath of a tragedy, a train derailment that occurred in Philadelphia in May 2015.

The train was carrying 238 passengers. When it derailed, eight people lost their lives. Over 200 were injured in that derailment. Fortunately, through funding from PAHPA's Hospital Preparedness Program, which we know by the acronym HPP, the Pennsylvania Department of Health and a regional healthcare coalition had long been working together to prepare local healthcare systems for emergencies that could cause a surge in patients.

When the train derailed, HPP funded systems were tracking bed availability in local hospitals and providing that information in real time to emergency responders who were at the scene, helping them to effectively triage patients, send them to hospitals that had the capacity to accept additional patients so they could begin to receive the care they needed.

Because these systems were in place before the train derailed, they were ready to protect both health and to save lives when seconds, literally seconds, counted.

Yet, health security threats are increasing in frequency and intensity due to a combination of factors including newly emerging infectious diseases, extreme weather events, and our aging infrastructure.

So now, more than ever, we must continue to build our Nation's resiliency by investing in countermeasure development, surveillance, and supporting state and local partners to reduce the impact of health events in the country.

So I would like to thank today's witnesses for their service. It is important to mention your service to the country, as well as your commitment to protecting America's public health.

We look forward to the hearing and grateful for the work that we can do today at this hearing.

Thank you, Mr. Chairman.

Senator BURR. Senator Casey, thank you.

Thank you for your continued help and work on this issue.

Let me just remind Members that this is the start of the reauthorization of PAHPA. Now, having been in Congress for 24 years, I realize that when you get involved in HHS legislation and FDA legislation, there is always a temptation to fix other things.

I want to encourage you to fight the urge. Let us keep this focused on perfecting PAHPA. It has been successful. We still have work to do, but if we become distracted and create a fight over changes within the FDA that have nothing related to this, or HHS, or somewhere else because the sheer geography that just PAHPA allows us to get into, we will lose the focus of what we are doing, and that is trying to make PAHPA even more effective in the future.

So with that, I would like to introduce our witnesses, which each have up to 5 minutes to give their testimony.

I am pleased to welcome today Dr. Robert Kadlec. Dr. Kadlec is the Assistant Secretary for Preparedness and Response at the Department of Health and Human Services. If he does not like the title, he was the one that created it.

It was with Dr. Kadlec's help that we created the ASPR position as part of PAHPA to establish a clear line of authority in the event of a public health emergency. The APSR is the person at HHS solely responsible for leading and coordinating the Federal medical and public health preparedness and response effort across all the agencies within HHS including FDA and CDC.

Dr. Bob, delighted to have you back today.

Next, we will hear from Dr. Scott Gottlieb. Dr. Gottlieb is the Commissioner of the Food and Drug Administration.

The FDA plays a critical role in our emergency preparedness and response capabilities through its review of medical countermeasures, including drugs, vaccines, diagnostic tests, and by ensuring these countermeasures are safe and effective.

Further, the 2013 reauthorization of PAHPA aimed to improve regulatory certainty and predictability for medical countermeasures under review at the FDA, while also providing the agency with the additional authorities to support rapid response to public health emergencies.

Scott, we are delighted to have you here and delighted to have you in that position at FDA.

Finally, we will hear from Dr. Stephen Redd. Dr. Redd is the Director of the Office of Public Health Preparedness and Response at the Centers for Disease Control and Prevention.

The CDC serves a number of roles under the PAHPA framework and has built strong relationships with state and local public health departments, an important aspect of preparing for, and responding to, emergency public health threats.

The CDC also works to make sure we have the information we need in advance of and during a public health emergency. As part of this effort, the CDC houses an expansive epidemiology laboratory capacity and is responsible for biosurveillance and public health data collection activities.

Again, we welcome all of you.

Let me just say at the beginning, I believe the hurdle that is in our way is not available innovation. I believe the hurdle that is in our way is government. Clearly defining what it is that our need is, and the certainty of a pathway for getting the approvals that we need for those to actually be deployed.

So I hope you will keep those in mind as you go through, not just your testimony, your questions, but more importantly in the roles that you carry out after leaving. Understand that you are on the frontlines at making this happen.

Dr. Bob, the floor is yours.

STATEMENT OF ROBERT KADLEC, MD, ASSISTANT SECRETARY FOR PREPAREDNESS AND RESPONSE, DEPARTMENT OF HEALTH AND HUMAN SERVICES, WASHINGTON, DC

Dr. KADLEC. Well, thank you, sir. Sorry for the false start there. I was excited to be here, sir. I was ready to go.

Good morning, Mr. Chairman, both of you, sirs and Senator Murray, and distinguished Members of the Committee.

I assumed this role 5 months ago just a week before Hurricane Harvey struck Texas. It has been an interesting experience so far and I have much to share from that experience.

I appreciate the opportunity to appear before you today as you prepare to consider the second reauthorization of PAHPA. This Committee championed the bipartisan effort to draft and pass this groundbreaking legislation and I want to thank you for your continuing commitment to this endeavor.

I am proud to have played a part in the original legislative process during my tenure with this Committee, and acknowledge the vision and leadership of Senator Burr and the late Senator Ted Kennedy.

This morning, I will share with you my perspective on the national security imperative of PAHPA, the mission and duties of ASPR, and my vision for areas of improvement.

The Constitution states that one of the Federal Government's fundamental obligations is to provide for the common defense, to protect the American people, our homeland, and our way of life. The strength of our Nation's public health and medical infrastructure, as well as the capabilities to quickly mobilize a coordinated national response to pandemics, attacks, and disasters are essential to save lives and protect all Americans.

Therefore, improving national readiness and response capabilities for 21st century threats is a national security imperative, as Senator Burr outlined earlier, and is the crux of my efforts as the ASPR.

The 21st century health security environment is increasingly complex and dangerous. It demands that we react with urgency. Having recently left my job with the Senate Select Committee on Intelligence, I know these threats all too well.

Terrorist organizations remain determined to attack the United States. State actors now directly threaten our homeland with nuclear weapons and have the means to employ both chemical and biological weapons.

Further, we have witnessed the increased frequency of naturally occurring disasters as well as disease outbreaks and are currently monitoring potential emerging infectious diseases that could cause a pandemic such as the H7N9 influenza strain circulating in China.

The bottom line is whatever happens, your constituents, the American people, expect our Federal Government to be ready to respond to save lives.

When APSR was originally established by PAHPA a decade ago, the objective was to answer a simple question: who is in charge of all Federal public health and medical preparedness and response functions? The approach adopted was based on the Goldwater-Nichols Act that created the Unified Combatant Commands at the Department of Defense.

APSR's mission is to save lives and protect Americans from these threats by recruiting the entire weight of the federal, medical, and public health assets and recruit support of the public health sector to support state and local activities and responses to help Americans in distress.

As APSR, I have four key priorities.

First, provide strong leadership. Focus on coordination, planning, and preparing for events that threaten the national health security.

Second, develop the national disaster healthcare system.

Third, advocate for CDC's sustainment of a robust and reliable public health security capabilities.

Last, but certainly not least, advance an innovative medical countermeasure enterprise.

Two areas of progress and opportunity I will elaborate on are operational healthcare readiness capacity and the medical counter- measures enterprise.

The importance of the national healthcare readiness and medical surge capacity was highlighted during this hurricane season. After Hurricanes Harvey, Irma, and Maria, ASPR led federal medical and public health response and recovery activities under the national response framework. We worked closely with FEMA, and state, and territorial health officials to augment healthcare with HHS disaster medical assistance teams, as well as V.A. and DOD assets.

We learned from these disasters that ASPR needs to update its incident command and deployable medical capabilities, as well as enhance our support for the healthcare infrastructure across the country.

As with medical countermeasures, the Nation's healthcare delivery infrastructure is mostly a private sector enterprise that must be effectively engaged in improving readiness.

To address the potential catastrophic medical consequences of the 21st century threats, we need a tiered regional system that is based on existing local healthcare coalitions and trauma centers that integrates all medical response capabilities, including Federal assets, as well as emergency medical services, the frontline of our response capabilities.

We must expand specialty care expertise and trauma, behavioral healthcare and chemical, biological, radiological nuclear response. And certainly, but not least, incentivize the healthcare system to integrate measures of preparedness into daily standards of care. I call this the foundation of a national disaster healthcare system.

The second area is our medical countermeasure enterprise, and I am grateful that Dr. Rick Bright behind me—Rick, why do you not wave to the crowd—who is the Director of BARDA, is joining me today.

BARDA was established as part of PAHPA and is a component of ASPR to bridge the so-called "valley of death" in the late stage development of vaccine, drug, and diagnostic development when many products historically languished or failed.

By using flexible, nimble authorities, multiyear advanced funding, strong public-private partnerships, and cutting edge expertise BARDA has successfully pushed many innovative products from advanced development to stockpiling FDA approval. To this date, 34 products have been approved by the FDA for the purposes of responding to disasters to the credit of Dr. Bright and his predecessor, Dr. Robin Robinson and the team at BARDA.

We have opportunities to further improve this enterprise by streamlining our internal decision-making processes, finding new ways to support innovation, promoting flexible, fast response capabilities, and increasing our collaboration with Federal interagency partners.

We also must work closely with our state and local partners, as well as the private sector to enhance the capability to quickly distribute and dispense medical countermeasures in an emergency.

In times of great challenge, we have the opportunity to build on the great progress made and further improve our national readiness and response capabilities.

I look forward to working with you and your staff. And thank you, again, for your bipartisan support and commitment to national security.

I am happy to answer any questions you have. [The prepared statement of Dr. Kadlec follows:]

PREPARED STATEMENT OF ROBERT KADLEC

Good morning Mr. Chairman, Senator Murray, and other distinguished Members of the Committee. I am Dr. Bob Kadlec, the Assistant Secretary for Preparedness and Response (ASPR) at the Department of Health and Human Services (HHS). I assumed this role 5 months ago, a week before hurricane Harvey struck Texas. I appreciate the opportunity to appear before you today as you prepare to consider the second reauthorization of the Pandemic and All-Hazards Preparedness Act (PAHPA), which expires at the end of this fiscal year.

Building upon years of incremental legislative changes in the prior decade, this seminal legislation transformed the Federal Government's medical and public health preparedness for threats to our national security. This Committee championed the bipartisan oversight and analysis that led to the drafting and passage of this groundbreaking legislation. I want to thank you for continuing that commitment here today.

I am proud to have played a part in that original legislative process, when during the 109th Congress, I was Staff Director of this Committee's Subcommittee on Bioterrorism and Public Health Preparedness, led by Senators Burr and Kennedy. In the decades before and after PAHPA was passed, I worked in various government capacities focused on biodefense and national security. I spent more than 20 years in the United States Air Force as an officer and physician, and served as Special Advisor for Counter Proliferation Policy within the Office of the Secretary of Defense during 9/11 and the 2001 anthrax attacks. I served two tours of duty at the White House Homeland Security Council, first as the Director for Biodefense then as Special Assistant to President Bush for Biodefense Policy from 2007 to 2009. Most recently before taking my current position, I served as the Deputy Staff Director for the Senate Select Committee on Intelligence.

This morning, I will share with you my perspective on the national security imperative of PAHPA, the mission and duties of ASPR, the status of our Department and our Nation's public health and medical preparedness and response capabilities, and my vision for areas of improvement. I welcome the opportunity to engage with you and your staff in the months ahead as you continue your oversight and legislative drafting.

The National Security Imperative

The Constitution states that one of the Federal Government's fundamental responsibilities is to provide for the common defense—to protect the American people, our homeland, and our way of life. The strength of our Nation's public health and medical infrastructure, and the capabilities necessary to quickly mobilize a coordinated national response to emergencies and disasters, are foundational for the quality of life of our citizens and vital to our national security. Therefore, improving national readiness and response capabilities for 21st century health security threats is a national security imperative and is my singular focus as the ASPR.

The 21st century health security environment is increasingly complex and dangerous; it demands that we act with urgency and singular effort: to save lives and protect Americans. Terrorist organizations such as ISIS and al-Qaida remain determined to attack the United States as we experienced first-hand in 2001. ISIS has demonstrated no compunction about using chemical and other unconventional weapons in attacks overseas. State actors, such as North Korea, have already threatened our homeland with nuclear weapons, and have the means to employ both chemical and biological weapons; the Syrian regime has already used chemical weapons against its own citizens.

Furthermore, we have witnessed the impacts of naturally occurring outbreaks such as influenza, Ebola, and SARS, and we are monitoring other potential emerging infectious diseases that could cause a pandemic, such as the H7N9 influenza strain circulating in China. 2018 marks the 100 year anniversary of the 1918 influenza pandemic, which killed more people than World War I. During that pandemic, more than 25 percent of the U.S. population became sick and 675,000 Americans, many of them young, healthy adults, died from the highly virulent influenza virus. Cyber-attacks like the WannaCry incident remind us that technological advancements have tradeoffs in the form of new vulnerabilities and risks, as our health delivery systems become more networked.

Finally, we face extreme weather events, such as the recent 2017 hurricane season in which Hurricanes Harvey, Irma, and Maria caused an unprecedented amount of damage, reminding us of the awesome destructive power of nature.

These are threats that most of us would rather not think about. However, when natural disasters, disease outbreaks, or attacks occur, the people expect our government to be ready to respond to save lives and protect Americans.

The ASPR Mission and Duties

When ASPR was originally established by PAHPA a decade ago, the objective was to create "unity of command" by consolidating all Federal nonmilitary public health and medical preparedness and response functions under the ASPR. This approach was modeled on the Goldwater-Nichols Act that created the Department of Defense (DoD) combatant commands; the impetus was the disorganized and fragmented response to Hurricane Katrina in 2005.

ASPR's mission is to save lives and protect Americans from 21st century health security threats. ASPR is, in effect, the national security mission manager for HHS. As such, on behalf of the Secretary of HHS, ASPR leads the public health and medical, preparedness, response and recovery to disasters and public health emergencies, in accordance with the National Response Framework (NRF) and Emergency Support Function No. 8 (Public Health and Medical Services). It is my responsibility to coordinate the Nation's medical and public health capabilities to help Americans during such events, whatever their cause. ASPR also coordinates with other components of HHS with respect to HHS's role in ESF No. 6 (Mass Care, Housing, and Human Services) and HHS's lead role as the coordinating agency with respect to the Health and Social Services Recovery Support Function.

ASPR coordinates across HHS, the Federal interagency, and supports state, local, territorial, and tribal health partners in preparing for and responding to emergencies and disasters. ASPR, in partnership with HHS agencies, works to enhance medical surge capacity by organizing, training, equipping, and deploying Federal public health and medical personnel and providing logistical support for Federal responses to public health emergencies. ASPR supports readiness at the state and local level by coordinating Federal grants and cooperative agreements and carrying out drills and operational exercises. ASPR oversees advanced research, development, and procurement of medical countermeasures (e.g., vaccines, medicines, diagnostics, and other necessary medical supplies), and coordinates the stockpiling of such countermeasures. ASPR manages the Biomedical Advanced Research and Development Authority (BARDA), Project BioShield, and the Public Health Emergency Medical Countermeasures Enterprise.

HHS and ASPR have made significant progress since PAHPA was enacted in 2006 and was reauthorized in 2013, which I will discuss shortly. The ASPR organization is filled with very capable, committed, and mission-driven staff; I am proud to lead them. It is my goal to further improve national public health and medical readiness and response capabilities, which have been developed by my predecessors who worked long hours to establish ASPR and build the capabilities that exist today. I aim to do that through four key priority areas:

First, provide strong leadership, including clear policy direction, improved threat awareness, and secure adequate resources.

Second, seek the creation of a "national disaster healthcare system" by better leveraging and enhancing existing programs—such as the Hospital Preparedness Program (HPP) and the National Disaster Medical System (NDMS)—to create a more coherent, comprehensive, and capable regional system integrated into daily care delivery.

Third, advocate for the sustainment of robust and reliable public health security capabilities, primarily through the Centers for Disease Control and Prevention (CDC), but also through other components of HHS, including an improved ability to detect and diagnose infectious diseases and other threats, as well as the capability to rapidly dispense medical countermeasures in an emergency.

Fourth, advance an innovative medical countermeasures enterprise by capitalizing on additional authorities provided in the 21st Century Cures Act, as well as advances in biotechnology and science, in order to develop and maintain a robust stockpile of safe and efficacious vaccines, medicines, and supplies to respond to emerging disease outbreaks, pandemics, and chemical, biological, radiological, and nuclear incidents and attacks.

The State of Public Health and Medical Preparedness and Response Capabilities

In 2006, when then Secretary of Health and Human Services Michael Leavitt testified before this Committee in advance of PAHPA's passage, he told Senators that we had the ability to "become the first generation in history to be prepared for a possible pandemic." At that time, HHS was closely watching the H5N1 influenza virus, and was concerned about the potential for another human influenza pandemic. Congress invested heavily by passing emergency supplemental appropriations bills, which were used to greatly expand our domestic vaccine manufacturing infrastructure, invest in new vaccine development, and provide funding to state and local governments to enhance medical and public health readiness.

Today, our capabilities are far greater than they were then; for example, we have sufficient domestic vaccine manufacturing capacity to produce bulk vaccine for every American within 6 months. However, we have exhausted the emergency supplemental funding balances at a time when we are now closely watching the H7N9 influenza virus circulating in China, and we are concerned with the ominous trends that we are seeing. While building domestic manufacturing capacity may be a onetime expenditure, maintaining that capacity as well as sustaining, testing, and strengthening the readiness of our medical and public health infrastructure at the state and local level requires continuous support and an enduring commitment to the Public Health Emergency Medical Countermeasures Enterprise.

Last month, a report by the public health organization Trust for America's Health found that half of states scored five or lower out of 10 on health emergency preparedness. Earlier in 2016, the National Health Security Preparedness Index from the Robert Wood Johnson Foundation found that health security metrics showed modest 1.5 percent improvement overall during 2016, reaching the highest level of out of 10 total;

however, levels of readiness varied significantly across the country. So, while we have made progress in the last decade, we still have work to do. Two areas of progress and opportunities I would like to highlight are our medical countermeasures enterprise, specifically BARDA, and our healthcare readiness capacity.

Medical Countermeasures Enterprise—BARDA

PAHPA established BARDA to bridge the so-called "valley of death" in late stage development of medical countermeasures where many products historically languished or failed. By using flexible, nimble authorities, multiyear advanced funding, strong public-private partnerships, and cutting edge expertise, BARDA has successfully pushed innovative medical countermeasures, such as vaccines, drugs, and diagnostics, through advanced development to stockpiling and FDA approval or licensing.

In the last decade, BARDA's strong partnerships with the National Institutes of Health, other HHS components, and biotechnology and pharmaceutical companies have led to 34 medical countermeasures approved or licensed by the FDA, which is a staggering accomplishment. BARDA has supported the development of 27 medical countermeasures against Department of Homeland Security (DHS) identified national security threats through Project BioShield, including products for smallpox, anthrax, botulinum, radiologic/nuclear emergencies, and chemical events. Fourteen of these products have been placed in the Strategic National Stockpile and are ready to be used in an emergency. BARDA also has supported the development of 23 influenza vaccines, antiviral drugs, devices, and diagnostics to address the risk of pandemic influenza. As a result of this progress, more medical countermeasures than ever before are eligible to be acquired for the SNS, thereby creating new challenges in terms of acquiring and maintaining sufficient quantities of medical counter-measures for identified threats.

We are supporting the development and stockpiling of many more novel medical countermeasures within the next few years, such as H7N9 influenza vaccines, next generation anthrax vaccines, enhanced smallpox vaccines, biodosimetry diagnostic devices, thermal burn radiation drug and skin replacement therapies, radiation cell therapies, new antibiotics, and new chemical antidotes.

We also have opportunities to further improve our national security medical countermeasures enterprise by streamlining our internal decision-making processes, finding new ways to support innovation, promoting flexible, fast response capabilities, and increasing our collaboration with Federal interagency partners, such as DoD and Department of Veterans Affairs (VA). We also must work closely with our state, local, territorial, and tribal partners, as well as the private sector to enhance the capability to quickly distribute and dispense medical countermeasures in an emergency—if we can't get these products to the right place, at the right time, then the enterprise has failed.

Healthcare Readiness to Respond

The 2017 hurricane season highlighted the importance of national healthcare readiness and medical surge capacity. ASPR led the public health and medical responses to Hurricanes Harvey, Irma, and Maria under the National Response Framework Emergency Support Function No. 8 mission. We worked closely with state and territory health officials in affected areas to augment care with NDMS teams, VA personnel and facility support, and DoD transportation, facilities, and clinicians. Personnel under the supervision of HHS treated over 36,000 patients, and HHS deployed over 4,500 personnel, evacuated nearly 800 patients, awarded over 200 contracts, and provided nearly 950 tons of equipment.

During the response, due to the combined efforts of ASPR and the Centers for Medicare & Medicaid Services (CMS), we utilized the innovative HHS emPOWER program to identify and treat at risk individuals requiring electricity-dependent medical and assistive equipment (e.g., ventilators, oxygen concentrators, feeding machines, intravenous infusion pumps, suction pumps, dialysis machines, wheelchairs). In one instance, ASPR teams used this data and worked with Urban Search and Rescue teams to identify all of the dialysis patients in the U.S. Virgin Islands and evacuate those patients for treatment since the local dialysis centers were destroyed. Despite our successes, we also learned that ASPR needs to improve its internal capabilities as well as enhance our support for the healthcare infrastructure across the country. As with medical countermeasures, the Nation's healthcare delivery infrastructure is mostly a private sector enterprise. We must better leverage and enhance existing Federal programs—such as the Hospital Preparedness Program and NDMS—to create a more coherent, comprehensive, and capable regional system integrated into daily care delivery I call this the foundation of a "national disaster healthcare system."

Conclusion

Through this second reauthorization of PAHPA, we have the opportunity to build on the great progress made and further improve our national readiness and response capabilities for 21st century health security threats. The Department looks forward to working with you in the months ahead to consider any legislative changes needed to achieve this objective. I am committing the entire ASPR team's grit, ingenuity, expertise, and perseverance to this mission. Thank you, again, for your bipartisan commitment to this national security imperative, and I look forward to continuing to work together to enhance our Nation's health security. I am happy to answer any questions you may have.

Senator BURR. Thank you, Dr. Bob. Dr. Gottlieb.

STATEMENT OF SCOTT GOTTLIEB, MD, COMMISSIONER, U.S. FOOD AND DRUG ADMINISTRATION, SILVER SPRING, MD

Dr. GOTTLIEB. Senator Burr, Ranking Member Murray, and Members of the Committee.

Thank you for the invitation to testify today about genome editing technology.

Our Nation has faced many emerging public health challenges and unfortunately, will face additional challenges in the future. Thankfully, our preparedness and the ability to respond to such challenges has improved greatly since the original enactment of the Pandemic and All-Hazards Preparedness Act.

Each emergency is unique. Many are the result of emerging infectious threats, but the technology for manipulating science for diabolical purposes is becoming more ubiquitous and widely understood. So we face new and pervasive risks.

2017 was marked by the risks posed by several extreme natural disasters, which caused significant devastation and human suffering. These tragedies tested our Nation's capabilities to respond. Today, I am going to focus my remarks on the impact of these storms on medical products manufactured in Puerto Rico and the actions we are taking to mitigate existing and potential product shortages.

The impact of Hurricane Maria showed the importance of Puerto Rico to our medical product manufacturing base, as well as the intricate and sometimes fragile nature of that supply chain.

I want to focus on the complexities of the saline shortage because it has stressed our system and I know that many of you are deeply and rightly concerned by this situation.

Saline solution has been in and out of shortage for several years. There are only a small number of primary manufacturers. So when one manufacturer lowers production, even for routine maintenance, there is stress on the entire system.

One of the largest manufacturers of I.V. saline is Baxter, and their primary sites for small volume bags are located in Puerto Rico. These sites struggled to regain power and return to full capacity following the storm when roads to some of the manufacturing plants were disabled.

We worked closely with Baxter in partnership with the Department of Homeland Security, and Puerto Rico authorities, and Bob—so thank you for your support, as well—to ensure that they were able to get back on the power grid on a priority basis to stabilize production.

We also worked with various saline manufacturers to find other manufacturing facilities globally that could help supply the U.S. until Baxter's Puerto Rico location was back up and running and the shortage was addressed.

To mitigate that shortage, we worked with manufacturers on the importation of saline from locations in Ireland, Australia, Mexico,

Canada, Germany, and most recently, Brazil. When we import from international facilities, generally, the manufacturers adjust their distribution to send some product to the U.S., but there is no actual increase in the total global production of product.

Baxter's manufacturing facilities in Puerto Rico are now stable and on the grid, although the power situation on the island is still fragile. We expect their return to normal production will improve the situation.

Before the storms hit, and in anticipation of the crisis, FDA also prioritized the approval of saline products by two manufacturers, Fresenius Kabi laboratories, and Grifols. Both should start production soon, and having these two additional manufacturers online will help increase the overall supply of saline produced and distributed in the U.S.

But this shortage has also had ripple effects. In order to find workarounds for the filled saline bags that were in shortage, providers have put various mitigation strategies in place. One strategy has hospitals compounding product themselves and this has caused an increased demand for empty I.v. bags. There have been signals indicating that this increased demand is putting pressure on the supply of empty I.v. bags. The FDA is taking steps to address that situation and determine which manufacturers could potentially increase capacity if necessary.

I have reached out to some of these medical device manufacturers personally to inquire about their capacity to increase production as demand for I.V. containers continues to increase.

The scope of the flu outbreak across the country has also added to the strain on this tight supply chain. The shortage, and the impact of the crisis in Puerto Rico, underscores the need to continuously elevate our preparedness.

There are going to be lessons learned from this episode, and already, we have made some key observations about our ability to detect device shortages. Since we lack authority to require notification of device shortages, we have had to depend on manufacturers and distributors reaching out to the FDA or had to seek them out proactively.

Our work in the shortage situation is an example of how the FDA has reacted in response to emergency situations. At the same time, we continue to work hard to improve our regulatory clarity and predictability for the development of medical countermeasures. That is an essential component of our national preparedness strategy.

Today, we released draft guidance on Material Threat Medical Countermeasure and Priority Review Vouchers which explains how the FDA is implementing the PRV program to incentivize the development of certain drug and biologics medical countermeasures. I look forward to working with Congress to continue to increase our readiness for emergencies, and look forward to answering your questions today.

[The prepared statement of Dr. Gottlieb follows:]

PREPARED STATEMENT OF SCOTT GOTTLIEB

Chairman Alexander, Ranking Member Murray, and Members of the Committee, thank you for the opportunity to appear today to discuss reauthorization of the Pandemic and All-Hazards Preparedness Act (PAHPA). PAHPA, which was passed in 2006 and reauthorized in 2013, is a key piece of legislation that—along with other significant legislative achievements such as the Project BioShield Act of 2004, the Public Readiness and Emergency Preparedness (PREP) Act (2005), and the 21st Century Cures Act (Cures Act) enacted in 2016—has served to significantly strengthen our country's preparedness for, and response to, public health emergencies involving chemical, biological, radiological, and nuclear (CBRN) threats as well as emerging infectious disease threats, such as the Zika virus and pandemic influenza.

The Pandemic and All-Hazards Preparedness Reauthorization Act of 2013 (PAHPRA), in particular, recognized the key role the Food and Drug Administration (FDA or the Agency) plays in emergency preparedness and response, and codified and built on FDA's ongoing efforts to augment review processes and advance regulatory science to enable FDA to better respond to public health emergencies. The provisions in PAHPRA—as well as in the other key pieces of legislation I mentioned—have provided FDA with essential tools that continue to support us in our mission to protect and promote public health.

FDA's Public Health Emergency Preparedness and Response Mission

FDA plays a critical role in facilitating preparedness for and response to CBRN and emerging infectious disease threats. These threats can and often do emerge without warning as was the case with the anthrax attacks of 2001, the 2009 H1N1 influenza pandemic, the 2014 Ebola outbreak in West Africa, as well as in the ongoing Zika virus outbreak.

FDA's role in facilitating preparedness for, and response to, CBRN and emerging infectious disease threats focuses largely on facilitating the development and availability of medical countermeasures—such as vaccines, therapeutics, and diagnostic tests—to respond to these threats. FDA works closely with its HHS and other U.S. Government partners through the Public Health Emergency Medical Countermeasures Enterprise (PHEMCE), as well as with regulated industry and non-governmental organizations (NGO's), to build and sustain the medical countermeasure programs necessary to effectively respond to public health emergencies. FDA is also committed to working closely with the Department of Defense (DoD) to facilitate the development and availability of medical counter-measures to support the unique needs of our Nation's warfighters. The Agency is already actively implementing the legislation enacted at the end of last year to further prioritize this critical work with DoD. Senior leadership at the Agency is lead ing these efforts, and we look forward to keeping Congress informed of our progress in these critical areas.

FDA's Medical Countermeasures Initiative (MCMi)—established in 2010—brought additional resources to FDA that enabled FDA to hire additional expert staff and to become more deeply and thoroughly engaged in medical countermeasure activities. This program continues to be key to establishing clear regulatory pathways for medical countermeasures, advancing medical countermeasure regulatory science to support regulatory decisionmaking, and advancing important policies and mechanisms to facilitate the timely development and availability of medical counter-measures. FDA's goal is to be modern and efficient in its regulation of safe and effective medical products, and that includes medical countermeasures.

FDA's operations within its medical countermeasures mission cover a broad range of activities vital to facilitating the development of, and access to, safe and effective medical countermeasures, including:

- Reviewing medical countermeasure marketing applications and approving those that meet standards for safety and efficacy;
- Providing regulatory advice, guidance and technical assistance to sponsors developing medical countermeasures, as well as to U.S. Government partners, international regulators, and international organizations such as the World Health Organization;
- Supporting efforts to establish and sustain an adequate supply of medical countermeasures, including averting supply disruptions when feasible and, in certain situations, allowing products to be used beyond their expiration dates when supported by appropriate scientific evaluation;
- Enabling access to medical countermeasures that are not yet approved for use—when necessary—through an appropriate mechanism, including through FDA's Emergency Use Authorization (EUA) authority;
- Proactively identifying and resolving regulatory challenges associated with medical countermeasure development and ensuring that FDA regulations and policies adequately support medical countermeasure development and enable preparedness and response activities;
- Fostering the professional development of FDA scientists to ensure that FDA personnel maintain the skills and abilities to support the medical counter-measure mission; and
- Supporting regulatory science to create the tools, standards, and approaches necessary to develop and assess the safety, efficacy, quality, and performance of medical countermeasures.

FDA is also a critical partner in preparing for, and responding to, natural disasters, as demonstrated by its ongoing 2017 hurricane recovery efforts, including its work in Puerto Rico following Hurricane Maria. FDA performs extensive preliminary work in advance of storms to help prepare for potential impacts. For example, FDA utilizes storm prediction data and firm registration data bases to prepare maps to identify FDA regulated firms, including those that manufacture critical products that could be impacted by the storms. Where necessary, FDA may take contingency steps to help ensure a continuous supply of critical medical product manufacturing. The most significant role that FDA plays comes after the storm, as facilities come back on line and may need remediation, and farmers seek to put crops or farmland that were damaged back into commercial use. FDA has supported the many pharmaceutical and medical device manufacturers in Puerto Rico to help address and prioritize recovery operations based on the potential for medical product shortages based on public health needs. Many of the requests FDA received were for infrastructure support, primarily getting a reliable source of power, and FDA worked with partners at the Department of Homeland Security to support getting critical manufacturing back online. Through product registrations and communications with manufacturers, FDA was able to identify the medically necessary products manufactured in Puerto Rico and determine which were the top public health priorities. FDA continues to be focused on storm-related shortage issues, including shortages of saline solution and amino acids, as well as the cascading increase in demand for other medical products, such as empty IV containers which are now being used in higher quantities for compounded products. FDA has been in direct communication with manufacturers, distributors, hospitals and other health care providers, including the Department of Veterans Affairs (VA), and we are assessing existing product supply, demand trends and manufacturer capacity to increase availability of the empty IV containers.

Fostering Innovation in Medical Countermeasure Development

At FDA, we fully appreciate that the development of medical countermeasures can present complex and unique challenges. For example, it is not ethical to conduct human studies for many of the high-priority threat agents. In these situations, the Animal Rule, which enables animal efficacy studies to substitute for efficacy trials in humans if the results can reasonably be extrapolated to the expected human use, can be used to facilitate the development and availability of medical counter-measures. PAHPRA recognized the importance of the Animal Rule; and in 2015, FDA finalized guidance for product development under the Animal Rule, incorporating the learnings of considerable product development experience and providing scientific and regulatory expectations for animal data intended to support medical countermeasure approval.

To date, 12 medical countermeasures have been approved under the Animal Rule, including inhalational anthrax therapeutics, a botulism antitoxin, antibiotics for the treatment and prophylaxis of plague, and treatments for acute radiation syndrome. These approvals underscore the critical role the Animal Rule and animal studies can play in advancing medical countermeasures for some of the most challenging threats. Of note, through the use of regulatory science, FDA was able to approve the inhalational anthrax therapeutics and the botulism antitoxin for use in children as well as adults, despite the fact that pediatric patients were not actually studied in clinical trials, due to ethical concerns.

However, for many threats there are not yet adequate regulatory science foundation, such as animal models to support medical countermeasure development or sufficient biomarkers to enable the extrapolation of data generated in animal models to humans. Without such tools, it is difficult to generate the data necessary to support regulatory decision-making.

FDA has established a broad and robust portfolio of cutting-edge research under MCMi's Regulatory Science Program to help develop these tools and promote innovation in the development of medical countermeasures. A few examples of projects include: supporting the development of organs-on-chips models to assess radiation damage in lung, gut, and bone marrow, and then using these models to test candidate medical countermeasures; collaborating to establish a publicly available genomic sequence reference data base for use by developers seeking to validate candidate multiplex in vitro diagnostic tests that could be used to diagnose multiple pathogens simultaneously; developing reference materials for developers to use to validate nucleic acid-based and serological diagnostic tests for Zika virus; supporting a project to identify and correlate biomarkers of host response to Ebola virus infection in animal models and humans to support medical countermeasure development; developing methods for obtaining safety and limited efficacy data from patients who receive medical countermeasures during public health emergencies; and establishing the Animal Model Qualification Program designed to support medical counter-measure development by promoting the development of animal models for use across multiple product applications, thereby minimizing duplication of effort and resources.

PAHPRA also provided authorities to ensure that FDA personnel are well-trained in how to review medical countermeasure applications for approval. Under these authorities, FDA has established a professional development program, including speakers' series and academic certifications, to ensure that FDA scientists are working through the regulatory challenges posed by new areas of science and technology as they relate to medical countermeasure development. FDA also has spent considerable energy and resources establishing an efficient approach to conduct and support training within the agency.

More recently, the Cures Act included several provisions that are intended to advance innovation in medical product development more generally, but will also help to facilitate the development of medical countermeasures, including the provisions to encourage novel trial designs, and to develop new antimicrobial drug products. Through the Cures Act, Congress also provided a new priority review voucher (PRV) program to help incentivize the development of material threat medical countermeasures. Under this program, FDA will award a PRV upon approval of a material threat medical countermeasure application provided that certain criteria are met. The PRV may in turn be used by the sponsor who receives it, or sold to another sponsor, who may then use it to obtain priority review for a product application that would otherwise not receive that benefit, enabling a developer to potentially bring a product to market sooner than otherwise possible—something that may be of great value to product developers. FDA plans to issue guidance to address medical countermeasure specific considerations with the intent to implement the program consistently with the other PRV programs, such as the Neglected Tropical Disease Voucher Program.

There are tremendous opportunities to continue to further the development of groundbreaking, innovative medical countermeasures, and the Agency intends to fully seize and build upon these opportunities. Toward that goal, this past July FDA announced the launch of a comprehensive Innovation Initiative aimed at making sure its regulatory processes are modern and efficient so that safe and effective new technologies, including medical countermeasures, can reach patients in a timely fashion.

Facilitating Access to Safe and Effective Medical Countermeasures

Enabling access to medical countermeasures when they are needed is a high priority for FDA. Amended and new authorities provided by Congress have enabled the Agency to further prepare for, and better respond to, emerging public health threats. For example, PAHPRA amended FDA's EUA authority to provide additional flexibility for issuing EUAs. These additional flexibilities have enabled FDA to better support responses to emerging health threats by issuing nearly 40 EUAs to enable the emergency use of *In Vitro* diagnostic devices for H7N9 Influenza virus, Enterovirus D68 (EV-D68), Middle East Respiratory Syndrome Coronavirus (MERS-CoV), Ebola virus, and Zika virus. FDA also issued an EUA to enable the emergency use of an autoinjector medical countermeasure to maintain preparedness for chemical threats, which has been critical for supporting both warfighter and first responder preparedness goals related to an emergency involving nerve agents. The authority for prepositioning medical countermeasures provided in PAHPRA also proved useful to allow the manufacturer to ship, and the U.S. Government stakeholders to receive, certain strengths of the unapproved autoinjectors that were not yet authorized for use under that EUA.

PAHPRA also provided FDA with several new streamlined authorities to facilitate the emergency use of approved medical countermeasures without the need for issuing an

EUA. For example, PAHPRA provided FDA with the authority to issue emergency dispensing orders (including mass dispensing at a point of dispensing (POD)) for approved medical countermeasures during an actual CBRN emergency without requiring an individual prescription for each recipient of the medical countermeasure, if permitted by state law or in accordance with an emergency dispensing order issued by FDA. FDA has used this authority to issue emergency dispensing orders to permit emergency dispensing of doxycycline and ciprofloxacin for post-exposure prophylaxis of inhalational anthrax, to ensure government stakeholders can rapidly provide these therapies in the event of an anthrax attack.[1]

Another new FDA authority created by PAHPRA is the explicit ability to extend expiration dating of eligible FDA-approved medical countermeasures stockpiled for use in CBRN emergencies, if the extension is supported by an appropriate scientific evaluation. This authority streamlines FDA's ability to authorize expiration dating extensions without the need to issue an EUA, which will enable faster response, and has been crucial to FDA's ability to support preparedness efforts. For example, when production stopped after quality issues were identified in the manufacturing process of autoinjectors used for the treatment of nerve agent and insecticide poisoning, FDA used this authority to help prevent shortages of auto-injector products to help ensure that the Nation's warfighters and first responders continue to have ready access to these products. FDA also used this authority to extend the expiration date of certain lots of doxycycline capsules held in strategic stockpiles by the Centers for Disease Control and Prevention, state and local public health, and other response stakeholders and issued draft guidance to provide recommendations to government stakeholders on testing that can be conducted to support future extensions, in order to help sustain preparedness levels.

The Cures Act also amended the EUA and related emergency use authorities to clarify their applicability to animal drugs. FDA encourages anyone interested in utilizing these authorities to contact FDA to discuss how to proceed.

Most recently, Congress passed H.R. 4374, legislation that amends FDA's EUA authority to enable FDA to issue EUAs for medical products to reduce deaths and mitigate injuries from agents that may cause imminently life-threatening and specific risks to United States military forces. Prior to the passage of this legislation, the EUA authority was only applicable to medical products to address CBRN threats. In addition, the legislation contains provisions codifying enhanced collaboration between FDA and DoD, in order to facilitate the development of medical products and countermeasures for the warfighter. FDA is working closely with DoD to implement these new and amended authorities as quickly as possible.

---

[1] The term "stakeholder(s)" means the public agency or its delegate that has legal responsibility and authority for responding to an incident, based on political or geographical boundary lines (e.g., city, county, tribal, state, or federal), or functional (e.g., law enforcement or public health range) or sphere of authority to prescribe, administer, deliver, distribute, or dispense oral doxycycline products in an emergency situation.

Conclusion

At FDA, we have made it a priority to proactively work with our private sector and government partners to help facilitate the translation of breakthrough discoveries in science and technology into innovative, safe, and effective medical countermeasures. FDA takes its responsibility seriously to help drive and foster innovation as part of advancing public health and our national security. Active FDA involvement is essential to encouraging industry engagement in medical countermeasure development. FDA remains deeply committed to working closely with its partners and continuing to use the authorities Congress provides to the fullest extent to help facilitate the development and availability of safe and effective medical countermeasures. We believe that partnership and innovation will continue to be key drivers to success in the medical countermeasure space and are taking steps to further empower FDA's scientific and clinical experts to drive the innovation necessary to help protect the Nation from the threats we may face.

FDA appreciates Congress's support in continually delineating, clarifying, expanding, and extending its authorities—and providing resources—to enable FDA to achieve its public health emergency preparedness and response mission. FDA stands ready to work with Congress and stakeholders to enable us to better achieve this critical work.

Thank you for inviting FDA to testify today. I am happy to answer any questions you may have.

Senator BURR. Thank you, Scott. Dr. REDD.

STATEMENT OF STEPHEN C. REDD, MD, RADM, DIRECTOR, OFFICE OF PUBLIC HEALTH PREPAREDNESS AND RESPONSE, CENTERS FOR DISEASE CONTROL AND PREVENTION, ATLANTA, GA

Dr. REDD. Senator Burr, Chairman Alexander, and Ranking Member Murray.

I am Dr. Stephen Redd, the Director of the Office of Public Health Preparedness and Response at the Centers for Disease Control. And I am pleased to be here to talk with you today about the role the CDC plays in public health preparedness and response, including those responsibilities under the Pandemic and All-Hazards Preparedness Reauthorization Act.

The CDC is the common defense of the country against health threats. Our work to prepare and respond to health emergencies require that we build on our day to day in two particular areas.

No. 1, our longstanding partnership with state and local health departments and;

No. 2, our medical, scientific, and program expertise.

I will describe the three pillars of our defense strategy: science, surveillance, and service.

First, the CDC has a unique collection of scientific expertise that exists nowhere else in the world. We have the ability to identify agents causing illness, whether that illness is caused by an infectious microbe, or a chemical, or a radiation exposure.

We are ready to respond to a broad range of threats including diseases like Ebola, small pox, and H7N9 influenza.

The CDC plays a key role in discovering new and emerging infectious diseases using advanced detection techniques to identify pathogens quickly and more accurately.

Every year, laboratories from all over the world send hundreds of thousands of specimens to the CDC for testing.

The second pillar enabling the CDC's common defense of the country is surveillance. Public health surveillance is the collection, analysis, and use of data to target public health prevention and response. It is basically making sure the best information is used to make the right decisions.

Examples of this work include what we do to track influenza, the National Syndromic Surveillance system and the Global Disease Detection Program.

Influenza is probably the greatest natural health threat we face. Influenza viruses change continuously and require vigilance to detect these changes. The CDC provides support to every state, to several major cities, and to a number of ministries of health throughout the world to conduct influenza surveillance and laboratory work.

With the National Syndromic Surveillance Program, the CDC collects deidentified health information on causes of emergency room, urgent care, and hospital visits. We, along with state and local health departments, use the data in real time to detect abnormal situations requiring public health response.

The CDC's Global Disease Detection Operation Center monitors 30 to 40 outbreaks every day across the globe, 24/7, and assesses the potential risk to the United States from these events. In addition to science and surveillance services, the final pillar is supporting the CDC's common defense of the country.

Let me focus on three particular programs, the Public Health Emergency Preparedness Program, the Strategic National Stockpile, and the Cities Readiness Initiative.

In each of these programs, the keys to success are the close collaboration between CDC and state and local public health departments, and the connection of these programs to CDC's scientific expertise.

The Public Health Emergency Preparedness grants go to every state and support staff, enable exercises to test and validate capabilities, and pay for laboratory and communications equipment.

The Strategic National Stockpile is a $7 billion repository of pharmaceuticals, medical supplies, and medical equipment that is available for rapid delivery to support responses to health emergencies.

The CDC's Cities Readiness Initiative enhances preparedness in the Nation's 72 largest cities where nearly 60 percent of the U.S. population resides. These funds are used to develop, test, and maintain plans to receive countermeasures from the CDC's Strategic National Stockpile and rapidly dispense them.

I would like to leave the Committee with three primary points about the CDC's role in public health emergency preparedness and response.

First, the CDC is the common defense of the country against health threats.

Two, CDC's preparedness work is built on a day to day foundation of our broad and deep scientific medical and program expertise.

Three, the CDC's longstanding partnerships with state and local health authorities are essential.

Thank you for the opportunity to testify today. [The prepared statement of Dr. Redd follows:]

PREPARED STATEMENT OF STEPHEN C. REDD

Chairman Alexander, Senator Murray, and other Members of the Committee. I am Rear Admiral Stephen Redd, Director of the Office of Public Health Preparedness and Response at the Centers for Disease Control and Prevention (CDC). I appreciate the opportunity to be here today to discuss CDC's public health preparedness and response mission, and the agency's role in implementing the Pandemic and All-Hazards Preparedness Reauthorization Act of 2013 (PAHPRA).

CDC provides for the common defense of the country against public health threats. Through our dedication to science, surveillance, and service, CDC focuses on protecting the public health of the Nation from threats such as emerging infectious diseases, natural disasters, and terrorism.

In carrying out the mission set forth under the Pandemic and All Hazards Preparedness Reauthorization Act, CDC draws on expertise from throughout the agency. CDC's expertise includes world-class laboratory testing, surveillance (for disease detection), epidemiology, guidance to healthcare providers, incident management, logistics, emergency risk communication, disease control programs, distribution of medical countermeasures, human and animal medicine, and responder health and well-being. Our multidisciplinary workforce enables an integrated national system that is nimble and prepared to detect and respond to any developing situation that could affect the health of people in the United States. In addition, CDC draws on its long-standing relationships and close collaboration with state and local partners to protect the health of communities across the country, and collaborates closely with the Assistant Secretary for Preparedness and Response (ASPR), the Food and Drug Administration (FDA) and other Federal partners.

CDC experts lead and staff every activation of the agency's Emergency Operations Center (EOC), ensuring response activities are effective and efficient. HHS/CDC has an emergency management program accredited by the Emergency Management Accreditation Program. CDC activated its incident management system for 67 responses over the last 16 years, between September 2001 and December 2017. During a response, CDC's EOC rapidly deploys scientific experts, coordinates the delivery of supplies and equipment to the incident site, monitors response activities, provides resources to state and local public health departments, and disseminates timely and accurate information within government, to health care providers, and to the public. During the agency's Zika and Ebola responses, CDC deployed over 1,700 and 3,700 staff, respectively. CDC also responds to public health events that do not require EOC support. In fiscal year 2017, CDC assisted state, local, and overseas public health authorities in 23 epidemiologic investigations of emerging infectious disease outbreaks as well as more than 20 environmental responses.

CDC Programs under the Pandemic and All Hazards Preparedness Reauthorization Act

The Pandemic and All Hazards Preparedness Reauthorization Act of 2013 (PAHPRA) reauthorized several public health preparedness programs. The discussion immediately below focuses on two of those programs: CDC's Public Health Emergency Preparedness cooperative agreement program (which includes the Cities Readiness Initiative (CRI)) and the Strategic National Stockpile (SNS). Later in the testimony I will discuss CDC's work related to a third PAHPRA program, bio-surveillance.

Public Health Emergency Preparedness Cooperative Agreement (PHEP) Program: The PHEP cooperative agreement program is the largest CDC state program and provided approximately $600 million to state, local, and territorial public health departments in 2017. The program developed the first playbooks for public health preparedness and response, and has been instrumental in integrating state and local health departments into their jurisdictions' emergency response structures. PHEP currently supports 62 awardees—including all 50 states, eight territories and freely associated states, and directly funded cities (New York City; Washington, DC.; Chicago; and Los Angeles). Funding is awarded according to a base plus population formula prescribed by statute, which ensures a minimum amount of funding to each awardee. These funds support preparedness and response staff, enable exercises to test and validate capabilities, provide for timely training, and pay for laboratory and communications equipment essential to maintaining preparedness. In addition, CDC personnel support PHEP awardees by helping to identify and address gaps in preparedness capabilities, providing planning resources to ensure the needs of at risk individuals are incorporated into response strategies, and improving response capabilities from experience gleaned during public health responses, most recently to Ebola and Zika.

Strategic National Stockpile (SNS): The SNS is the largest federally owned repository of vaccines, drugs, medical supplies, Federal Medical Stations, and medical equipment available for rapid delivery to support federal, state, and local response to health security threats. The SNS was created in 1999 to ensure the Nation's readiness against public health emergencies by ensuring delivery of lifesaving medical countermeasures (MCMs) during deliberate or naturally occurring outbreaks and other events that threaten public health. Since its inception, SNS products and staff have been deployed more than 100 times for events ranging from natural disasters to infectious disease outbreaks. CDC works with the HHS Assistant Secretary for Preparedness and Response and with other Federal agencies through the Public Health Emergency Medical Countermeasures Enterprise (PHEMCE) to prioritize Federal investments in medical countermeasures based on analysis of risk, benefits to the American people and sustainability of the MCM pipeline.

Management of the SNS and deployment of its assets are complex endeavors which rely on a broad range of scientific expertise, surveillance systems, public health communications systems, and state and local partners. The SNS ensures that the right medical countermeasures and supplies are available when, where, and in the quantity needed to stop or slow a public health emergency and save lives. And, scientific experts ensure that medicine and supplies expeditiously get to our public health partners at the state and local levels, who have had the necessary training, exercises, and clinical guidance to effectively and efficiently receive those assets from the SNS and get them to those who need them.

Cities Readiness Initiative (CRI): CRI, funded through the PHEP cooperative agreement, enhances preparedness in the Nation's largest population centers, where nearly 60 percent of the population resides. The 72 cities (at least one in every state) use CRI funds to develop, test, and maintain plans to quickly receive medical countermeasures from the SNS and distribute them to local communities. This program, through reliance on local boots on the ground, enables effective response to large-scale public health emergencies needing life-saving medications and medical supplies.

Public Health Preparedness through Science, Surveillance and Service

In carrying out its public health mission CDC's subject matter experts from across the agency collaborate to detect and respond to emerging threats that could affect Americans' health.

Science

Exceptional and world-renowned scientific expertise and world-class laboratories ensure CDC is ready and able to respond to a broad range of threats, including highly hazardous and infectious diseases like Ebola, smallpox, and H7N9 influenza. For example, CDC's research on the smallpox virus helps find better drugs to treat the disease, stop the virus from spreading, make safer vaccines, and improve tests to detect the virus. Additionally, CDC's global influenza capacity-building efforts helped facilitate the rapid detection of the novel Asian linage influenza A (H7N9) virus in 2013. Most human infections resulted from exposure to infected poultry, but CDC assesses that the virus poses the greatest pandemic risk of all influenza viruses not yet circulating among humans, and is working with global health partners to monitor that virus and detect changes in it that could trigger a pandemic. CDC has developed two candidate vaccine viruses and shared them with vaccine manufacturers, for use in BARDA-supported vaccine production and in clinical trials by NIH's National Institute of Allergy and Infectious Disease. If the H7N9 virus develops the capacity to spread among humans, an effective vaccine would be key for preventing a pandemic.

CDC plays a critical role in discovering new and emerging infectious diseases, using advanced molecular detection techniques that combine next-generation genomic sequencing, high-performance computing, and epidemiology to identify pathogens faster and more accurately. Laboratories from all over the world send specimens to CDC, often in cases where the cause of illness is unknown. Annually, CDC receives hundreds of thousands of specimens to examine and helps diagnose hundreds of cases of unexplained illness or death. Through advanced molecular detection investments, CDC is seeing improvements in faster detection of outbreaks (catching them when they are smaller) and in faster development of diagnostics, applying these technologies in dozens of areas such as foodborne disease, influenza, antimicrobial resistance, hepatitis, pneumonia, and meningitis. CDC shares genetic sequencing technologies with state and local health departments, and funds them to acquire new technology that helps them to respond quicker and more efficiently at a local level.

CDC is critical to preparing for the next influenza pandemic. In an influenza emergency, CDC's public health and infectious disease experts use advanced molecular detection techniques to identify disease strains that could cause a pandemic, release recommendations for the prevention, diagnosis, and treatment of disease, and provide communication to the Nation about the pandemic. For example, each human case of infection with a new animal influenza virus represents the potential for a pandemic. CDC receives and studies viruses like these in its laboratories to better understand where and how they spread and the nature of illness they cause. This informs development of clinical and public health recommendations before and during emergency responses. In the event of an influenza pandemic, CDC's scientific experts use the best epidemiologic and laboratory data available to update or develop guidance to inform purchasing, distribution, and use of medical counter-measures including vaccines, antiviral drugs, respirators or masks, and ventilators. CDC also develops and evaluates solutions to lessen the impact of an influenza pandemic through non-pharmaceutical interventions or actions that people and communities can implement to help slow the spread of influenza, such as staying home when ill, coordinating school closures, and postponing mass gatherings.

CDC has longstanding collaboration with countries and institutions around the world. These strategic partnerships coupled with forward deployment of our scientists stationed in more than 60 countries enable CDC to identify new pathogens, assess risks, and devise effective control measures. Our partnerships provide the platforms for timely sharing of laboratory specimens, innovations and distribution of diagnostic materials and technologies to prevent epidemics, and promptly respond to disease outbreaks before they cross international borders.

Vector-borne diseases present another preparedness challenge, as we saw in the Zika emergency. CDC is one of the Nation's public health authorities on vector-borne diseases, like Zika, plague, and dengue. CDC scientists who specialize in vector-borne disease have deep expertise in entomology, microbiology, virology, veterinary medicine, zoology, and public health that does not exist elsewhere. These experts develop diagnostic tools and clinical guidance, as well as methods of treatment, prevention, and vector control, in order to slow the spread of these diseases. For example, CDC scientists have determined that a natural plant ingredient called nootkatone effectively repels and kills the mosquitoes and ticks that can spread disease. Nootkatone appears to work differently than available insecticides, and it could help fight mosquitoes that are resistant to existing insecticides.

CDC's scientific experts protect people from environmental health threats like contaminated water, radiation, and chemical emergencies. To do so, CDC identifies the environmental exposures that make people sick, investigates how those exposures are transmitted in the environment, and finds ways to eliminate the threat to people's health. For example, CDC's radiation guidelines help public health officials and clinicians prepare for, and respond to, radiation emergencies and treat exposures.

The list of CDC's scientific expertise is much longer than I have detailed, including myriad chronic diseases and also includes foundational scientific expertise critical to effective public health impact such as in the areas of workforce, laboratory systems, and data sciences.

Surveillance

Public health surveillance—the collection, analysis, and use of data to target public health prevention and intervention activities—is the foundation of public health practice. CDC monitors health surveillance information around the clock to detect and track diseases and protect Americans. As one example, following 9/11, CDC made investments in enhancing syndromic surveillance—using health-related data based on patient symptoms that precede diagnosis—as an early warning system for bioterrorism. This system now allows officials to detect a much wider range of health threats—from opioid overdoses to chemical spills to disease outbreaks. Moreover, CDC collects, analyzes, and interprets human, animal, environmental, and food surveillance data, in order to identify and respond to potential health threats before they become emergencies. In aggregate, CDC's specialized surveillance systems provide prompt situational awareness and early warning for unknown or unexpected threats. CDC's surveillance activities directly support states in their primary responsibilities in protecting the public's health. Surveillance data, collected in collaboration with domestic and international partners, inform CDC's threat assessments and ensures response actions are at the right speed, scope, and scale to protect Americans.

CDC supports integrated disease surveillance activities at the state and local level through funding and provision of surveillance tools and services. The following are examples of the surveillance systems and support that CDC provides to state, local, and territorial public health departments to develop and strengthen their surveillance activities:

- *National Notifiable Diseases Surveillance System (NNDSS):* NNDSS is a nationwide system that enables all levels of public health—local, state, territorial, Federal, and international—to collect and share data on approximately 100 diseases and conditions that are required to be reported in all 50 states, and keeps them under continuous surveillance. This system provides comprehensive, timely, and high-quality data for public health decision-making, enabling CDC programs to work with state partners to better monitor disease occurrence, identify potential outbreaks, recognize emerging trends, track the impact of public health interventions, and respond..
- *Influenza Surveillance*: Influenza viruses are constantly changing, and, thus, require continued vigilance to protect the United States and the rest of the world from both seasonal and pandemic influenza threats. Influenza surveillance, both epidemiologic and virologic, is at the core of influenza preparedness. The surveillance platforms used year round to combat seasonal influenza threats serve as the foundation for pandemic influenza surveillance. CDC provides support to every state, and several major municipalities and territories, to conduct influenza surveillance and laboratory work. For many decades, CDC has served as an

international leader in global influenza surveillance. We have partnered with more than fifty countries to establish, maintain, and expand influenza surveillance and laboratory capacity, in order to find influenza viruses where they emerge as quickly as possible to mitigate their potentially devastating impact on the United States. Domestic funding supports seasonal influenza surveillance through a network of interrelated systems that provide data on where influenza and influenza-like illnesses, hospitalizations, and deaths occur.

- *National Syndromic Surveillance Program (NSSP):* CDC, through state and local collaborations, collects deidentified health information on emergency room, urgent care, and hospital visits, as well as pharmacy and laboratory data. This investment has revolutionized public health surveillance to include this new type of data collection on top of traditional type and methods of data collection. States and local public health departments use the syndromic data to detect and characterize abnormal situations meriting further public health investigation. This strengthens local public health capacity to detect, respond to, and manage, outbreaks and other critical public health events. CDC has negotiated access to the data to enable situational awareness at regional and national levels. The series of three recent hurricanes presents a poignant example that demonstrates the usefulness and flexibility of this asset. Before the hurricanes, CDC and ASPR had begun establishing a mechanism to share National Disaster Medical Assistance Team (DMAT) data during mass gatherings. As the hurricanes hit, CDC and ASPR established data flow mechanisms and rules, and in 2 days put in place a system to receive hourly data from DMATs, resulting in timely information that helped responders target communities at greatest need for public health interventions.
- *Vector-Borne Surveillance:* CDC operates systems that allow for national and state-based monitoring of specific vectors, such as ticks and mosquitoes, which carry diseases and pose risks for outbreaks. These systems monitor laboratory documented cases of disease, allowing for the early detection of outbreaks and helping decisionmakers determine when and how to act in the interest of the public's health. State, territorial, city, and local health departments populate CDC's surveillance systems to inform vector control and management activities.
- *Antibiotic Resistance Surveillance:* Beginning in fiscal year 2016, Congress recognized the large and growing threat of antibiotic resistance and appropriated funding to CDC to detect and respond to resistant pathogens, prevent the spread of resistant infections, and collaborate with partners to encourage innovation for new prevention strategies. CDC has multiple surveillance systems that can detect and track resistant threats across healthcare, food, and the community. One important investment begun in 2016 is CDC's Antibiotic Resistance Laboratory Network (ARLN), which supports nationwide laboratory capacity to rapidly

detect antibiotic resistance in healthcare, food, and the community, and inform local responses to prevent spread and protect people. The ARLN includes seven regional laboratories, the National Tuberculosis Molecular Surveillance Center, and laboratories in 50 states, five cities, and Puerto Rico. The ARLN is vital to detecting new and emerging resistant pathogens, including those that are untreatable, to trigger infection control response measures to prevent spread. The ARLN collects actionable data on threats including the "nightmare bacteria," carbapenem-resistant Enterobacteriaceae (CRE), Candida auris, and Neisseria gonorrhoeae; some strains of these pathogens have become resistant to all or nearly all available antibiotics. In addition, samples from the ARLN can be made available to researchers to support innovations in antibiotic and diagnostic development.

- *Global Disease Detection:* CDC's Global Disease Detection (GDD) Operations Center monitors outbreaks 24/7 across the globe, assesses their potential risk to the United States and communities around the world, and improves global public health surveillance. The GDD Operations Center monitors approximately 30–40 public health threats each day, including outbreaks, disasters, poisonings, and chemical, radiological, or nuclear events. Since 2007, CDC has tracked more than 170 unique diseases globally and identified outbreaks in more than 190 countries. This tracking provides the agency with critical early warning and response capabilities.
- *Global Polio Surveillance:* CDC, as part of the Global Polio Eradication Initiative, supports polio surveillance to track potential cases and circulating viruses and to effectively target polio immunization efforts. The goal of these efforts is polio elimination in every country and eventual worldwide eradication, and we are closer than we have ever been to achieving that monumental accomplishment. In 2017, the Global Polio Eradication Initiative identified just 20 wild poliovirus cases worldwide, down from 350,000 cases in 1988 when the global eradication initiative began. The global polio surveillance system, coupled with the CDC-supported Global Poliovirus Laboratory Network (comprised of 145 laboratories around the world), also detects and assists in the diagnosis of other epidemic prone diseases such as measles, rubella, and yellow fever.

Taken together, these surveillance systems provide an early warning alert, allowing CDC to protect the health of Americans through rapid, evidence-based action.

Providing Public Health Services

State and local public health agencies are the cornerstones of preparedness and response. When states are prepared to respond, communities are better protected and more resilient in the face of threats. CDC has long-established relationships with state and local officials, and coordinates with them effectively and efficiently during public health emergency responses. CDC also collaborates with foreign ministries of health to protect global health security that directly impacts United States health security. Examples of CDC's critical support of state, local, and foreign health agencies to ensure they are ready to respond to emergencies include:

- 24/7 public health consultation and disease expertise.
- Enabling a quality public health laboratory system while maintaining critical laboratory infrastructure and specimen testing support.
- Managing and delivering medical countermeasures.
- Public health workforce development that complements preparedness-specific provision of guidance, training, and exercises to ensure jurisdictions are ready to detect and respond to an emergency.

In the event of an outbreak, bioterrorist attack, or chemical or radiological release, laboratory capacity is essential to quickly detect, diagnose, and treat those who are impacted. CDC's Laboratory Response Network (LRN) maintains an integrated network of state and local public health, Federal, and international laboratories that can respond to all types of public health threats. The linking of state and local public health laboratories, and veterinary, agriculture, and water-and food-testing laboratories is unprecedented and provides for training, rapid testing, timely notification, and secure messaging of laboratory results. With the LRN, CDC has developed and deployed tests to combat our country's most pressing infectious and non-infectious health issues, from Ebola to Zika to ricin toxin to nerve agents. CDC ensures the Nation is able to respond to influenza pandemics, vector-borne or vaccine-preventable disease outbreaks, other emerging infectious disease threats, and environmental health threats by supporting planning efforts among health departments, hospitals, and emergency responders. CDC tests its pandemic influenza response capabilities with federal, state, and local partners through virtual tabletop and functional exercises. CDC evaluates and improves its response plans based on lessons learned from previous responses and exercises. CDC supports state and local health departments directly during vector-borne and environmental health incidents by developing and evaluating novel repellents and other prevention tools; improving and deploying diagnostic tools and tests; responding to toxic health threats; and providing unique expertise and training regarding radiation.

The existing public health system, its people, networks and resources, form the basis for response to health emergencies. For example, CDC's National Center for Immunization and Respiratory Diseases funds state infrastructure awards, manages vaccine shortages, prevents disease outbreaks and responds early and rapidly should they occur, and stands ready to respond quickly and comprehensively to other urgent emergencies requiring vaccination such as a pandemic or biologic attack. CDC also funds state and local public health agencies through the Epidemiology and Laboratory Capacity for Infectious Diseases cooperative agreement (ELC). This funding allows jurisdictions to strengthen their basic epidemiologic and laboratory capacity to address infectious disease threats. Multiple CDC programs use the ELC platform to protect the public health and safety of the American people by supporting health departments to effectively detect, respond to, prevent, and control a wide range of known and emerging (or reemerging) infectious diseases. These CDC programs and others provide ongoing support to prevent, prepare for, and respond to public health emergencies.

An outbreak that starts in another country can hit our shores in a matter of hours. Strengthening global health security protects Americans' health. New diseases, like MERS and influenza H7N9, can emerge without warning and have the potential to cause widespread infection and fear. CDC works with 31 Global Health Security Agenda partner countries to help them build the core public health capacities necessary for identifying and containing outbreaks before they become epidemics that could affect us all. This work is focused on strengthening four critical areas: surveillance, laboratory, workforce development, and rapid response capability. In addition, CDC medical and public health officers staff United States Quarantine Stations that are located at 20 ports of entry and landborder crossings where the majority of international travelers arrive. These health officers are the first line of defense to prevent the introduction and spread of infectious diseases.

Conclusion

I want to leave the Committee with three primary points about CDC's role in public health emergency preparedness and response.

- CDC is the common defense of the country against threats to public health,
- CDC's preparedness work is built on a foundation of our broad and deep scientific, medical, and programmatic expertise, and
- CDC's longstanding partnerships with state and local public health authorities are essential to the health security of our country.

Through the three interconnected pillars of science, surveillance, and service, CDC plays a critical role in working to ensure that the United States is ready to respond to public health emergencies. CDC has over 70 years of experience in bringing top scientific expertise to health emergencies and remains a trusted partner in the United States and around the world. CDC stands ready to do its part to protect the health and well-being of the American public and save lives. We cannot necessarily predict the next disaster, but we know that being prepared protects health, saves lives, and prevents economic losses.

Thank you for the opportunity to testify.

Senator BURR. D. Redd, thank you very much.

You won the award for getting the closest to the 5 minutes of all our witnesses today.

[Laughter.]

Senator BURR. The Chair would recognize himself and the Ranking Member, and then Senator Alexander, Senator Casey, and then Members in the order of attendance to today's hearing.

Dr. Bob, my first question is simple. Are we prepared for public health threats we face?

Dr. KADLEC. Sir, I would have to say equivocally for some, but not all.

I think the reality is when this concept of PAHPA first came up in 2005, we had witnessed the terrorist attacks of 9/11. We were anticipating potentially a pandemic and we had just experienced Katrina. But those are all in the rearview mirror in terms of the threats that we are prepared to deal with.

Quite frankly, if you had to look at Nation State threats that we are considering today, or multiple Nation States that are willing to use terrible weapons against, both physical as well as potentially cyber, I think we are not prepared. And quite frankly, those are the things that keep me up at night as well as a pandemic that could emerge again from Asia. As well as the risks that have come up that Dr. Gottlieb identified with synthetic biology tools now that allow nefarious people to do unimaginable things potentially.

So I think we have a long way to go. We have done very well in some areas; again, a compliment to the effort that was done by the Federal Government in support of state and local authorities. And again, for those three hurricanes nearly consecutively, I think that was a great commitment of effort by everyone.

But there is no time to rest on our laurels in that respect.

Senator BURR. The statute is very clear on BARDA's specific and targeted medical countermeasure mission to ensure that BARDA is staying focused in bringing forward the countermeasures we need to protect the American people from a range of chemical, biologic, radiologic, and nuclear threats. All of BARDA's work should be tied to this threat context.

Why is it important that BARDA's mission not be diluted by matters or mandates that would require BARDA work on areas outside of those tied to threats specifically?

And how does the comment of 34 innovations out of BARDA relate to a focus on its mission?

Dr. KADLEC. Yes, sir.

Well, I think the key thing here is to remember what the mission was originally. And again, BARDA was only part of the puzzle here.

Project Bioshield, which was a 10-year advanced appropriation, was another critical element of that formula of success, which was a guaranteed market to manufacturers should they get across the finish line.

But the key issue that you have raised, sir, is that we cannot boil the ocean. Quite frankly, the BARDA model works. The resources that have been given to BARDA to date have been somewhat limited. We have had, literally in some circumstances, to rob Peter to pay Paul given events that have transpired with Ebola and other events.

We do not have a sustained level of funding necessarily, a line item for pandemic influenza, for example. That would give us great confidence that we would have a sustained, uninterrupted funding stream.

So the answer is arguably, you could do more things, but the answer is you cannot do more things with limited resources. If we focus on the national security mission which, I think, is vital— again, vital to the role of BARDA—then I think we have to stick to our lane and highlight the fact that right now, to use a defense analogy, we are operating with about half an aircraft carrier of resources to basically do this mission. A national security mission to basically protect 320 million people and that is a challenge.

Senator BURR. Dr. Gottlieb, in your experience, what is working well in the agency's review of medical countermeasures? And what challenges have you seen in the medical countermeasure pipeline?

Dr. GOTTLIEB. I think we are doing a much better job now. I look at this over a 15 year period.

I came into the agency shortly after the animal rule was implemented back in 2002. Between my two tours at the agency, I think we are doing a much better job at leaning in with respect to trying to bring some of these technologies forward; trying to look at ways that we can lean forward and develop the animal models that are going to form the basis of some of the product approvals; trying to put out perspective guidance and talk to manufactures and provide more regulatory clarity.

I think there are still challenges around the incentives in this market. Frankly, I think having been on the other side of this in the private sector, the prospect of being able to commercialize something just for stockpiling purposes sometimes is not enough of an incentive to offset the enormous capital costs of some of these endeavors.

I think we are also looking at, we focused on some of the immediate dangers, some of the pathogens we knew and we are developing countermeasures on them. I think we are looking at a future where it is going to be much easier to bioengineer some of these things in ways that we cannot fully anticipate and create very new risks.

Senator BURR. Senator Murray.

Senator MURRAY. Well, thank you very much to all of you.

In the wake of Hurricane Irma, as hospitals were evacuating, the top priority was protecting vulnerable populations including people and individuals with disabilities, and children, and pregnant women.

In every public health emergency, we have to pay unique attention to people with functional needs that put them particularly at risk. That is true for preparedness planning and for emergency response, including, for example, making sure that there is adequate medical countermeasure development and dosing guidance for children and pregnant women.

PAHPA actually acknowledges that there must be specific attention paid to at risk individuals, and we want to build on that last authorization, because I think we can do better.

So I wanted to ask each of you to briefly describe your agency's efforts to meet the needs of all people. And, what more can we do to ensure that when it comes to public health preparedness, we are prepared for everyone?

Dr. Redd, let me just start with you, and if we could, just go down the panel.

Dr. REDD. Thank you for that question.

Let me just highlight a couple of things that we are doing at the CDC.

First of all, our guidance through the Public Health Emergency Preparedness Program requires that states have a plan for persons with functional needs. So that is part of the planning process.

We also work closely with the American Academy of Pediatrics and the American College of Obstetrics and Gynecology, depending on what the emergency is, but work with them to make sure that those needs are being covered.

I would also say in the stockpile that we have made progress in procuring products that are needed to treat children.

For example, there are 100,000 treatment courses of Oseltamivir in suspension form that are intended, or targeted, for children.

Senator MURRAY. What could we do better?

Dr. REDD. I think there is always more work to do.

I think that we need to make sure that these plans are exercised and that we have actually covered all the bases. That they are not just written on paper, but that we actually are able to execute the plans that we have made.

Senator MURRAY. Dr. Gottlieb.

Dr. GOTTLIEB. I would just highlight that PAHPA gave us new authority to put forward, to your point, treatment guidelines that can help guide the applications of some of these therapeutics, particularly with respect to pediatric dosing, which we have used. We have approved 12 drugs under the animal rule; 7 have been approved with pediatric dosing requirements.

I think this is something that we can continue to do better. I think one of the ways that we are going to do that is to have better development of animal models that have better natural histories associated with the pathogens in those animal models that allow us to predict what the therapeutic impact is going to be on a pediatric population.

So, this is some basic research that we need to do to develop those models that are going to, then, allow us to extrapolate into a pediatric population; and other populations, for that matter, other vulnerable populations, to your point, and allow us to have dosing guidelines for those populations.

Senator MURRAY. Is there anything we can do within PAHPA to help improve that?

Dr. GOTTLIEB. I think to Senator Burr's point as well, I think this, as a scientific basis, still needs further development. PAHPA gave the agency resources and we have developed discrete expertise in this area as a result of the legislation.

I think that is a place where we can continue to make more investment.

Senator MURRAY. Okay. Dr. Kadlec.

Dr. KADLEC. Thank you, ma'am, for the question.

I would just like to highlight during the hurricanes, we actually did some very specific things around people with functional disabilities.

I do not know if any of the Members have heard of emPOWER. It is a program that allows us to basically identify, in the CMS data base for Medicare, people who are dependent on durable medical equipment.

Based on requests from states, we can provide actually very specific information where these people live by ZIP Code and by address. In cases like Irma, Florida was able to do a reverse 9–1–1 call to those people at risk well before any evacuation orders went out to the general public to advise them that they should consider leaving before things got worse.

In the cases of Maria, we actually used that data to identify, on the islands St. Thomas and St. Croix, people who were dialysis dependent. And after the storm passed, we were able to basically link up with the urban search and rescue teams, and actually recover dialysis dependent people, and basically evacuate them to safety. So there is that part of it.

One of the limitations currently is that it is only for Medicare data. The State Medicaid data is limited. We can do that if we have access to that and provide the same information. So that is one area that we could probably benefit from working with you all to see how we can have the states work collaboratively to use that information prospectively.

To add to the points that were made by the other gentlemen, clearly BARDA has looked at specific products for pediatric patients, as well as people with immune-compromise, and there are products that are in the stockpile today that are to benefit both of those populations.

One of the areas, and I highlighted it in my testimony, is on the National Disaster healthcare System. One of the specific areas we would like to do is take the learnings or lessons learned from Ebola where we created a national Center of Excellence at Nebraska University for infectious disease and replicate that for other very important trauma-related or disaster-related areas like pediatrics.

We think that that would be a way where not only can you create the necessary, if you will, critical mass of expertise, but also teach through telemedicine and through teleconsultations to provide support during disasters.

The last area I would like to do, and a shout out to our V.A. colleagues, is the V.A. was a very significant contributor to our response to Harvey. HHS responded and took care of 36,000 patients. The V.A. provided care to 21,000 patients, many of those were V.A. beneficiaries, but some of those, many of those were families of V.A. beneficiaries. And then a larger number were actually the general public.

The V.A. has unique capabilities as it relates to geriatric populations, and that is one area that we can probably benefit from in terms of utilizing some of their expertise.

Senator MURRAY. Thank you very much. Senator BURR. Chairman Alexander.

The CHAIRMAN. Thanks, Mr. Chairman.

Dr. Kadlec, Dr. Gottlieb, let us talk about the flu. This is the 100th anniversary of the 1918 influenza pandemic that killed an estimated 50 million people worldwide; 600,000 in the United States.

According to the Centers for Disease Control, year in and year out, between 12,000 and 56,000 Americans die as a result of seasonal flu.

We heard last week in our opioids hearing that opioids kill more Americans than car accidents. And those statistics that I just read would suggest that in a severe year, so could the flu.

Dr. Collins, the head of the National Institutes of Health, has made the prediction before our Committee that if we keep up our investments in biomedical research—which Senator Blunt, and Senator Murray, and the rest of us have been doing pretty well the last 3 years—that we may have a universal flu vaccine, as well as a vaccine for Zika, within the next decade.

Dr. Fauci at NIH has said that the most effective method for protecting Americans against another pandemic influenza is to encourage and invest in the development and stockpiling of influenza vaccines that will broadly protect against the virus.

Well, in Tennessee right now, the hospitals are filling up with people with the flu. So Dr. Kadlec and Dr. Gottlieb, if researchers at NIH, or any partners with them, discover a platform technology that could speed the development of a universal flu vaccine, what would BARDA do to support the advanced research and development of that technology?

Dr. Gottlieb, what is the FDA ready to do to encourage the use of that technology for new and innovative vaccines?

I have 3 minutes.

Dr. KADLEC. Chairman, I will be very brief, then, in the sense that BARDA has an integrated portfolio with NIAID. So once a product gets through Phase 2a clinical trials, it would be transitioned over to BARDA, which would take the advanced development through to fruition. So that part of it is done.

They have the capacity to basically identify manufacturers who could produce that either in eggs, or tissue cell culture, or emerging technologies.

The CHAIRMAN. Dr. Gottlieb.

Dr. GOTTLIEB. Yes. I will just quickly add, we already have, in development, vaccines that might be universal flu vaccines that, presumably, could elicit a T-cell response and could achieve what you are outlining.

We continue to provide advice to clinical developers and manufacturers on the proper pathway for looking at trying to bring those new technologies through.

I would point to one place where the legislative suite that we have adopted to try to address some of these biological threats has been helpful in the development of manufacturing capacity. That could greatly aid in the scope of these new vaccines, particularly cell-based manufacturing, which we have made a lot of investments in, as you know, that could provide the proper platform for the development of these vaccines.

The CHAIRMAN. Dr. Gottlieb, this is a related matter.

We are all concerned about Puerto Rico and the impact of the hurricane there. I think you told me at one point that maybe one-third of the economy of Puerto Rico has to do with medical technology.

Is that right?

Dr. GOTTLIEB. That is about right. It is about 30 percent.

The CHAIRMAN. And many of those facilities, as you described, were destroyed.

Are they rebuilding in Puerto Rico, or are they rebuilding other places, or do you know yet, because that could have a major effect on Puerto Rico's future?

Dr. GOTTLIEB. Right. And we are obviously very concerned about the situation in Puerto Rico for a host of reasons, not the least of which is that the Puerto Rican economy is very dependent upon that skilled manufacturing base.

I am happy to tell you that all of the facilities that we are concerned about—that produce product that we were worried could go into shortages if the facilities continued to remain offline—are now back on the grid.

So the facilities themselves actually did not sustain a lot of damage. It was the power grid and the infrastructure in between the facilities to try to move equipment in and off the island, and that sustained a lot of the damage. The facilities actually were fairly hardened.

But the ones we were worried about are back on the grid. There are still some facilities that are not on the grid, but they have such redundant electric generation capacity that we do not really have concerns about the product supply coming out of facilities.

So the situation now looks a lot better than it did 4 months ago. The CHAIRMAN. Mr. Chairman, I think my time is about up, and

I will give the rest of it back. Senator BURR. Senator Casey.

Senator CASEY. Thank you, Mr. Chairman.

I wanted to start with the reference that I made earlier to the train derailment in Philadelphia as an example of good preparation. Part of that has its origin in the fact that it happened in an urban area where you have not just the resources, but you have hospitals and the healthcare infrastructure, which is close by way of distance, as well as by way of coordination.

I represent a state that has 48 rural counties out of a total of 67 counties. So we have a lot of small towns and rural areas where you do not have the institutional capacity necessarily. In the event of an emergency, that could be exacerbated by distance and other challenges, so you have this type of gap or potential gap, where some communities may be particularly vulnerable.

I would start with Dr. Kadlec and then go to Dr. Redd.

In terms of the Hospital Preparedness Program, the so called HPP, as well as PHEP, how do those programs attempt to close the gap in preparedness among states and regions?

Dr. KADLEC. Thank you, sir, for the question.

I think the point is that the way we are structuring it right now, we are trying to actually build healthcare or promote healthcare coalitions which are collections of hospitals, as well as other entities like emergency medical services. So you can build a regional.

That is why we would like to expand that effort to basically do it so not only would it cover specific regions within a state, but statewide and across states so that you can develop a much stronger backbone, if you will, to do this.

I think the idea of basically building out the National Academy of Sciences' study on trauma systems is worthy of reviewing because it highlights the important role that has a foundational capability for the country. Not only for day to day routine activities, but for these extraordinary events, train derailments that happen not only in Pennsylvania, but in the State of Washington, as an example, become a central piece of that.

My interest in this is seeing how we can leverage all those pieces together with some of the Federal assets the V.A. identified. Madigan Army Medical Center was a critical first responder in the train derailment in Washington State.

The thing is, how do we basically build, forge a public-private partnership for those purposes that can basically strengthen it? So not only do you have the transport mechanisms with emergency medical services, but also telemedicine and teleconsultation that would be available from this specialty services, these Level I trauma service hospitals or Level I expert hospitals like Nebraska to basically deal with a range of topical areas.

Senator CASEY. Doctor, before moving to Dr. Redd, I just want to inject another question.

This is an authorizing Committee and a reauthorization process. But I want to specifically ask, in light of the question I posed, are there additional authorities you need or additional dollars?

Dr. KADLEC. Sir, I would suggest both. We have a $3.3 trillion healthcare system for which, right now, we invest approximately $250 million annually for preparedness and resilience. I think it just highlights the fact that it is kind of a drop in the bucket.

I do not think it is necessarily the role of the Federal Government to pay for the whole bill, but certainly, we need to look at a variety of incentives, whether that is through CMS reimbursements, whether that is through insurance programs, or tax benefits that would incentivize hospitals to do it.

Our conversations with some of the outside partners, we held kind of a listening session with 35 stakeholders last week, including hospital associations. They are all willing and we have the hospitals volunteering to help. I think they are just looking for a means to do this in a way that is mutually beneficial.

Senator CASEY. Thank you, doctor. Dr. Redd, I only left you 45 seconds. Dr. REDD. I will be brief.

We actually met with selected state health officials last spring to ask this exact question that you asked. Are there things that we should be doing differently to support rural health departments?

The conclusion was, it was a little bit surprising to me that the capabilities needed for rural districts and urban are largely the same: detection capability, communications, incident command or the structure to run responses. But there are additional, as you mentioned, there are additional layers of challenge with transport and access to medical care.

I think that this is an issue a little bit beyond emergency response and I think the idea of telemedicine as a tool is a great idea. But it is essentially a question of, how do we make sure that those communities have access to medical care during and not during emergencies?

Senator CASEY. Thank you, Mr. Chairman. Senator BURR. Senator Isakson.

Senator ISAKSON. Thank you, Senator Burr.

Thank you for your work on pandemics and on BARDA for a long period of time. It is very valuable. The Committee has worked on it a long time.

I appreciate Chairman Alexander and Senator Murray, and the work that they have done.

Thanks, Dr. Kadlec, for calling out the V.A.

As Chairman of the Veterans Committee in the Senate, I have learned a lot of things about our delivery system and capabilities in terms of V.A. healthcare, which is the second largest employer in the United State Government. A lot of people do not realize that, but that is how big and pervasive the V.A. is, and they provide significant healthcare to seniors by virtue of their delivery system.

Your callout for them and what they did in Houston, Houston has appreciated it.

Also, I would say that most of the research dollars that are invested by the U.S. Government in control groups are through the V.A. because you have a control group of patients where you can do a good research sample. Our veterans, and our Veterans Administration, provide a great service in terms of that, which brings me to Admiral Redd.

You have your emergency preparedness grant that you give to the local governments. When we had the incident we had happen in Hawaii last week, where we had a false alarm on a missile attack, which was rather unsettling to the people of Hawaii and, quite frankly, it was unsettling to me. That is an emergency grant challenge you want to make sure you do not ever have with a pandemic where you get the wrong information going out from a designated agency at the wrong time.

Do we concentrate a lot on that to protect ourselves from bad information getting out on pandemics or on diseases?

Dr. REDD. I think that really gets to one of the core requirements that we have, which is to be sure that the information we are providing is as valid as it can be. And if we are not certain, but we believe people need to know, we make sure that those caveats are expressed.

It really gets to some of the basic principles of risk communication to tell people what we know, what we do not know, and what we are doing to find out those things that we do not know.

Senator ISAKSON. Dr. Gottlieb, I appreciate your mention of Priority Review Vouchers.

Senator Casey and I worked on PRV's for rare diseases that affect children and successfully passed legislation. I think the first drug has been approved now and put on PRV. It was issued by the department, and we appreciate that.

Your use of that to expand the use of PRV's to encourage the development of drugs that are either very costly to develop or hard to develop is very important.

How do you intend to use that to expand the development in terms of new pharmaceuticals?

Dr. GOTTLIEB. Well, as you know, the PRV program provides an additional incentive for manufacturers to try to develop products for these purposes. And so, I think it is one of the tools that Congress contemplated to try to address some of the challenges that we have already talked about that I mentioned, which is that sometimes this is not a typical market where you have the usual market-based incentives to try to make the capital investments to develop these products.

There is work going on to look at what impact the PRV's have had. We have implemented the program. We have seen sponsors come forward and be awarded these PRV's and sell them in the secondary market as a way to try to recoup some of the cost of the investment.

Senator ISAKSON. On that same subject, I have done a lot of work on a disease called Batten's, which is an incurable disease of young people. I had a personal situation that piqued my interest in my district when I was in the House, and I have remained interested in that.

It is a very difficult disease for which there is no cure, but with the gene therapy development and the delivery system of pharmaceuticals to specific parts of the body, and the brain in particular, there is hope and promise for that.

Do you issue guidance letters to research hospitals or research facilities to give them guidance on how they can test or develop to work on a breakthrough drug for a disease like Batten's?

Dr. GOTTLIEB. Senator, I think one of the areas of the most promise right now that we are looking on when we look across our portfolio is what is going on, as I said, with biologics with respect to cell based therapies, machine based therapies where we have the ability to cure inherited disorders, devastating inherited disorders that were not treatable just a short time ago.

We are going to be putting out this starting probably this spring, maybe a little earlier, a suite of products with specific guidance on how sponsors can address certain disorders with gene therapy to try to provide as much regulatory clarity as possible.

We are going to look at some of the more common disorders first, but we are going to try to work through some of these rarer diseases to make sure that product developers have a lot of clarity around what the pathway forward would be.

Senator ISAKSON. I commend you on the leadership you have shown in that effort already and plan to support you in any way we can to help you do that in the future.

Thank you very much. Thanks to all of you for testifying. Senator BURR. Senator Smith.

Senator SMITH. Thank you very much, Senator Burr, and Chair Alexander, and Senator Murray.

I am so pleased to be able to serve on this Committee. Thank you very much.

I would like to come back to something that Senator Murray and, I think, several others have talked about, which is the importance of a connection and support to local public health organizations.

In the past year in Minnesota, we have dealt with three infectious disease outbreaks: measles, multidrug resistant tuberculosis, and also syphilis. And all of these outbreaks have required a really immediate response, as well as a sustained response, as we have gone forward.

Minnesota has traditionally, as I am sure you know, invested heavily in emergency preparedness and dealing with infectious diseases, probably because of our history in agriculture more than anything.

But in these particular situations, the financial resources that we had were not enough and so, we turned to the CDC for support. And, of course, no fault of yours, there were no resources there.

What we did is we moved forward with the state legislature to pass an emergency public health response account so that we could respond quickly because speed is of the essence when you are dealing with these kinds of outbreaks.

My question is in what ways do you think that an emergency response fund would strengthen our federal and state efforts during an outbreak or after a disaster?

Maybe if you could just talk a little bit about that, that would be helpful.

Dr. REDD. Thank you very much.

I think that resources are critical in responding to an emergency. We had lengthy delays, both in the Ebola response and in the Zika response before funding became available, and I think that hindered what we were able to accomplish.

There has been discussion both in Congress and in the Administration about how to do that, and I think that those discussions will continue. But I think something along those lines would be quite helpful.

Let me mention one thing that we have done specifically once funds are available to make sure that they are used more quickly. We had a Notice of Funding Opportunity that we opened to our grantees through the Public Health Emergency Preparedness program and allowed them to apply for funds. There were no funds in this award, but we have an approved, but unfunded, grant mechanism so that we do not get delayed at the Federal level once funding is appropriated.

Senator SMITH. Thank you.

Dr. KADLEC. Senator Smith, if I could just add.

There exits already in authorizing language for a fund for HHS that has $57,000 in it. Obviously, it is not an authorization problem.

But I just want to highlight the fact that, yes, there is a fund that is needed. It should be a fund that necessarily is managed by the Secretary and based on a public health emergency. There can be, if you will, distribution of funds from that, and that it can be used across HHS, or to fund states and locals in a way that would be rapid.

Obviously, there is going to be a need for, it would be like the medical equivalent of the disaster relief fund, I think. But I think there would be, obviously, a requirement to notify Congress in those sorts of situations on a basis of reporting back on some occasions to make sure the funds are being spent appropriately.

Senator SMITH. Right. Thank you.

Essentially, we need to make sure we have good accountability. Dr. KADLEC. Right.

Senator SMITH. That the funds are being spent the way they are supposed to be spent——

Dr. KADLEC. Yes, ma'am.

Senator SMITH ——which I would completely agree with.

I realize that this is an authorizing question and not an appropriating discussion here, but Dr. Kadlec, if such a fund were to be made available, what would you advise in terms of the level of funding that would be necessary to have this actually be workable? Dr. KADLEC. Well, ma'am, I would have to back in a firm number, but I think what you probably looked at is what happened with Ebola or the original pandemic influenza appropriations, which are on the order of $2.5 to $3.5 billion.

Again, what you need to hedge is the opportunity for Congress to weigh in fully, and again, on the basis of time. So obviously, there are a lot of factors to be considered in there, but there is a rich, historical record that could probably be drawn upon to identify an appropriate level that would get us through the initial crisis to the point where Congress can basically perform its fiduciary responsibilities.

Senator SMITH. Right. Thank you very much.

Senator Burr, I was struck by what you said about how we need to stick to our knitting on this Committee and not expand too much. And also how important it is to think about the processes that we have in place with this authorized legislation, to make sure that it works well.

I appreciate your comments. I think it gives us some good food for thought as we consider how we can respond as quickly as possible when there is an emergency.

Thank you.

Senator BURR. We, again, welcome you to the Committee. Senator Young.

Senator YOUNG. Well, thank you, Chairman.

The World Organization for Animal Health estimates that roughly 60 percent of known human diseases are transmitted from animals to people. They are of so called zoonotic origin.

Every year, an average of five human diseases appear such as Ebola, HIV, and new strains of influenza; three of which are zoonotic.

In my home State of Indiana, we suffered considerable losses in the widespread bird flu outbreak, one that led to the destruction of 400,000 turkeys. And this followed in 2015 and the outbreak that led to the loss of 48 million poultry.

Dr. Kadlec, what are we doing now to prevent the spread and transmission of diseases from animals to human beings?

Dr. KADLEC. Well, sir, I have to say that, quite frankly, we need to do more.

The one health concept that you are outlining is an important one. Influenza is not the only disease that is of zoonotic importance that has pandemic potential; SARS and MERS are examples of others.

But I think I need to really defer to Admiral Redd to talk about the role of the CDC here and their role of surveillance because, quite frankly, they are on the cutting edge to ensure that you can recognize those events rapidly as they have in Iowa, I think.

Senator YOUNG. Thank you. Admiral.

Dr. REDD. Thank you, Dr. Kadlec and Senator Young.

We are working very closely with USDA on this issue and particularly on influenza. We were really joined at the hip in the response to this importation of these avian influenza viruses.

Our role was to make sure that we understood the biology and that if any human infections occurred, that those were rapidly detected and treated, and to protect workers in the process of the culling that was going on.

Senator YOUNG. You, no doubt, do the best you can with the resources and authorities you have.

No. 1, how are we doing with respect to tracking and then the responding to these situations and preparing for the next one?

Then secondarily, speak to any additional authorities or resources you might need to optimize your efforts.

Dr. REDD. I think that given the strategy that we have, which is a reactive one, I think we are doing well at detecting and containing importations.

Senator YOUNG. That predicate caught my attention. Dr. REDD. Yes.

Senator YOUNG. Given that our strategy is a reactive one. Dr. REDD. Right.

I think that the ability to prevent importation of influenza viruses that could be transmitted by migratory waterfowl, for example.

Senator YOUNG. Yes, sir.

Dr. REDD. It is very challenging.

I think there is a lot being done on the animal health side. I think that it is a challenge and the basic strategy is to identify and limit, to the extent possible, to one flock or as small an area as possible. And through that process to prevent human infection should the virus have the capability to be transmitted or to be infectious to humans.

Dr. GOTTLIEB. If I may, just for 15 seconds.

I would also talk about the importance of thinking about animal drugs in our approach. And Cures, as you know, extended the EOA authority to animal drugs. We might also contemplate trying to think about how we create incentives for the development of animal drugs to target some of these threats including maybe a break through therapy designation for animal drugs or other kinds of creative policy approaches to make sure that that is a part of our approach as well.

Senator YOUNG. Well, thank you.

I look forward to working with each of you. I will probably have some follow-up questions I will submit in writing, and hopefully we can improve our current systems for dealing with these matters.

Senator YOUNG. Dr. Gottlieb, you just once again mentioned incentives in the animal context, but I would like to pivot to our antibacterial resistance threats.

Every year, at least 2 million people in the U.S. acquire serious bacterial infections that are resistant to one or more types of antibacterial drugs.

However, as I understand it, there are very few companies that are developing new antibiotics, and those that are focused on the most serious bacterial threats are even fewer.

Is additional action needed to immediately incentivize the development of drugs to combat this growing global problem? And if so, what might new incentives look like? And what might we do as Members of Congress to provide those incentives?

Dr. GOTTLIEB. Senator, thank you for the question.

As you know, Cures created a number of new vehicles, and some incentives, for development in this space. We are encouraged by the early interest we are seeing in those pathways, things like the LPAD pathway. I think we are going to have more information soon on how well they are working.

I mean, we can always contemplate additional policy steps, and I would be happy to talk to your office and work with you on that. I think that this is an area, to your point, that we need to think about what more we can be doing.

But Congress has done, taken some steps recently that we are very encouraged by. We are seeing a lot of good, early interest in them.

Senator YOUNG. Thank you. Senator BURR. Senator Kaine.

Senator KAINE. Thank you, Mr. Chair, and thanks to the witnesses.

I have great confidence in this Committee's ability to work on this PAHPA reauthorization in a bipartisan way. I have two observations and a concern. So an observation is this and some of you have alluded to it, and Senator Isakson's questions alluded to it. One of the tasks of emergency preparedness is to prepare for attack, and you have talked about chemical and biological. Senator Isakson talked about the incident in Hawaii this weekend.

I just want to say for the record and for the public. The prospect of nuclear war is being discussed with a lot of frequency in this building to a degree that I have not seen in the time I have been in the Senate.

I am on the Armed Services and Foreign Relations Committees. We have had a series of hearings, even open, where there has been discussion about the prospect of land war on the Korean peninsula. We had an Armed Services hearing recently where a witness volunteered in public—and it was sort of a non sequitur, why he would bring it up as a Member of the Administration—about what the likely cost of reconstructing Kansas City would be after a nuclear attack.

I noticed an article in "The New York Times" a few days ago. "The C.D.C. Wants to Get People Prepared for Nuclear War." That was supposed to happen yesterday.

"On January 16, the Centers for Disease Control and Prevention will present a workshop titled 'Public Health Response to a Nuclear Detonation,' for doctors, Government officials, emergency responders, and others whom, if they survive, would be responsible for overseeing the emergency response to a nuclear attack."

Quote, "'While nuclear detention is unlikely,' the C.D.C. stated on its Website, 'It would have devastating results and there would be limited time to take critical protection steps. Despite the fear surrounding such an event, planning and preparation can lessen deaths and illness.'

Quote, "'Join us for this session of Grand Rounds to learn what public health programs have done on a Federal, state, and local level to prepare for a nuclear detonation. Learn how planning and preparation efforts for a nuclear detonation are similar and different from other emergency response planning efforts.' "That is off the CDC Website.

The article goes on to say, "The agenda for the day includes, 'Preparing for the Unthinkable,' to 'Roadmap to Radiation Preparedness,' and, 'Using Data and Decision Aids to Drive Response Efforts.'

I understand the CDC rescheduled that, canceled it from yesterday, and had a roundtable on the flu instead, but this is a realistic discussion about these prospects. And then add to it the "Dr. Strangelove" like incident over the weekend where a state sent out a mass e-mail telling people there was a ballistic missile incoming to Hawaii, which occasioned 38 minutes of panic.

Then on Tuesday, the Japanese state broadcaster, NHK, put out a warning that North Korea had fired a nuclear missile and urged Japanese citizens to take cover. That was retracted within a very few minutes.

There is a lot of discussion, some very intentional and some frightening, about the prospect of nuclear war that is happening, and this is in the provenance of your agencies.

I just want to put that on the record that that is sort of a normal area for discussion these days. I find it incredibly frightening and the normality of it I find incredibly frightening.

The second observation I want to make is this. This is a discussion about national security. We are involved in a budget debate right now. Right now, the spending bill ends January 19 and one of the points of argument is whether we might fund defense accounts over the budget caps of nondefense accounts.

You are about national security. You are about national defense and all of your agencies are funded through the nondefense accounts of the Federal budget.

Any suggestion that we would increase defense budgeting, but hold the line and put nondefense agencies subject to their caps, would not really fund the national security priorities that you are here about, and that is something we have got to grapple with.

Here is my question.

I am very worried about this Hawaii incident because in a time of heightened tension, we know from history that wars often start accidentally. There is a miscommunication and a misunderstanding; there is an overreaction. That is how World War I started. That is how most wars start.

I know there is going to be a hearing later in the week, I think, on the House Armed Services Committee about this. I am sure that there is an investigation at the state level. But part of the responsibility—and Dr. Kadlec, I guess this is mostly directed to you—part of the responsibility in the emergency preparedness and response side is accurate communication. As a former mayor and Governor, that depends heavily upon communication between Federal, state, and local officials.

As you approach this thought of thinking about reauthorization in this climate where things can sometimes be pretty tense, how do you look at that state, local, and Federal coordination effort, especially as it deals with the communication of accurate information, and knocking down inaccurate information?

As quickly as you can.

Dr. KADLEC. Well, sir, we take it very seriously, No. 1.

No. 2 is the experience we had with the hurricanes, particularly Hurricane Maria, I think, highlighted some of the challenges. In my testimony, I identified some of the incident command issues that we have to address, which really is not only information out, but information in.

I think the issues that we need to work with—not only with our CDC brethren, but with state and local authorities, as well with FEMA; I met with them just as of yesterday—talking about, how do we integrate our efforts closer so that we have better information exchange on these kinds of issues? Whether they are hurricanes, pandemics, or whatever it is that, quite frankly, you need to kind of think through, learn through not only experience, as we did with the hurricanes, but exercises, as we did.

Sir, just to highlight one thing, since I have been around the block on these sets of issues. Going back to 2000, it has been a routine practice in the U.S. Government, the Federal Government at least, to exercise the idea of a nuclear detonation. Most concerning then was terrorism as a matter of an improvised nuclear device.

It is not necessarily new. Obviously, the context is different.

But I think the point here, though, to your issue is it does require a closer lash up with our Federal partners on these issues to make sure that we have good cross lateral, horizontal flow of information, as well as with our state and local folks.

We are investigating with FEMA just as another example of how we can basically work together in bed both our health and disaster people in state and local state EOC's to, again, work more seamlessly with our state colleagues.

We are looking at all kinds of options right now to that effect. Senator KAINE. I appreciate it.

Mr. Chair, thank you for letting me go over.

I hope you will follow the investigation of the Hawaii incident for your own purposes because for purposes of having good information and that coordination, I suspect there will be some lessons that will come out of that that would be relevant to other circumstances as well.

Thank you, Mr. Chair.

Senator BURR. Thank you, Senator Kaine. Senator Collins.

Senator COLLINS. Thank you, Mr. Chairman.

I want to applaud you for your leadership in this area.

More than a decade ago, we established a Port Security Program that led to radiation portal monitors being installed at our major ports so that they could screen incoming and outgoing cargo, trucks, and individuals for radiological material.

I contrast that port security effort with what I perceive to be a real vulnerability in our ability to detect and effectively and quickly respond to an attack using biological or chemical agents.

Dr. Kadlec and Dr. Redd, I would like you both to address the level of preparedness that we have to respond and detect, first of all to detect, a biological or chemical attack and to respond to it. I would like specifically to know whether cities have used some of the Federal funds that the Admiral referred to, to install sensors that would be able to detect these agents.

I would also like you both to comment on the preparedness of our hospitals to cope with the victims of a biological or a chemical attack.

I remember being in Israel many years ago and being so impressed with their preparation and their ability to convert their hospitals to respond to that kind of attack.

Dr. Kadlec, why do we not start with you and then Admiral Redd?

Dr. KADLEC. Thank you, Senator Collins. I think one of the issues, and again, I have some insights on this historically.

But currently, the biologic program run by the Department of Homeland Security provides area protection for cities. So I think there is a real desire.

I have met with the new WMD, I do not know, directorate, Assistant Secretary over at DHS about improvements we can make to our chemical and biological attack kind of detection.

Quite frankly, our capabilities are fairly still limited and primitive, quite frankly. And I think there is a sincere desire on the part of DHS and HHS between ourselves to basically do improvement to do that.

To your second issue, how well prepared we are. Certainly, we have a Strategic National Stockpile that can address many, but not all, of these threat agents. So there is work to do there in terms of some of the development and procurement we need to do on those issues.

But one of the critical areas that collectively the CDC and our office are considering is really on the last mile of distribution.

As mentioned by Senator Murray, we can move Strategic National Stockpile resources anywhere in the country within 12 hours. The question is from that point forward getting it into the hands and into the mouths of every American person who is at risk is a significant challenge that, I think, collectively, we need to work on.

But now, I will defer to Admiral Redd for his comments.

Dr. REDD. Thank you. I think this is a really important question. If we are attacked in this way, the effectiveness of our response will depend on the speed and the scale with which we respond.

I think that the way that a biological attack would manifest itself would probably be different than a chemical attack. A chemical attack would primarily require a local, a near-instantaneous local response.

The CDC's Strategic National Stockpile has deployed antidotes for nerve agents. Over 1,000 different locations have pallets of these antidotes that are available to supplement the treatment that would be available immediately.

We also have and getting ever better capability to determine exactly which toxin has been used. So there is a laboratory element that the CDC is also responsible for.

On the biological side, we have made great strides with the laboratory response network. Every state has at least one laboratory that is able to use advanced techniques to diagnose these infections. There are a total of 150 laboratories around the world, including laboratories that can test food, can test water, and environmental samples from animals.

So looking to the future, thc tcchnology of whole genome sequencing is something that we need to continue to push out that would allow very rapid——

We talked about faster and more accurate. This is actually more information than we can get from current technologies; things like resistance to antibiotics or relationships of certain organisms to other, "where did it come from?" kinds of questions.

Senator COLLINS. Thank you.

Dr. KADLEC. Ma'am, can I just add one thing? Senator COLLINS. Yes.

Dr. KADLEC. To your question about how our hospitals would do. Senator COLLINS. Yes.

Dr. KADLEC. I think it was noted by the Chairman that even a bad flu seasons, as the current one we have, is overwhelming our hospital system.

Senator COLLINS. Exactly. That is one reason that I asked the question.

Thank you.

The Chairman [presiding]. Thanks, Senator Collins.

Senator Jones, welcome. We are glad to have you a part of this Committee. I acknowledged your new membership a little earlier, but we are glad to have you here. This is a Committee that has many different points of view, but works well together. So this is another subject that we intend to have some bipartisan success on.

Senator JONES. Thank you.

The CHAIRMAN. Senator Warren.

Senator WARREN. Thank you, Mr. Chairman.

So we are here today to talk about PAHPA, the framework for our response to all sorts of emergencies: natural disasters, accidents with hazardous materials, terrorist attacks, pandemics, you name it.

I returned, just a few days ago, from a trip to Puerto Rico and I know some of my colleagues have also been to Puerto Rico recently.

During my trip, it was clear that nearly 4 months after the storm, the crisis in Puerto Rico is a daily reality for tens of thousands, hundreds of thousands of people.

Dr. Kadlec, you are the top official in charge of preparedness and response at HHS. What is the biggest thing you have learned from the situation in Puerto Rico and the U.S. Virgin Islands about how we need to strengthen our preparedness and response capabilities?

Dr. KADLEC. Well, thank you, ma'am.

I think there are a couple of levels to go here.

One is improving the resilience of our innate hospital healthcare structure. That is one area.

The other thing is really the resilience of our public health system, which is a separate piece, but a related piece.

In Puerto Rico in particular there were, in the initial stages— after that terrible devastation that literally devastated the whole island and every life was touched—it was very difficult for the local public health and medical infrastructure.

There are some incredible heroic stories of doctors, nurses, laboratorians who basically responded, public health officials, who left their families, left their houses in disarray and basically went to respond to help their neighbors and their communities. But I think that is one piece of this that needs to be addressed, what happens before the storm.

The second piece is, how quickly can we move in? We had deployed teams to Puerto Rico in advance of both Irma and Maria to be available once the storm passed, both storms passed, to basically respond quickly. But even so, with the level of devastation, that was a huge piece of it. And a huge piece of it was the lingering devastation, not only the loss of communications and electricity, but also the damage to the ports and the airfields that limited some of the movement.

So I think one of the lessons learned was you want to go in aggressively before the storm, if you can. We literally put peoples' lives at risk from our response teams, including people from Massachusetts, Massachusetts One, that responded to all three storms.

Senator WARREN. Yes.

Dr. KADLEC. They are great people and, again, representative of your constituents from other states around the country that responded.

But also, there is a piece of this that we have to somewhat remove some of the dependencies in the responses. Seeing how we can move quicker and faster, if that is possible. A lot of it was dependent on being able to transport through air or barge, again, responding to an island is a tough one.

Senator WARREN. So I appreciate this and I am glad we are trying to think about what we need to do and what we need to do better, and to acknowledge heroic efforts, but we need a better structure here.

But to apply these lessons, we also need good data. We need to know not just what we got right or what we got wrong, but when we got it right, when we got it wrong, by how much, and what kind of difference it would make on the ground.

One of the things that struck me during my trip last week was how sketchy the data are. For example, I met with the Federal and Puerto Rican officials at FEMA's field office and they said, "No more issues with potable water." No waterborne diseases, all the water is drinkable. And I asked this specifically. Turn on the taps. You hold a glass under it. The water will be drinkable, is drinkable, everywhere on the island. It sounds great.

Not so much though.

I met with the Massachusetts State Police volunteers who told me that they had observed raw sewage in the water. At the public health center that I visited in Loiza, they said they still do not have potable water, no drinkable water for their patients. They said they serve 100,000 people and that none of them have drinkable water.

We heard the same kind of contradictions when it came to statements about how many people lacked power.

Dr. Kadlec, I get that public health emergencies are really challenging circumstances, and it is hard to get good data. But how does HHS and other agencies collect data in a way that is reliable so that you can deploy your resources effectively, hold yourselves accountable to get the job done that needs to be done?

Dr. KADLEC. Well, ma'am, we learned a lot from the experience in Puerto Rico and we are trying to rectify that.

Because of the loss of communications, cell towers, and the like, the ability to get information either from local authorities or local hospitals or clinics was practically nil.

We literally went to the point, at one time, to basically use runners from the National Guard who would have satellite phones to basically go to hospitals and clinics to report information out.

But that is a major consideration and lesson that we are still learning that we have to address because it is a major shortfall. Because if you were to add, again, a terrible event like this, a terrible earthquake or a nuclear or radiological event, you could imagine that the circumstances would be even more challenging.

But that is an area of great, intense concern, quite frankly, and work that we have to do.

Senator WARREN. I am very concerned about this and I do not have time. I am out of time now, so I cannot ask Rear Admiral Redd and Dr. Gottlieb about their work in Puerto Rico.

But Senator Cassidy and I sent a letter to Chairman Alexander signed by seven other Members of this Committee asking for a hearing on the recovery efforts in Puerto Rico and the U.S. Virgin Islands, and I hope we will be able to hold that hearing.

Puerto Rico might not be on the front pages anymore, but it is a humanitarian crisis and we have a moral, and a constitutional, responsibility to exercise oversight responsibilities here. Thank you.

Thank you, Mr. Chairman.

The CHAIRMAN. Thank you, Senator Warren. Senator Cassidy.

Senator CASSIDY. Well, thank you.

Dr. Kadlec, I am going to put you on the payroll, man. Earlier, you were responding to Senator Smith regarding a possible bill. We have that bill.

The Public Health Emergency Fund, actually stimulated by conversations with Dr. Frieden. He said that in the Ebola crisis, "There were ten different authorizations that had to be signed off on," before he could get somebody to travel immediately to Africa. Kind of crazy.

And, "I kept on contrasting the authorization process we were going through, which was cumbersome and slow with that before and after Katrina." Before Katrina, FEMA had to come to get the initial dollars. After Katrina, Congress recognized that is not the best way, so there is a pot of money that can immediately be accessed. And if it goes over that, then they come back and get another authorization.

Senator Schatz and I have put together a bill that, one, waives these contracting requirements for that immediate period so you can actually deploy people.

Second, based upon—and Dr. Kadlec this is where you nailed it— the previous 14 years of public health emergencies, we take the average of that expenditure and we make those dollars available upfront to be immediately drawn down.

Still accountability; GAO is going to do a report and make sure that the CDC has not used it to go to Hawaii for a conference as opposed to Africa to fight Ebola. No offense, Dr. Redd. But still, the point being that we would have the accountability built in, but we think it is a good bill.

Now, let me move onto something different.

Dr. Redd, I was struck speaking to people after Zika hit that in retrospect—and of course, everything in retrospect, if I could do things in retrospect I would be a millionaire on the stock market— but in retrospect, you could have predicted what was going to happen because supposedly Brazil was flying in folks from the South Pacific to work on their Olympic stadiums that Zika had been breaking out in the South Pacific where these workers were coming from. Brazil is like a Petri dish for Zika, and you could have predicted it.

Now, of course, it is retrospective. But the thought occurs to me with Big Data, we can actually put in travel patterns. We can put in areas of receptivity. We can put in where there are outbreaks and make some, at least, first blush guess as to where the next epidemic is going to be.

Is that just me, "would that not be great," sort of thing or is this something practical? And if it is practical, is the CDC doing it?

Dr. REDD. I agree with your overall statement.

I think another way of looking at this is that the pathway that Zika followed was very similar to Chikungunya just a few years before where it existed in the Pacific and then caused big outbreaks in Brazil and South America.

Another point that is the same is when we had outbreaks in the Caribbean, we knew locations of lots of travel to the U.S. and where the vector was, the Aedes aegypti mosquito lived. It is the same place that we have seen small dengue outbreaks in the past. Senator CASSIDY. So, can we use this predictively? Because if we could use it predictively, if we could see, "Well, Brazilians are going to be having this problem. Let us go down there and encourage them to spray for mosquitoes," et cetera. Dr. REDD. I think it is hard to do that.

I think that the vector is very resilient and there were some questions——

Senator CASSIDY. Now, I was just giving the example of spraying the mosquitoes as a concrete action. But what I am asking about is not the vector of resilience.

Can we use Big Data just to look at travel patterns where there is an outbreak and guess where there might be a spread of such an outbreak?

Dr. REDD. I think we can. I think the challenge is what do you do with that information. And is there a way to use that, for example, to have prevented the Zika outbreak in Miami-Dade County?

I think that the things that you do——

Senator CASSIDY. So you were ahead of us. What you use the information is different than if you can actually acquire the information.

If it is practical and right, if you will, to acquire the information, are we putting such systems in place?

Dr. REDD. Well, just to take the Zika example, there was a lot of communication with Texas and Florida, Louisiana, the Gulf Coast areas that have the Aedes aegypti mosquito recognizing that——

Senator CASSIDY. Okay. You are still after me because that is after it hit Brazil and after we knew that there was going to be travel from Brazil up.

I am actually trying to go proactively before that in that we could see the Brazilians were bringing in lots of workers from the South Pacific and therefore, it was predictable that whatever was breaking out there was going to breakout here.

Now, that is taking the battle to the enemy, if you will. Are we doing that?

Do we have a worldwide kind of map—and I have seen such a map of hotspots of infectious diseases—overlaid with travel patterns to guess whether or not? And I understand the CDC has worldwide outposts.

So again, I am asking something closer to the point—— Dr. REDD. Sure.

Senator CASSIDY ——than whether it gets to Texas.

Dr. REDD. I think the quality of information is variable. I do not think we have——

For example, I think the information we have about influenza is much better than we have about all the vector-borne, all the mosquito-borne diseases that are out there where we know what viruses are circulating in China because of the known importance of influenza and the risk it poses for a global pandemic.

Senator CASSIDY. Now, I have seen maps—and I am overtime, and I will stop after this—but I have seen maps put out by the CDC and the World Health in which it shows, "Oh, yes. Here is this and there is that." And it is a hotspot of a particular virus.

Can that not be, again, overlaid with travel patterns?

Dr. REDD. Well, there are parts of the world that some of the discussion earlier about the number of zoonotic diseases that are detected that cause infections in humans, there are certain parts of the world that are more prone to those emergences.

I think, again, your question is, how do we use that information? We certainly do have travel maps of where people travel to and from. We have information about where various diseases occur at variable degrees of granularity. I think those two things do go together.

I think how we would use that to take a preemptive action is really, I think that is the question that you are getting at.

Senator CASSIDY. Okay. I yield back. The CHAIRMAN. Senator Murphy.

Senator MURPHY. Thank you very much, Mr. Chairman.

This is incredibly informative. Thank you to all of the witnesses. I want to raise two concerns that I have emanating from conversations I have had with companies in Connecticut that operate in the pandemic response field.

The first is regarding response to an influenza outbreak and this is for either Dr. Kadlec, I think, or Dr. Redd.

Dr. Kadlec, in your testimony, you write that we have sufficient domestic vaccine manufacturing capacity to produce a bulk vaccine for every American within 6 months.

But I want to ask either of you about the question of vaccine delivery. This comes from conversations with a manufacturer in Connecticut, BD, which is one of the bigger syringe manufacturers.

My understanding is that if you needed to get a vaccine to everybody, you would need about 600 million drug delivery devices. Now, BD is one of the biggest manufacturers, but it would take them 6 years to do 600 million units.

What are your thoughts on preparation to make sure that we not only have the right amount of vaccine, but the right amount of vaccine delivery devices?

Dr. KADLEC. Well, thank you, sir.

That is one of the issues, and then problems, that has to be addressed, quite frankly, and I have my Director from BARDA, if he wants to make a comment. He is welcome to at this point.

But I think part of the strategy we are looking at also is, how can we innovate and either have better delivery devices? Or specifically, can we make better vaccines that only require one dose? Remember, the 600 million doses are for two per person.

The third thing is there are maybe new vaccine technologies that allow you to do it orally, or intranasally, or a variety of other means beside subcutaneously with a needle. So I think all those issues are being evaluated and pursued.

But yes, there are some very significant shortfalls and there are other disposables as well that are a matter of concern when you get into that kind of circumstance.

Rick, do you have anything? Senator MURPHY. I am sorry.

Dr. KADLEC. I just wanted to make sure if I left something out, if Dr. Bright could offer it.

Dr. REDD. I think this is a modeling problem. Particularly from the supply standpoint, making sure that we are tapping into the existing commercial market, and we are able to leverage that system in addition to stockpiling what that market cannot produce.

Senator MURPHY. Dr. Kadlec, back to you, and my second concern.

BARDA, as we have talked about, is such a wonderful model and working with industry, you have developed 34 approved medical countermeasures, 23 influenza vaccines.

Again, coming back to a company that BARDA has worked with in Connecticut, Protein Sciences, which as you may know, has come up with an innovative way to develop a vaccine; not the traditional egg-based vaccine, but a recombinant DNA technology mechanism. They raised the issue of how you make sure that having spent the money to develop these vaccines, there is a market so that they can continue to develop processes and make sure that they are available.

What is the responsibility of BARDA, or HHS or, I guess, if the CDC wants to weigh in, on how you make sure that the money being spent on research ends up on a marketable vaccine? And that you are working with companies to make sure that a bridge market exists so that they are available in the case that you need them for a pandemic.

Dr. KADLEC. Well, clearly, that is one of the factors that goes into this public-private partnership. And I would also invite Dr. Gottlieb because it has been the case with the PRV's, like with the vouchers, if you get through that you can get some benefits. But we need to look at the whole variety of incentives to not only get companies into the market, but keep them in the market and keep them viable going forward.

There is this issue of "the second valley of death," which has been raised at some point in time that once you have delivered your vaccine—and if you do not get either the opportunity to replenish or use that technology for some other commercial purpose— that the company may still be at risk, and you may still basically be confronted by the limitations that you do not have the producer. So these are issues that are still pretty thorny and, quite frankly, that is one of the areas, I think, that probably deserve a little more consideration during your reauthorization.

Senator MURPHY. I do not mean to keep Dr. Gottlieb out of this conversation.

You raised this in some of your earlier testimony, some of the market disincentives here and I would love to hear your thoughts. Dr. GOTTLIEB. Yes, I think you raise a very valid point, Senator. If you are talking about a countermeasure that does not necessarily have a dual use for another public health application, you only market is going to be in preparedness and presumably the only market is going to be for stockpiling. And if it is not something that turns over a lot, so you are not going to have to constantly replenish your stockpile.

Depending on what you are developing, the cost of capital to try to develop that product might be too high to justify the investment. I saw this when I was on the other side of this equation.

We have tried to offset some of that with the PRV's, but I will say that the value of the PRV's in the marketplace have diminished as we had more PRV's. So the value of the incentive has also gone down over time.

So I think this is something we should all contemplate. Senator MURPHY. Thank you.

Thank you, Mr. Chairman.

The CHAIRMAN. Thank you, Senator Murphy. Senator Murkowski.

Senator MURKOWSKI. Thank you, Mr. Chairman. Appreciate the discussion here this morning.

Dr. Kadlec, you recognized, in response to Senator Warren's question, the challenge that Puerto Rico faced after the devastating hurricanes. I mean, it is difficult in an island area where you are not connected, where you are remote.

Well, that brings it close to home to me. We are not an island in Alaska, but we are not connected to the continental United States, and we are really big, and we do not have a lot of roads. It was just about 75, 78 years ago that we had a diphtheria outbreak in Nome and we were able to deliver the serum by dogsled.

We are not doing that anymore, thankfully.

But it does speak to the reality of how to respond when you have an outbreak, and your ability to move in quickly is limited either because of weather or just access limitations.

We were reminded of this at 9/11 when all the airspace was shutdown, when you now have 80 percent of your communities that have no way to get things in and out. A major earthquake that can take out a major port that serves access or airports. And so, for us particularly in Alaska, we had to be our own little island when it comes to response.

But when you are trying to get stockpiles of vaccines or the like, that makes it very, very challenging. And I do not recall whether it was you, Dr. Kadlec or Admiral Redd, mentioned that you can get stockpiles, I believe, of vaccines anywhere in the United States within 12 hours.

Did I hear that correctly? [All nod in assent.]

Senator MURKOWSKI. Should I be worried in a small, remote, not accessible by road, shut out by weather? We cannot even get a state trooper in for 3 days into certain of our villages at certain points in time.

What can you do to assure me that we can be that responsive in our more rural areas? That is one part of the question.

The other part is when it comes to infrastructure itself.

Several years back, we had the first sizable cruise ship going through the Arctic. We had all kinds of emergency preparation drills and it was not because we were most fearful of an oil spill from a ship that might hit the ice. But an issue on a ship where you now have 500 passengers who need some level of healthcare and there is no healthcare facilities to be had in the region.

So for purposes of how we can be responsive when there is a public health crisis, whether it is an outbreak or some kind of a disaster, manmade, natural, or otherwise, what assurances can you give us from these rural states?

I will turn to Dr. Kadlec and you, Admiral. Dr. KADLEC. Well, thank you, ma'am.

That is a challenge. I think the reality is the Strategic National Stockpile can get anywhere to be delivered to the state authorities within 12 hours.

Senator MURKOWSKI. So that would get to?

Dr. KADLEC. To Anchorage, for example. And then, it is really the state's responsibility to basically get those products, or those vaccines, or drugs to the last terminal mile to those people who need them.

That is an issue, quite frankly, I think ASPR and the CDC share concern, that that is an area where concerted work has to be done because there are other places in the country that probably would have similar challenges.

Admiral Redd, do you want to?

Dr. REDD. Yes, I think this is a very challenging scenario and I think that if it were a challenge to move product to a location, there would be other challenges as well; understanding the problem of the disease in that location.

We might have telecommunication, but access to laboratories, access to epidemiologic investigation, those would also be things that would be limited.

I think this probably needs to be thought of as a broader set of capabilities that are needed to assure the protection of these populations. Not just the stockpile, but medical care and really situational awareness as to what is happening in those locations.

Senator MURKOWSKI. Well, and it is something, of course, that we clearly think about.

The last thing I am going to leave you with. The State of Alaska just conducted an Alaska Health Impact Assessment. It was a framework based on the current National Climate Assessment predictions and the impact to Alaska as a state that is seeing the impact of climate change as warming temperatures. You might not feel it here on the East Coast, but it is warmer back home.

It outlines some of the potential health effects that could be coming our way several decades out. We recognize that.

But one of the concerns, of course, is infectious diseases that are particularly associated with vector borne. Usually, we are able to freeze those nasty mosquitoes and they cannot move these levels of outbreaks.

But it is something that, as we think about public health emergencies, we are so focused on the here and the now, and the disaster of the day, but I do think it is important that we be thinking long term about the changes that might be headed our direction.

Thank you, Mr. Chairman.

The CHAIRMAN. Thank you, Senator Murkowski. Senator Jones.

Senator JONES. Thank you, Mr. Chairman.

Once again, thank you for your kind welcome to this Committee. To kind of follow-up on, I think, Senator Casey may have highlighted it and Senator Murkowski was talking about the rural health areas.

I can understand the challenges when there is a pandemic and you need to get access, but I have a state that is also very rural, but we have roads. We have the ability to get serum in and things like that. But yet, we are in Tornado Alley. We are in Hurricane Alley. It comes through.

My concern is the preparedness for healthcare delivery on an immediate basis when you have those disasters because in Alabama, like so many other states, rural healthcare is disappearing, and that is a real challenge.

So I would like to have you address what is being thought about, what is being done to prepare for those types of emergencies for those communities that do not have the daily healthcare that they have got, so that immediate healthcare needs can be given to them. Dr. KADLEC. Sir, I would just say one of the areas I touched in my written testimony is on this idea of creating a National Disaster Healthcare System, really taking advantage of the nascent trauma system that we have in our country that clearly needs to be amalgamated or, if you will, kind of unified.

We would like to basically use the Hospital Preparedness Program as a means to do that. It certainly would need more resources to do that. But basically expand the regional coalitions to not only cover states, but regions, Mississippi, Alabama, that part of the country where you can actually share resources and basically do better coordination, mutual aid in those kinds of situations. Build the kind of relationships where you know about bed availability, work with the EMS systems in terms of transportation to basically identify the appropriate places to take people with different injuries or different kinds of casualties to the right place to ensure their survival.

There is a lot that can be done and quite frankly, we think by regionalizing this will help. Because Alabama has a few major cities, Mobile, clearly there are some great facilities there, as well as other parts of the state, as well as adjacent parts in Mississippi. If you can build that coalition on a regional basis, you can probably address some, but not all, of those issues.

Dr. REDD. This is a little bit beyond preparedness, but one of the things we had done at the CDC is to examine rural health. The way that we have done that as a first step is to actually examine the data that we have.

There are a series of publications on issues related to rural health in our in-house journal, "The Morbidity and Mortality Weekly Report," and we would be happy to get those to you to define the problem.

Senator JONES. Okay, that would be great.

I also was going to ask a similar question about citizens with disabilities.

Do you have specific guidelines, things that you do to take care of those with disabilities, whether it is a physical disability, a mental disability, or whatever?

Dr. KADLEC. Sir, we have a program at HHS and the ASPR that basically uses CMS data, Medicare data to basically identify people in different regions or in states by ZIP Code, by home address, even by phone number to identify people who are dependent on durable medical equipment.

So in advance of a hurricane, for example, we provide the states, like in the case of Florida and, I believe, in Alabama too prior to Norm, before that hit that we identified people who would be at risk to power outages or who need probably special assistance if they needed to be evacuated. That is one piece of the problem.

Quite frankly, we do not have that data from Medicaid from individual states. So that would be another way to enhance that if we could get data on that.

But that is just one way to basically preidentify people at risk and it goes a long way to basically take care of folks.

Senator JONES. All right.

Dr. REDD. Just three quick things. Senator JONES. Sure.

Dr. REDD. We require our state grantees to include a section on vulnerable populations in their emergency response plans. So that is one thing.

The second is that we work with professional associations—predominantly, I am thinking more of the American Academy of Pediatrics, the American College of Obstetrics and Gynecology—when there is an emergency to make sure that we are addressing those populations.

Also, when we activate our operations center for an emergency response, there is a functional desk on vulnerable populations to try to deal with the kinds of issues that come up.

Senator JONES. Great, thank you. Thank you, gentlemen. Thank you for your testimony.

Thank you, Mr. Chairman.

The CHAIRMAN. Thank you, Senator Jones.

Senator Casey, do you have any questions or concluding remarks you would like to make?

Senator CASEY. Mr. Chairman, just some concluding remarks, and I will read through them quickly.

I want to thank our witnesses, obviously, for their insights and expertise today and their ongoing as part of the Federal Government to develop and maintain the necessary public health preparedness capabilities.

I will have some questions for the record in addition to the ones I asked already.

Senator CASEY. Next week, we look forward to hearing from non- governmental stakeholders about how we can continue to strengthen our readiness for future public health emergencies and keep the American public safe.

As we heard today, preparedness is continuous and must evolve to face new and different types of threats. I remain committed to ensuring we sustain the progress we have already made in preparing for public health emergencies, while continuing to work to anticipate the next threat.

We have a strong, bipartisan history of working together on this Committee to improve our communities' ability to respond to all manner of public health threats, and I look forward to continuing that tradition in the months ahead.

Mr. Chairman, I want to thank you for your work on this, as well as Ranking Member Murray and Senator Burr, of course.

Thank you.

The CHAIRMAN. Thank you, Senator Casey.

Senator Casey is exactly right. This is one of the many areas that this Committee has effectively worked on, both in the authorization and reauthorization of legislation to prepare our country for the unexpected disaster that might occur to us.

A lot of progress has been made and I want to thank Senator Casey and Senator Burr, especially, for their leadership over the years in this area.

As he indicated, we will be having our second hearing on this topic next Tuesday, January 23 working with Senator Murray, Senator Casey, Senator Burr, and others. We hope to be able to write legislation revisiting this Act, and mark it up in Committee this spring, and present it to the Senate for bipartisan action.

I thank the witnesses for coming today. The testimony has been very helpful. The attendance has been good.

The hearing record will remain open for 10 days. Members may submit additional information within that time, if they would like. The CHAIRMAN. Our Committee will meet again tomorrow on a different topic at 10 a.m. for a hearing entitled, "Reauthorizing the Higher Education Act: Financial Aid Simplification and Transparency."

We have been working for more than 4 years on taking a new look at the Federal Government's relationship to our colleges and universities. There are 6,000 of them. Our major role is that we appropriate about $34 or $35 billion a year in grants for students to attend colleges. There is more than $100 billion of new student loans each year.

In connection with all of that money, there is a lot of opportunity and a lot of need for us to take a look at accreditation, innovation, simplification, getting through the jungle of red tape, another whole set of activities.

That will be our major focus during this year and we hope also to have that bipartisan legislation to the Senate floor sometime this spring.

Thank you for being here today.

The Committee will stand adjourned.

[Whereupon, at 12:08 p.m., the hearing was adjourned.]

INDEX

A

access, vii, 13, 16, 22, 37, 38, 74, 111, 112, 154, 156, 160, 234, 240, 257, 260, 261, 270, 277, 281, 298, 299, 300
agencies, 5, 11, 12, 13, 15, 21, 22, 38, 39, 40, 41, 88, 94, 98, 99, 110, 112, 113, 118, 119, 120, 121, 122, 124, 126, 128, 134, 137, 141, 145, 147, 154, 159, 160, 163, 175, 180, 183, 187, 190, 192, 193, 196, 201, 202, 206, 208, 209, 215, 220, 222, 226, 236, 240, 244, 250, 266, 272, 273, 288, 293
agriculture, 26, 272, 284
airports, 8, 10, 22, 62, 103, 173, 216, 298
anthrax, 109, 118, 120, 121, 131, 135, 138, 142, 144, 146, 147, 151, 154, 155, 157, 159, 165, 174, 178, 190, 194, 195, 197, 198, 210, 223, 240, 248, 252, 256, 259, 261
antibiotic, 118, 120, 121, 123, 125, 128, 133, 143, 144, 158, 168, 169, 185, 214, 219, 224, 233, 235, 236, 270
antibiotic resistance, 123, 125, 128, 143, 144, 158, 168, 169, 233, 235, 270
antibody, 149, 150, 151, 229
antiretrovirals, 11
antitoxin, 157, 259
antitrust, 27
antiviral agents, 149, 231, 232
antiviral drugs, 12, 25, 135, 214, 226, 232, 252, 268
appropriations, 15, 16, 17, 22, 88, 89, 90, 131, 136, 185, 186, 204, 209, 217, 251
assessment, 15, 30, 36, 104, 178, 182, 183, 191, 195, 198, 203, 206, 213, 216
assessment tools, 195
assets, 69, 170, 191, 193, 198, 202, 218, 246, 247, 266, 280
authorities, 3, 5, 8, 9, 13, 30, 34, 38, 61, 63, 69, 70, 73, 77, 87, 88, 89, 90, 95, 97, 100, 115, 130, 131, 135, 136, 139, 145, 146, 154, 160, 161, 164, 173, 185, 188, 207, 219, 220, 236, 241, 244, 247, 251, 252, 254, 259, 260, 261, 262, 264, 265, 268, 273, 281, 286
authorized programs, 7
autoimmune disease, 149
avian, 94, 95, 96, 152, 157, 181, 213, 232, 286
avian influenza, 95, 96, 152, 157, 213, 286
awareness, 59, 100, 108, 134, 218, 250, 269, 270, 299

B

bacteria, 118, 120, 121, 128, 133, 143, 149, 151, 168, 197, 214, 219, 224, 231, 234, 240, 271
bacterial infection, 214, 219, 287
bacterial pathogens, 214, 230
barriers, 108, 164, 173, 233, 234, 236
basic research, 148, 229, 230, 233, 277
bilateral, 95, 98
bioinformatics, 96
biological attacks, vi, vii, 117, 118, 120, 123, 125, 132, 138, 139, 144, 155, 187, 211, 212, 222, 225, 235
biological weapons, 155, 189, 246, 249
biomarkers, 154, 158, 159, 209, 259
biosafety, 98, 121, 129

biotechnology, 135, 238, 251, 252
bipartisan commitment, 137, 253
blood, 21, 39, 85, 160, 181, 191
blood supply, 160
bloodstream, 31
border crossing, 144
botulism, 144, 147, 157, 259
breakdown, 170
breathing, 4, 20, 45, 62, 84, 85
bubonic plague, 127, 142
business environment, 204
business model, 164, 205, 206
business partners, 186
businesses, 24, 25, 26, 67, 68, 88

C

candidates, 149, 150, 152, 157, 169, 197, 218, 220, 225, 226, 227, 228, 229, 231, 232, 233, 234
Centers for Disease Control and Prevention (CDC), v, vi, 2, 3, 4, 5, 6, 7, 8, 9, 11, 13, 14, 15, 16, 17, 19, 20, 21, 22, 32, 40, 43, 44, 47, 49, 50, 51, 52, 53, 54, 55, 56, 57, 58, 59, 63, 65, 73, 81, 82, 94, 96, 97, 98, 99, 100, 104, 105, 106, 110, 112, 113, 118, 119, 120, 121, 122, 124, 125, 126, 127,128, 129, 130, 134, 138, 139, 140, 141, 142, 143, 144, 145, 146, 147, 151, 157, 158, 159, 165, 166, 167, 168, 169, 170, 171, 172, 173, 174, 175, 176, 177, 178, 181, 182, 183, 184, 188, 189, 190, 191, 192, 193, 194, 195, 196, 198, 199, 200, 209, 210, 213, 215, 216, 221, 222, 223, 224, 229, 234, 237, 239, 241, 244, 246, 251, 261, 262, 263, 264, 265, 266, 267, 268, 269, 270, 271, 272, 273, 274, 276, 284, 286, 288, 289, 290, 291, 294, 295, 296, 297, 299, 301
challenges, 35, 36, 61, 63, 91, 99, 106, 125, 129, 131, 135, 136, 153, 155, 156, 157, 182, 191, 202, 206, 209, 215, 223, 224, 227, 228, 233, 239, 241, 252, 254, 257, 258, 259, 275, 280, 282, 289, 299, 300
chemical, 11, 124, 125, 131, 135, 138, 139, 140, 141, 143, 144, 148, 149, 152, 153, 155, 189, 193, 196, 214, 219, 238, 246, 247, 249, 251, 252, 256, 260, 263, 268, 269, 271, 272, 274, 287, 290, 291
childcare, 39, 50
children, 118, 120, 138, 142, 157, 158, 166, 178, 186, 187, 223, 259, 276, 282
China, v, vi, vii, 1, 2, 3, 4, 5, 6, 7, 8, 9, 10, 12, 15, 19, 21, 23, 24, 25, 26, 27, 30, 31, 32, 34, 35, 36, 37, 38, 39, 43, 45, 47, 48, 49, 51, 54, 55, 56, 58, 61, 62, 67, 68, 71, 72, 73, 75, 89, 91, 92, 93, 94, 95, 96, 97, 98, 99, 100, 101, 102, 103, 104, 105, 106, 107, 108, 111, 112, 113, 118, 120, 130, 133, 189, 213, 223, 233, 246, 249, 251, 296
Chinese government, 24, 25, 27, 93, 97, 98, 102, 104, 105, 107
cities, 24, 92, 103, 138, 140, 141, 143, 191, 221, 263, 264, 265, 266, 271, 290, 301
citizens, 7, 14, 16, 22, 34, 51, 62, 75, 133, 176, 217, 249, 288, 301
clarity, 40, 204, 255, 275, 283
climate, 114, 289, 300
climate change, 114, 300
clinical symptoms, 101
clinical trials, 22, 150, 157, 206, 214, 218, 219, 220, 227, 231, 232, 233, 234, 259, 267, 279
collaboration, 5, 12, 13, 21, 40, 91, 94, 95, 105, 106, 140, 145, 147, 151, 154, 169, 174, 184, 196, 206, 214, 215, 216, 219, 228, 235, 247, 252, 261, 263, 264, 268, 269
communities, 43, 50, 51, 68, 69, 91, 130, 136, 139, 140, 141, 144, 145, 146, 154, 159, 183, 199, 216, 218, 240, 241, 265, 266, 268, 270, 271, 272, 280, 281, 292, 298, 300, 302
community, 3, 5, 6, 14, 19, 39, 41, 47, 48, 49, 50, 53, 54, 58, 64, 68, 69, 72, 74, 82, 83, 94, 96, 98, 99, 104, 115, 131, 143, 144, 160, 162, 165, 173, 216, 218, 270
Congress, iv, 14, 15, 16, 17, 22, 24, 26, 39, 67, 68, 69, 75, 87, 89, 90, 92, 108, 109, 110, 112, 113, 114, 115, 117, 118, 121, 123, 124, 125, 127, 130, 134, 135, 137, 144, 154, 161, 164, 165, 198, 204, 206, 207, 208, 210, 211, 222, 224, 235, 236, 237, 238, 240, 241, 244, 248, 251, 255, 257, 260, 261, 262, 270, 282, 284, 285, 287, 294
consent, 126, 129, 161, 167, 170
constituents, 68, 123, 246, 292
control measures, 5, 6, 10, 268
conversations, 30, 202, 209, 281, 294, 296
cooperation, 5, 21, 54, 93, 94, 95, 96, 98, 105, 107, 112
cooperative agreements, 94, 134, 215, 216, 221, 250
coordination, 59, 74, 89, 99, 111, 112, 131, 145, 154, 170, 171, 194, 199, 203, 209, 246, 280, 289, 290, 300

coronavirus, v, vi, vii, 1, 2, 3, 4, 5, 6, 7, 8, 9, 10, 11, 12, 13, 14, 15, 16, 17, 19, 20, 23, 24, 29, 30, 31, 34, 35, 43, 44, 47, 51, 53, 55, 56, 57, 58, 59, 61, 67, 71, 73, 74, 77, 83, 87, 91, 92, 97, 99, 100, 101, 102, 104, 105, 107, 108, 111, 112, 113, 114, 115, 154, 160, 232, 233, 260
cost, 59, 89, 104, 113, 171, 191, 203, 206, 228, 234, 283, 287, 298
cost saving, 191
COVID-19, v, vi, vii, 23, 43, 44, 45, 46, 47, 48, 49, 50, 51, 52, 53, 54, 55, 56, 58, 61, 62, 64, 65, 67, 68, 69, 71, 72, 73, 74, 75, 77, 82, 83, 84, 85, 86, 87, 88, 89
critical infrastructure, 50, 150
cyber-attack, 133
cybersecurity, 124, 125

D

daily care, 134, 137, 250, 253
data analysis, 96
data collection, 241, 245, 270
database, 96, 159, 234
deaths, 31, 32, 39, 40, 50, 56, 67, 72, 92, 93, 96, 100, 104, 123, 125, 233, 261, 270, 288
decision-making process, 120, 247, 252
Department of Agriculture, 68, 192, 202
Department of Commerce, 69
Department of Defense, 12, 53, 88, 134, 153, 155, 190, 192, 202, 246, 250, 256
Department of Health and Human Services (HHS), v, vi, 2, 3, 5, 6, 7, 8, 9, 12, 13, 14, 15, 16, 17, 21, 22, 40, 43, 63, 73, 74, 75, 77, 81, 83, 94, 95, 113, 118, 120, 127, 130, 132, 133, 134, 135, 136, 137, 139, 141, 145, 146, 148, 153, 155, 167, 170, 183, 186, 188, 189, 190, 191, 192, 193, 194, 195, 196, 197, 198, 201, 202, 203, 204, 205, 208, 210, 211, 212, 215, 216, 221, 222, 226, 237, 239, 244, 247, 248, 250, 251, 252, 253, 256, 265, 266, 278, 284, 290, 292, 293, 297, 301
Department of Homeland Security, 6, 8, 62, 75, 88, 124, 126, 135, 190, 202, 214, 252, 254, 258, 290
Department of Justice, 135
Department of the Treasury, 68
detection, 10, 11, 35, 59, 96, 99, 102, 103, 119, 120, 122, 131, 138, 140, 142, 143, 146, 168, 171, 173, 174, 181, 188, 189, 191, 263, 264, 267, 270, 281, 290
developing countries, 105, 177, 231
disaster, 68, 69, 70, 88, 134, 137, 146, 217, 246, 247, 250, 253, 274, 278, 284, 289, 299, 300, 302
diseases, vii, 2, 3, 5, 9, 10, 11, 17, 21, 29, 38, 44, 58, 63, 72, 77, 92, 99, 109, 118, 119, 123, 124, 125, 126, 133, 135, 136, 140, 142, 143, 144, 146, 147, 148, 149, 153, 155, 162, 165, 176, 180, 181, 182, 188, 189, 190, 191, 196, 202, 203, 204, 207, 215, 216, 229, 230, 231, 232, 233, 243, 246, 249, 251, 263, 264, 267, 268, 269, 270, 271, 273, 282, 283, 284, 285, 293, 296, 300
distribution, 11, 39, 53, 65, 88, 140, 157, 171, 192, 195, 210, 212, 215, 222, 255, 264, 268, 284, 290
doctors, 12, 58, 102, 105, 110, 122, 173, 288, 292
draft, 124, 125, 126, 142, 185, 245, 255, 261
drug delivery, 296
drug discovery, 234
drug resistance, 96
drug treatment, 89
drugs, 11, 12, 13, 15, 58, 130, 131, 132, 135, 158, 159, 162, 167, 169, 172, 174, 219, 233, 244, 252, 261, 266, 267, 276, 282, 286, 287, 299
due process, 63, 64

E

early warning, 35, 143, 190, 209, 269, 271
economic activity, 23, 25, 68
economic consequences, 59
economic development, 67, 69, 87
economic downturn, 24
economic growth, 24
economic implications, vii, 67, 68
economic incentives, 88
economic losses, 146, 274
egg, 157, 175, 176, 213, 223, 226, 227, 228, 297
emergency, 1, 2, 3, 5, 11, 13, 14, 16, 17, 21, 22, 35, 36, 39, 40, 47, 50, 53, 65, 69, 70, 74, 75, 85, 87, 89, 108, 109, 111, 113, 114, 118, 119, 120, 122, 123, 131, 134, 135, 137, 138, 140, 141, 142, 144, 145, 152, 154, 159, 160, 161, 167, 173, 176, 177, 178, 181,183, 187, 190, 192, 194, 196, 203, 204, 207, 215, 216, 220, 230, 232, 240, 241, 243, 244, 247, 251, 252, 254, 255, 256, 260, 261, 262, 263, 264, 265, 266, 267, 268, 270, 272, 273, 276, 280, 281, 282, 284, 285, 287, 288, 289, 299, 301
emergency management, 137, 215, 265
emergency physician, 178

emergency preparedness, 87, 161, 187, 232, 244, 251, 256, 262, 264, 273, 282, 284, 287, 289
emergency response, 5, 21, 40, 134, 137, 138, 140, 144, 145, 241, 265, 268, 272, 276, 281, 284, 288, 301
employees, 2, 24, 99, 110, 154, 159, 179, 199, 200
environment, 154, 159, 199, 246, 249, 268
environmental factors, 56
environmental regulations, 159
epidemic, 3, 15, 19, 22, 30, 31, 33, 34, 35, 36, 37, 38, 39, 40, 68, 73, 93, 97, 99, 100, 101, 102, 103, 104, 105, 106, 107, 108, 109, 111, 112, 113, 114, 115, 124, 125, 147, 151, 160, 177, 184, 190, 239, 240, 271, 295
epidemiologic, 30, 35, 56, 145, 193, 265, 268, 269, 273, 299
epidemiological investigations, 34, 35
epidemiology, 35, 95, 140, 141, 142, 176, 245, 264, 267
equipment, 11, 15, 25, 27, 39, 88, 89, 135, 136, 137, 138, 140, 145, 253, 263, 264, 265, 266, 277, 279, 301
evidence, 9, 10, 20, 30, 31, 33, 34, 36, 40, 62, 103, 187, 214, 239, 241, 271
exercises, 115, 134, 138, 140, 141, 194, 221, 250, 263, 265, 266, 272, 289
expertise, 95, 108, 113, 114, 115, 130, 132, 135, 138, 139, 140, 141, 142, 144, 146, 150, 170, 171, 178, 187, 215, 216, 231, 247, 252, 253, 262, 263, 264, 266, 267, 268, 272, 273, 274, 277, 278, 302
exposure, 30, 34, 43, 48, 50, 54, 63, 65, 103, 121, 131, 143, 151, 152, 154, 157, 159, 214, 223, 261, 263, 267
extreme weather events, 133, 243, 249

F

families, 8, 75, 172, 203, 239, 240, 241, 278, 292
family members, 2, 51, 62, 113
FDA approval, 13, 131, 135, 141, 151, 152, 192, 195, 247, 252
fear, 33, 104, 113, 115, 240, 273, 288
Federal Emergency Management Agency, 210
Federal funds, 290
Federal Government, 121, 122, 123, 124, 126, 127, 130, 239, 245, 246, 248, 249, 274, 281, 289, 302, 303
fever, 4, 10, 20, 24, 32, 44, 45, 56, 62, 72
fiduciary responsibilities, 285
financial, 35, 67, 144, 150, 284
financial resources, 284
financial support, 35, 144
first generation, 251
first responders, 177, 178, 195, 221, 261
fiscal year, 144, 145, 149, 170, 215, 248, 265, 270
flexibility, 7, 16, 17, 22, 26, 185, 260, 270
flights, 8, 10, 21, 25, 38, 63
Food and Drug Administration, 2, 6, 129, 149, 155, 158, 188, 190, 205, 228, 235, 237, 241, 244, 254, 256, 265
funding, 12, 13, 15, 16, 17, 22, 40, 74, 90, 99, 108, 113, 114, 119, 121, 130, 135, 136, 137, 140, 144, 149, 152, 164, 189, 190, 193, 194, 195, 200, 202, 203, 204, 208, 209, 210, 214, 215, 216, 219, 220, 221, 223, 226, 240, 243, 247, 251, 252, 265, 269, 270, 273,275, 284, 285
funds, 16, 22, 39, 75, 114, 138, 140, 141, 143, 171, 197, 214, 219, 223, 234, 264, 265, 266, 267, 273, 284, 285

G

genome, 58, 96, 254, 291
global demand, 72
global economy, 59
global leaders, 112
global response, vii, 72, 91, 109, 110
global scale, 239
governments, 25, 94, 95, 97, 98, 99, 231
grants, 69, 134, 138, 217, 221, 241, 250, 263, 303
guidance, 2, 9, 21, 47, 50, 51, 52, 54, 65, 123, 140, 141, 142, 156, 160, 170, 178, 215, 236, 255, 257, 258, 260, 261, 264, 266, 268, 272, 275, 276, 283
guidelines, 6, 32, 223, 268, 276, 277, 301

H

health, 2, 3, 5, 6, 7, 9, 10, 13, 14, 15, 16, 17, 19, 21, 22, 25, 29, 30, 34, 35, 36, 37, 38, 39, 40, 43, 45, 47, 49, 50, 51, 52, 53, 59, 63, 64, 67, 68, 69, 77, 85, 86, 92, 93, 94, 95, 97, 98, 99, 100, 102, 103, 104, 105, 106, 109, 110, 113, 118, 119, 127, 128,130, 131, 132, 133, 134, 135, 136, 137, 138, 139, 140, 141, 142, 143, 144, 145, 146, 152, 153, 159, 161, 163, 173, 174, 176, 178, 187, 191, 192, 193, 194, 199, 202, 203, 209, 214, 215, 216, 217,

221, 223, 230, 232, 238, 240, 241, 243, 244, 245, 246, 247, 249, 250, 251, 253, 256, 258, 260, 262, 263, 264, 265, 266, 267, 268, 269, 270, 271, 272, 273, 274, 281, 285, 286, 289, 300, 301
health care, 6, 14, 15, 17, 21, 43, 45, 49, 92, 99, 102, 104, 105, 109, 110, 113, 145, 191, 215, 216, 221, 258, 265
health care professionals, 92, 105
health care system, 14, 15, 17, 102, 105, 113, 216, 221
health condition, 49
health effects, 68, 300
health information, 143, 223, 263, 270
history, 6, 21, 30, 114, 123, 186, 251, 284, 289, 302
House of Representatives, 29, 91, 117, 155, 187, 222, 224, 235
Hubei Province, 1, 8, 21, 30, 48, 51, 61, 63, 72, 75
human, 4, 30, 31, 34, 56, 72, 94, 96, 114, 133, 140, 142, 143, 149, 151, 157, 158, 160, 178, 186, 191, 196, 202, 203, 205, 208, 214, 229, 230, 232, 233, 235, 239, 251, 254, 258, 264, 267, 269, 285, 286
human exposure, 143
human health, 202
hurricanes, 69, 128, 130, 216, 270, 274, 277, 289, 298

I

identification, 6, 14, 30, 52, 103, 138, 143, 229, 231, 233, 234
immune response, 150, 151, 229, 230
immune system, 169, 227, 232
immunization, 149, 213, 230, 271
immunogenicity, 166, 227
improvements, 118, 120, 137, 181, 198, 215, 267, 290
in vitro, 12, 13, 159, 233, 259
individuals, 5, 7, 8, 9, 21, 30, 31, 32, 33, 38, 39, 63, 70, 101, 113, 142, 158, 172, 173, 183, 198, 200, 226, 238, 240, 241, 253, 266, 276, 290
industrial chemicals, 152
industry, 11, 12, 13, 15, 27, 50, 59, 70, 88, 89, 118, 120, 130, 136, 146, 149, 150, 151, 152, 155, 161, 163, 164, 171, 174, 185, 192, 203, 204, 205, 206, 208, 209, 220, 227, 228, 230, 231, 234, 235, 240, 256, 262, 297
infection, 4, 5, 6, 10, 20, 21, 30, 32, 33, 34, 35, 40, 43, 44, 45, 54, 56, 61, 63, 64, 143, 151, 158, 165, 177, 196, 223, 226, 229, 232, 268, 271, 273, 286
infectious agents, 138
infectious diseases, vii, 10, 11, 12, 16, 29, 95, 100, 118, 119, 123, 125, 129, 130, 133, 135, 136, 140, 142, 144, 146, 147, 148, 149, 153, 155, 157, 176, 180, 181, 188, 189, 190, 191, 196, 202, 204, 207, 214, 215, 216, 219, 224, 225, 228, 230, 231, 232, 243, 246, 249, 251, 263, 264, 267, 273, 284, 296, 300
influenza, 4, 9, 10, 12, 20, 31, 39, 51, 94, 95, 96, 97, 118, 120, 130, 131, 133, 135, 136, 144, 152, 154, 155, 157, 158, 162, 175, 176, 180, 181, 189, 196, 204, 208, 212, 213, 214, 217, 223, 225, 226, 227, 228, 229, 230, 232, 233, 239, 246, 249, 251, 252, 256, 263, 267, 269, 272, 273, 278, 285, 286, 296, 297
influenza a, 10, 31, 158, 162, 225, 229, 232, 233, 270, 285, 296
influenza vaccine, 96, 135, 136, 152, 157, 176, 212, 213, 217, 223, 225, 226, 227, 228, 229, 232, 252, 278, 297
influenza virus, 94, 96, 133, 154, 196, 208, 213, 214, 225, 227, 228, 230, 232, 249, 251, 267, 268, 270, 286
information exchange, 161, 289
information sharing, 59, 218, 241
information technology, 144
infrastructure, 69, 94, 95, 97, 112, 127, 128, 132, 136, 144, 152, 176, 189, 195, 202, 216, 217, 231, 243, 245, 247, 249, 251, 253, 258, 272, 273, 279, 280, 292, 299
intellectual property, 27, 206, 208
investment, 25, 34, 35, 38, 131, 152, 165, 202, 204, 208, 218, 219, 229, 233, 270, 277, 283, 298
isolation, 5, 6, 10, 21, 30, 37, 39, 62, 63, 64, 86
issues, 2, 8, 11, 53, 55, 68, 69, 88, 94, 95, 99, 105, 106, 118, 120, 124, 125, 127, 170, 175, 180, 187, 194, 195, 198, 200, 210, 214, 241, 258, 261, 272, 289, 290, 293, 297, 298, 301

L

labor market, 68
laboratory tests, 34, 189
law enforcement, 50, 261

leadership, 40, 41, 106, 111, 112, 126, 131, 134, 135, 183, 185, 192, 210, 226, 239, 245, 246, 250, 257, 283, 290, 302
learning, 4, 20, 124, 168, 293
legislation, 114, 115, 118, 120, 124, 126, 184, 241, 242, 244, 245, 248, 256, 261, 277, 282, 285, 302, 303
loan guarantees, 69, 88
loans, 25, 68, 69, 88, 89, 303
local authorities, 274, 289, 293
local government, 5, 24, 25, 99, 113, 221, 251, 282

M

management, 7, 15, 50, 52, 68, 106, 118, 120, 124, 125, 127, 140, 145, 182, 183, 191, 192, 193, 194, 195, 196, 198, 209, 264, 265, 270
manufacturing, 25, 27, 53, 68, 89, 136, 157, 192, 203, 204, 205, 206, 212, 213, 217, 226, 227, 228, 251, 254, 255, 258, 261, 279, 296
medical, 5, 8, 11, 13, 14, 15, 23, 25, 26, 27, 31, 32, 33, 37, 38, 39, 40, 45, 46, 49, 50, 59, 62, 65, 68, 83, 84, 85, 87, 89, 97, 101, 104, 105, 109, 110, 112, 113, 114, 119, 120, 122, 129, 130, 132, 133, 134, 135, 136, 137, 138, 139, 140, 141, 144, 146, 148, 149, 152, 153, 154, 155, 156, 157, 158, 159, 160, 161, 163, 170, 171, 172, 178, 182, 185, 188, 192, 193, 194, 196, 197, 202, 214, 215, 216, 217, 218, 219, 220, 221, 222, 226, 229, 230, 232, 238, 239, 240, 241, 244, 245, 246, 247, 248, 249, 250, 251, 252, 253, 254, 255, 256, 257, 258, 259, 260, 261, 262, 264, 266, 268, 272, 273, 274, 275, 276, 277, 279, 280, 281, 284, 292, 297, 299, 301
medical assistance, 113, 247
medical care, 45, 46, 50, 83, 109, 281, 299
medical expertise, 138
medicine, 113, 115, 136, 140, 168, 264, 266, 268
meningitis, 31, 143, 144, 267
Middle East, 3, 19, 31, 35, 56, 57, 96, 143, 154, 160, 232, 260
Middle East Respiratory Syndrome (MERS), 3, 12, 19, 31, 35, 36, 48, 49, 56, 57, 58, 72, 96, 101, 104, 143, 154, 160, 173, 232, 233, 260, 273, 285
military, 14, 24, 27, 87, 88, 97, 137, 153, 156, 159, 168, 202, 206, 210, 261
monoclonal antibody, 12, 147, 150, 151, 167, 229
morbidity, 10, 133, 139, 162, 226, 232
mortality, 10, 55, 56, 67, 109, 114, 139, 214, 226, 232
mortality rate, 55, 56, 109, 214
mosquitoes, 172, 268, 270, 295, 300
mucous membrane, 152
mutations, 56, 125

N

National Institutes of Health, 6, 22, 72, 97, 129, 130, 135, 148, 188, 192, 209, 214, 224, 225, 252, 278
National Response Framework, 133, 250, 253
national security, 14, 16, 22, 88, 126, 131, 133, 135, 136, 137, 154, 161, 192, 196, 202, 204, 208, 214, 238, 245, 246, 247, 248, 249, 250, 252, 253, 262, 275, 288
National Security Council, 2, 74, 110, 111
natural disaster, 127, 133, 139, 249, 254, 258, 264, 266, 292
negative consequences, 128, 178
novel coronavirus, v, vi, vii, 1, 2, 3, 4, 5, 6, 7, 8, 9, 10, 11, 12, 13, 14, 15, 16, 17, 19, 20, 21, 22, 23, 29, 30, 34, 35, 43, 44, 61, 71, 73, 91, 92, 100, 101, 102, 103, 104, 105, 107, 108, 111, 114
nuclear weapons, 189, 246, 249
nucleic acid, 159, 259
nurses, 110, 122, 173, 292

O

occupational health, 85
officials, 3, 4, 7, 20, 21, 24, 26, 30, 34, 64, 92, 93, 102, 103, 106, 108, 110, 123, 125, 127, 130, 136, 143, 144, 194, 198, 200, 202, 218, 241, 247, 253, 268, 269, 272, 281, 288, 289, 292, 293
operations, 24, 25, 35, 77, 156, 199, 200, 204, 257, 258, 301
opportunities, 25, 160, 215, 217, 221, 234, 247, 252, 260
oversight, 22, 63, 89, 118, 119, 120, 121, 178, 186, 187, 188, 197, 198, 199, 200, 248, 294

P

pandemics, vi, vii, 29, 35, 37, 99, 117, 122, 127, 132, 138, 139, 155, 162, 184, 187, 211, 212, 222, 225, 228, 232, 235, 239, 246, 251, 272, 281, 282, 289, 292

pathogens, 3, 15, 19, 99, 122, 123, 124, 125, 126, 138, 142, 144, 149, 150, 158, 159, 165, 173, 181, 188, 191, 197, 198, 203, 214, 218, 219, 223, 229, 230, 231, 232, 233, 234, 259, 263, 267, 268, 270, 275, 277
pharmaceutical, 10, 11, 27, 96, 124, 126, 135, 193, 202, 203, 233, 252, 258, 268
platform, 96, 136, 148, 149, 152, 163, 165, 175, 204, 205, 206, 218, 223, 228, 229, 230, 232, 233, 273, 278, 279
pneumonia, 1, 19, 30, 31, 44, 54, 55, 56, 73, 92, 93, 99, 100, 102, 103, 143, 267
pneumonia cases, 1, 19, 92, 99
policy, 14, 30, 37, 58, 64, 67, 87, 91, 95, 103, 106, 108, 113, 123, 134, 202, 205, 250, 286, 287
population, 99, 104, 133, 140, 141, 143, 162, 173, 189, 208, 218, 223, 239, 249, 264, 265, 266, 277
portfolio, 154, 158, 204, 208, 219, 220, 229, 230, 232, 233, 259, 279, 283
positive relationship, 38
potential benefits, 191
preparation, iv, 15, 77, 109, 110, 123, 125, 243, 280, 288, 290, 296, 299
preparedness, 2, 6, 14, 37, 51, 74, 88, 99, 105, 106, 109, 111, 112, 114, 115, 118, 119, 122, 126, 127, 130, 131, 132, 133, 134, 136, 137, 138, 139, 140, 141, 145, 153, 155, 156, 157, 187, 204, 212, 216, 218, 221, 224, 226, 228, 229, 230, 231, 233, 239, 241, 243, 244,246, 247, 248, 249, 250, 254, 255, 256, 257, 260, 261, 262, 264, 265, 266, 268, 269, 272, 273, 276, 280, 281, 290, 292, 298, 300, 301, 302
prevention, 6, 17, 21, 35, 56, 94, 95, 97, 102, 143, 144, 151, 169, 173, 263, 267, 268, 269, 270, 272
private sector, 129, 136, 154, 161, 184, 186, 203, 208, 236, 247, 252, 253, 262, 275
procurement, 17, 130, 134, 170, 171, 180, 192, 194, 195, 196, 202, 204, 209, 210, 215, 216, 219, 222, 223, 250, 290
protection, 63, 64, 105, 110, 138, 139, 164, 166, 172, 178, 202, 225, 226, 227, 229, 288, 290, 299
public assistance, 70
public awareness, 228
public health, 1, 3, 5, 14, 15, 17, 21, 29, 30, 34, 35, 38, 40, 47, 49, 50, 51, 53, 54, 63, 67, 68, 69, 70, 74, 77, 88, 92, 94, 95, 96, 97, 98, 99, 100, 102, 104, 105, 106, 115, 118, 119, 120, 122, 124, 125, 126, 127, 128, 130, 132, 133, 134, 136, 137, 138, 139, 140, 141, 142, 143, 144, 145, 146, 147, 149, 150, 152, 153, 154, 155, 159, 160, 161, 162, 163, 170, 173, 181, 183, 187, 189, 191, 192, 193, 194, 197, 198, 201, 202, 203, 204, 209, 213, 214, 215, 216, 217, 220, 221, 223, 229, 230, 232, 235, 238, 239, 240, 241, 243, 244, 245, 246, 248, 249, 250, 251, 253, 254, 256, 258, 259, 260, 261, 262, 263, 264, 265, 266, 267, 268, 269, 270, 271, 272, 273, 274, 276, 283, 284, 288, 292, 293, 294, 298, 299, 300, 302
Public Health Emergency, 2, 3, 7, 9, 14, 16, 22, 33, 71, 73, 98, 100, 114, 124, 126, 134, 138, 140, 141, 149, 155, 191, 194, 203, 224, 229, 230, 250, 251, 256, 263, 265, 266, 276, 284, 294
Public Health Emergency of International Concern (PHEIC), 1, 2, 3, 33, 36, 47, 71, 73, 98, 100, 105, 229
public interest, 91
public policy, 91
public safety, vii
public support, 10, 124, 126
public-private partnerships, 114, 130, 135, 163, 220, 247, 252

Q

quality of life, 133, 249
quantification, 214

R

radiation, 138, 152, 157, 159, 240, 252, 259, 263, 268, 272, 290
radiation damage, 159, 259
raw materials, 23, 26, 27, 39
recombinant DNA, 226, 228, 297
recommendations, iv, 30, 37, 73, 91, 96, 105, 119, 121, 127, 128, 171, 178, 180, 195, 198, 201, 202, 212, 261, 267
recovery, 69, 130, 133, 136, 218, 221, 246, 250, 258, 294
requirements, 2, 5, 7, 8, 9, 12, 24, 62, 63, 64, 77, 88, 90, 100, 131, 135, 136, 159, 160, 192, 196, 198, 203, 204, 207, 208, 210, 214, 218, 220, 276, 282, 294
researchers, 4, 20, 58, 98, 103, 112, 124, 126, 151, 172, 227, 228, 233, 234, 271, 278
resistance, 98, 128, 143, 158, 168, 169, 172, 177, 185, 197, 233, 234, 267, 271, 287, 291

resources, 17, 29, 34, 35, 36, 37, 38, 39, 41, 69, 74, 90, 99, 104, 111, 122, 128, 129, 134, 136, 137, 140, 142, 145, 146, 150, 156, 159, 161, 163, 194, 195, 196, 202, 206, 208, 209, 221, 224, 236, 241, 250, 257, 259, 262, 265, 266, 273, 275, 277, 280, 284, 286, 291, 293, 300
respiratory illness, vii, 32, 43, 44, 45, 56
respiratory pathogens, 3, 19, 99
response, vii, 2, 3, 5, 7, 9, 11, 13, 14, 15, 16, 17, 22, 25, 26, 29, 30, 33, 34, 35, 37, 38, 40, 51, 54, 58, 64, 69, 70, 72, 74, 75, 87, 88, 91, 94, 95, 96, 97, 99, 100, 102, 103, 104, 106, 107, 108, 109, 110, 111, 112, 113, 114, 115, 119, 121, 122, 124, 125, 128, 130, 131, 133, 134, 135, 136, 137, 138, 139, 140, 141, 142, 143, 144, 145, 146, 148, 150, 151, 153, 155, 156, 157, 159, 160, 161, 162, 163, 164, 166, 167, 170, 174, 176, 178, 183, 189, 190, 192, 193, 195, 196, 197, 198, 199, 203, 207, 210, 214, 215, 216, 217, 218, 221, 223, 224, 226, 229, 230, 231, 232, 239, 240, 243, 244, 246, 247, 248, 249, 250, 252, 253, 255, 256, 257, 259, 261, 262, 263, 264, 265, 266, 269, 271, 272, 273, 278, 279, 284, 286, 289, 291, 292, 296, 298
restrictions, 2, 5, 7, 9, 10, 24, 25, 33, 38, 52, 73, 98, 113, 198
risk, 3, 6, 7, 10, 14, 19, 21, 30, 31, 34, 43, 49, 50, 52, 54, 55, 59, 63, 64, 73, 86, 100, 113, 114, 118, 120, 123, 125, 135, 140, 143, 144, 148, 150, 157, 165, 183, 191, 192, 194, 196, 202, 203, 204, 205, 206, 208, 209, 213, 220, 234, 241, 252, 253, 263, 264, 266, 267, 271, 276, 277, 282, 291, 292, 296, 298, 301
risk assessment, 50, 118, 192, 203
risk management, 59
risks, 26, 35, 63, 99, 133, 184, 196, 206, 249, 254, 261, 268, 270, 274, 275
rules, 62, 63, 93, 106, 129, 185, 204, 270
rural areas, 97, 169, 280, 299
rural counties, 280

S

safety, 64, 119, 121, 124, 126, 154, 156, 159, 160, 166, 178, 179, 188, 193, 198, 199, 201, 206, 207, 227, 239, 257, 259, 273, 277
science, vii, 108, 113, 114, 115, 135, 136, 141, 154, 156, 157, 158, 161, 171, 178, 180, 183, 188, 199, 201, 207, 209, 240, 241, 251, 254, 256, 257, 259, 262, 263, 264, 274
security, 14, 16, 22, 35, 36, 37, 98, 106, 108, 118, 120, 124, 125, 130, 131, 132, 133, 134, 135, 136, 137, 139, 153, 163, 170, 174, 188, 194, 198, 199, 202, 204, 208, 214, 217, 221, 243, 246, 249, 250, 251, 253, 266, 272, 273, 275, 290
security threats, 130, 132, 133, 134, 135, 137, 214, 217, 221, 243, 249, 250, 253, 266
sequencing, 58, 72, 96, 102, 103, 142, 143, 149, 151, 229, 267, 291
services, iv, 17, 24, 25, 26, 50, 68, 85, 88, 134, 137, 150, 221, 234, 247, 263, 269, 280
severe acute respiratory syndrome, 3, 19, 23, 53, 71, 91, 92, 232
smallpox, 131, 135, 142, 144, 147, 151, 154, 157, 159, 165, 178, 197, 198, 199, 252, 267
spending, 17, 24, 26, 111, 170, 190, 193, 214, 288
stockpiling, 25, 87, 134, 135, 188, 195, 215, 222, 247, 250, 252, 275, 278, 297, 298
supply chain, 15, 23, 25, 26, 59, 67, 68, 69, 70, 87, 89, 213, 254, 255
supply disruption, 156, 257
surveillance, 29, 31, 32, 34, 35, 37, 39, 59, 73, 92, 94, 95, 96, 97, 99, 122, 128, 138, 140, 143, 144, 146, 172, 173, 176, 193, 215, 243, 263, 264, 265, 266, 269, 270, 271, 273, 274, 286
symptoms, 3, 4, 5, 8, 9, 10, 19, 20, 22, 31, 32, 33, 35, 44, 45, 46, 49, 54, 56, 72, 101, 104, 269

T

target, 128, 143, 149, 165, 226, 231, 234, 263, 269, 270, 271, 286
technical assistance, 7, 68, 69, 144, 145, 150, 156, 160, 216, 257
technical support, 105
techniques, 157, 226, 227, 228, 291
technological advancement, 133, 208, 249
technologies, 13, 131, 136, 149, 152, 163, 165, 169, 175, 176, 181, 182, 190, 191, 204, 205, 206, 208, 209, 213, 218, 220, 226, 228, 229, 230, 232, 233, 260, 267, 268, 275, 279, 291, 297
technology transfer, 27
territorial, 51, 134, 140, 141, 171, 210, 221, 246, 250, 252, 265, 269, 270
terrorism, 189, 264, 289
terrorist attack, 124, 126, 137, 198, 274, 292

testing, 6, 12, 13, 21, 31, 32, 34, 38, 40, 53, 58, 72, 97, 102, 103, 104, 105, 109, 112, 123, 125, 140, 143, 150, 173, 174, 175, 181, 191, 206, 207, 213, 226, 230, 231, 235, 251, 261, 263, 264, 272
therapeutics, 12, 37, 40, 109, 110, 113, 114, 129, 146, 148, 149, 150, 152, 153, 155, 157, 208, 209, 217, 218, 219, 229, 230, 231, 232, 233, 234, 236, 256, 259, 276
therapy, 39, 40, 97, 102, 286
threat assessment, 119, 120, 214, 269
threats, 11, 35, 98, 106, 109, 111, 118, 119, 120, 122, 124, 125, 126, 127, 128, 129, 130, 131, 132, 133, 135, 138, 139, 140, 141, 142, 143, 144, 148, 149, 152, 153, 154, 155, 157, 158, 159, 160, 161, 162, 163, 172, 173, 174, 181, 188, 189, 192, 196, 200, 202, 203, 204, 208, 209, 214, 215, 218, 229, 230, 232, 238, 239, 240, 241, 244, 246, 247, 248, 249, 251, 252, 254, 256, 259, 260, 261, 262, 263, 264, 267, 268, 269, 270, 271, 272, 273, 274, 279, 286, 287, 302
training, 34, 35, 95, 96, 97, 119, 120, 134, 140, 152, 174, 176, 178, 194, 195, 210, 216, 221, 250, 259, 265, 266, 272
transmission, 2, 4, 5, 6, 7, 9, 10, 17, 20, 21, 30, 31, 33, 34, 36, 39, 44, 50, 51, 63, 72, 74, 86, 92, 94, 96, 100, 101, 103, 104, 109, 143, 174, 226, 232, 285
transparency, 105, 106, 107, 163, 171, 206
transport, 6, 21, 25, 216, 221, 280, 281, 293
transportation, 24, 25, 50, 83, 101, 103, 136, 253, 300
treatment, 5, 10, 12, 21, 46, 49, 56, 59, 62, 97, 98, 101, 104, 109, 110, 114, 123, 125, 141, 143, 150, 151, 157, 158, 178, 182, 216, 219, 229, 231, 234, 253, 259, 261, 267, 268, 276, 291
trial, 147, 149, 150, 151, 160, 164, 166, 167, 220, 227, 229, 230, 231, 232, 260

U

U.S health officials, 3
U.S. Centers for Disease Control and Prevention, 3, 19, 73, 94
U.S. economy, 68
United States, vii, 1, 2, 3, 5, 6, 7, 8, 9, 11, 13, 14, 16, 17, 19, 21, 25, 26, 27, 29, 30, 34, 39, 43, 44, 47, 48, 49, 50, 51, 52, 55, 61, 62, 63, 64, 68, 71, 72, 73, 75, 87, 91, 93, 94, 95, 97, 98, 105, 106, 115, 118, 120, 129, 132, 133, 140, 143, 144, 146, 153, 155,157, 167, 168, 174, 177, 195, 196, 211, 216, 222, 224, 228, 229, 235, 237, 239, 240, 246, 248, 249, 261, 263, 264, 269, 271, 272, 273, 274, 278, 298, 299
United States Public Health System, vii

V

vaccinations, 145, 147, 214
vaccine, 5, 13, 21, 22, 39, 40, 45, 49, 50, 54, 56, 58, 72, 95, 96, 101, 104, 109, 121, 123, 125, 131, 136, 142, 144, 147, 149, 150, 151, 152, 157, 163, 164, 165, 166, 175, 176, 195, 196, 200, 207, 208, 212, 213, 214, 217, 218, 219, 223, 225, 226, 227, 228, 229, 230, 231, 232, 233, 240, 247, 251, 267, 272, 273, 278, 296, 297
virus infection, 49, 159, 229, 259
viruses, 32, 33, 48, 56, 57, 59, 71, 95, 100, 118, 120, 149, 181, 196, 214, 218, 226, 231, 232, 233, 263, 267, 268, 269, 271, 286, 296

W

wildfire, 121
wildlife, 202, 203
withdrawal, 110, 112
witnesses, 126, 127, 128, 129, 161, 168, 174, 187, 238, 239, 243, 244, 274, 287, 296, 302
workers, 6, 21, 25, 36, 39, 43, 50, 65, 68, 105, 109, 110, 121, 122, 128, 172, 175, 177, 286, 294, 295
workforce, 35, 69, 98, 140, 144, 176, 217, 264, 268, 272, 273
World Health Organization (WHO), 1, 2, 3, 5, 7, 8, 9, 10, 19, 31, 33, 34, 36, 47, 56, 58, 59, 71, 72, 73, 74, 92, 93, 94, 96, 97, 98, 100, 104, 105, 112, 150, 151, 156, 160, 161, 176, 229, 240, 257
worldwide, 3, 19, 25, 36, 49, 67, 97, 271, 278, 296
Wuhan City, 1, 30

Y

young people, 283
young women, 172, 173